The Humanities in Asia

Volume 6

Editor-in-Chief
Chu-Ren Huang, Hong Kong, Hong Kong

This book series publishes original monographs and edited volumes in the humanities on issues specific to Asia, as well as general issues in the humanities within the context of Asia, or issues which were shaped by or can be enlightened by Asian perspectives. The emphasis is on excellence and originality in scholarship as well as synergetic interdisciplinary approaches and multicultural perspectives. Books exploring the role of the humanities in our highly connected society will be especially welcomed. The series publishes books that deal with emerging issues as well as those that offer an in-depth examination of underlying issues.

The target audience of this series include both scholars and professionals who are interested in issues related to Asia, including its people, its history, its society and environment, as well as the global impact of its development and interaction with the rest of the world.

The Humanities in Asia book series is published in conjunction with Springer under the auspices of the Hong Kong Academy of the Humanities (HKAH). The editorial board of The Humanities in Asia consists of HKAH fellows as well as leading humanities scholars who are affiliated or associated with leading learned societies for the humanities in the world.

More information about this series at http://www.springer.com/series/13566

Bernadette Watson · Janice Krieger
Editors

Expanding Horizons in Health Communication

An Asian Perspective

Hong Kong Academy of the Humanities
香 港 人 文 學 院

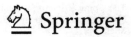

Editors
Bernadette Watson
Hong Kong Polytechnic University
Hong Kong, Hong Kong

Janice Krieger
University of Florida
Gainesville, FL, USA

ISSN 2363-6890   ISSN 2363-6904   (electronic)
The Humanities in Asia
ISBN 978-981-15-4391-3   ISBN 978-981-15-4389-0   (eBook)
https://doi.org/10.1007/978-981-15-4389-0

This Springer imprint is published by the registered company Springer Nature Singapore Pte Ltd.
The registered company address is: 152 Beach Road, #21-01/04 Gateway East, Singapore 189721, Singapore

Acknowledgements

The co-editors would like to acknowledge the assistance of a number of reviewers who provided valuable input to help complete this book. Those people are

Hong Kong, SAR
Louise Cummings
Phoenix Lam

Dennis Tay
Margo Turnbull
Wendy Wong

USA
Jordan Alpert
Maggie Pitts
Yulia Strekalova
Debbie Triese

Australia
Cindy Gallois
Liz Jones

Everyone has worked very hard to ensure this book is published. However, a special acknowledgement and thanks goes to Dr. Margo Turnbull (co-author of one of the chapters but also IRCAHC Postdoctoral Fellow) who has worked tirelessly with Janice and me to see the book to completion. Thank you so much Margo. In addition, we want to thank Ivy WU's expertise in making the book come together, literally.

Prologue

The Vision for This Book

This edited volume is part of *The Humanities in Asia* series. All the books in the series highlight areas in which Asia's approach and views can provide new insights to current Western opinions. Our book concentrates on health concerns in Asia so we can elucidate opportunities for health communication scholarship. In keeping with the spirit of this book series, the authors come from wide-ranging disciplines and feature both researchers and health providers. The book seeks to be comprehensive by focusing on well-being which includes diverse aspects of physical and mental health. The chapters also seek to be inclusive of different philosophies for maintaining well-being with research coming from fields of both Chinese Traditional Medicine and Western Medicine. We also investigate the challenges around disseminating public health information so that comprehensible messages are sent to the public to enable them to make informed health decisions. It is timely and appropriate that this text on well-being and health is brought to the public arena by the humanities. In so doing, it serves to build an understanding of two strong cultures.

How the Book Came About

This conception of this book coincides with the creation of the International Research Centre for the Advancement of Health Communication (IRCAHC), previously the International Research Centre for Communication in Healthcare. The new, renamed and rebranded Centre seeks to bring together different research disciplines and to connect both researchers and practising clinicians so that each can learn from the other and share their knowledge. The long-term aim of IRCAHC is for health providers, who experience the day-to-day problems in health care, to have a forum in which to share their understanding and experiences with health communication scholars. The Centre hopes to become a hub connecting sister centres around the globe. This book marks the commencement of this endeavour with Professor Janice Krieger, Director of the STEM Translational Communication Center (STCC) in the College of Journalism and Communications at the University of Florida. The end result being that scholars and practitioners can use their specific expertise to work towards improving patient care delivery and safety. Indeed, the IRCAHC logo statement is *connecting communities.*

To start this process of interdisciplinary connection, the inaugural symposium of IRCAHC was entitled *Expanding Horizons in Health Communication* and was held at The Hong Kong Polytechnic University in January, 2018. It brought together scholars from different disciplines and countries—the USA, Australia and Hong Kong. The symposium highlighted the gap in health communication research between Eastern and Western cultures. While both cultures have much to offer in the health domain, the West has tended to dominate the research across matters of health communication and health practice.

We invited speakers representing a wide range of health communication interests. The Symposium presentations were inspiring and gave insights into the potential to better understand the synthesis between the two cultures with respect to health communication and delivery of patient care. Following the symposium, it was clear to the co-editors of this book that we had to promote the research papers presented to a wider audience. This realisation led to the beginnings of the current edited book. The book's purpose is to break down cultural and linguistic barriers and to promote intellectual exchange in the area of health communication. However, we also recognised that we should not limit the book to the Symposium contributions as not all voices who had something important to say had presented at the symposium. To address this, we put a call for papers out to other scholars who might have relevant research or practice. The end result is this collection of rich, diverse chapters which position the health communication research in Asia in ways that have previously been neglected.

We have divided the book into three parts. The first part focuses on mental health and these chapters explore very different contexts in this domain. In the second part, we investigate more traditional areas of health communication. This is the largest part of the book and includes a range of different research studies focusing on health provider and patient communication. Many of the chapters in this part position communication from an Eastern perspective while some compare Western Medicine (WM) and Traditional Chinese Medicine (TCM). The final part examines other important, but distinct, areas of health and communication and is a celebration of the range of topics the edited book embraces. Topics include the role of teamwork in residential aged care and how safety can sometimes be compromised. Health policy and information dissemination is tackled by examining a diverse set of countries and finally a software analytical tool is used to interpret Cantonese data. We now briefly visit each part to provide a flavour of the book's content.

Health Communication and Mental Well-being in Asia

In Hans Ladegaard's chapter, we hear about the traumas experienced by some migrant workers in Hong Kong. The experiences of these domestic migrant workers are harrowing. They have come to Hong Kong in order to improve the economic situation of their families who remain in the worker's native home. Ladegaard gives us insights into their suffering and how these workers have managed to deal with difficult and challenging personal experiences in a foreign country. This is an area that merits more research and attention and we hope that our book may assist this future work. Staying with mental health, Tay, Huang and Zeng examine how pictures can be used as a stimulus in counselling sessions. They presented clients with two images in two conditions described as either fixed or free. In the free condition, participants interpreted the picture without any direction. In the fixed condition, the participants were provided with a concept to link to the image. The findings from their study suggest that when clients are given a concept on which they can focus, it results in more linguistic expression which has implications for counsellors. Specifically, they can use this knowledge to assist clients to learn from and move forward from the issues they are trying to address. The third chapter in this part investigates adolescent mental health. Harrison and Lam examine the perspectives of counsellors and their adolescent clients in the school context. Adolescent mental health problems are a growing concern globally and have not been well researched in Hong Kong. These authors use interview data with both counsellors and students to better understand their journeys through the different stages of counselling. Importantly, they unpack the barriers and facilitators experienced by clients and counsellors and provide data that expands current knowledge. Such information can be used by educators to assist in directing school counselling policy. The final chapter brings together physical and mental health. Chan discusses the importance of emotional counselling and the psychosocial needs of oncology patients in a ward environment with the associated ongoing time constraints and nurse shortages. Chan's chapter focuses on the Chinese culture where emotional expression is often not openly expressed with respect to feelings about personal health and the importance of family support. Interestingly, the study explores two different perspectives. We see the patients' perspectives in recorded interview videos and audio-taped nurse responses in nurse–patient communication. Chan's findings suggest that even though nurses work in a highly pressured environment, they are still able to respond appropriately to the emotional needs of their patients.

Health Communication in Patient–provider Contexts in Asia

The chapter by Wong, Loong and Lee introduces the fact that many patients in Mainland China and Hong Kong use a blend of Western medicine (WM) and Traditional Chinese Medicine (TCM.) They specifically examine how patients with colorectal cancer handle the two medical approaches in the treatment of their illness. From their interviews with patients, these authors found that the motivations and expected outcomes differed according to whether the patients participated in WM or TCM. They found that patients had firm beliefs in the efficacy of TCM because it provided them with some level of mental support. Although TCM is not always the first line of attack for cancer patients in these areas, it is clear that there is a legitimate role for TCM treatment. The authors suggest that more effort should be made to improve the standards of traditional medicine practitioners. Currently, TCM practitioners are not well regulated by the Chinese government. Still on the topic of WM and TCM, Jin Ying's chapter examines how the two approaches differ in their style of consultation. The data were collected from Mainland China and consisted of audio recordings of actual medical consultations. Jin Ying found that while there are similarities across the consultation process, there were also clear differences. For example, the ending of the consultation represented a more social exchange in TCM compared to the more dismissive conclusion in the WM exchanges. In line with this finding, Jin Ying found that TCM patients were able to produce frame shifts during their interactions that were not evident in the WM consultations. These differences highlight both the different expectations and behaviours by both patients and doctors across the two approaches. The next chapter by Yip and Zhang again explores TCM. The authors of this study, also drawing on data from Mainland China, observed five specific moves that occur in medical interactions. Of interest in their chapter is the co-construction of the medical consultation experience by both the doctor and patient and the sharing of the interaction between the two players. This finding links nicely with Jin Ying's observation of patient empowerment in TCM consultations. Yip and Zhang discuss how TCM is not asymmetrical as is so often observed in WM. Their chapter gives insight into how TCM and WM differ in the pattern of relationship dynamics. Together these two chapters showcase current research across these two types of doctor and patient consultations.

The next chapter in this part moves away from doctor and patient interactions and into the area of health consultations. Schoeb and Yip examine how Chinese patients in Hong Kong and their physiotherapists manage discussions about exercise regimens. They note differences between clients from Western cultures compared to their Eastern counterparts. The latter, they observe, are less willing to ask questions of their physiotherapists. These authors identify the different conversational techniques used by physiotherapists when they instruct their patients on exercise routines that are directly aimed at helping clients engage more actively with their treatment. Schoeb and Yip highlight the importance of a multi-modal approach to instructing patients on exercise and note how both verbal and non-verbal communication play distinctive roles in the treatment process. The final chapter in this part draws on new data collected in Singapore and discusses miscommunication and clinical handover. We note that there has been much work around the world concerning clinical handover (handoff in the United States) and the problems associated with ensuring the right information is provided and acted upon. Ang and Della's chapter presents a study with a large sample of 49 shift-to-shift handovers that were video recorded. They organised their observations around the dimensions of information, structure and interaction. Their findings reflect global issues in terms of ensuring accountability and responsibility of care. They noted that at times there was a lack of clarity. Specifically, they observed the use of native language which was not understood by all participants in their study and highlighted how this is problematic for accurate, timely patient care. Their use of video meant that non-verbal communication could be analysed alongside the verbal. One finding from this analysis was a lack of immediacy on the part of the nurse towards the patient which, they observe, may affect rapport. They suggest that nurses need to reframe handover as a key component of patient safety and not as a task of handing over patient information. It is indeed valuable to note how communication problems with handover—globally recognised as a weak link in patient care—are also evident in Singapore.

Health Communication in Organisational, Campaign and Informatics Contexts

The final part of the book moves to a broader conception of health communication across Eastern and Western cultures. Della, Ma, Roberts, Zhou, Michael and Dhaliwal investigate the safety culture across two aged care facilities in Singapore. This is an under-researched topic especially in Asia where aged care nurses come from many different cultural backgrounds. They tested the validity of a modified survey tool on factors around patient safety culture. Their study demonstrates the importance of open communication between care provider staff who manage and negotiate the needs of their residents. Their findings reveal how good teamwork and cooperation facilitate the achievement of a culture of safety. They note that even good teamwork needs to ensure problems that arise are resolved in ways that do not pose risks to safe care. Establishing a tool that can assess the patient safety culture across different countries is an important step forward to highlight issues that may adversely impact on residents in aged care settings. The chapter by Raisa, Bylund, Islam and Krieger is a systematic review into the role that health communication and information provision play to both treat and prevent disease in Bangladesh where there are large health disparities in the population. From their chapter, we learn that there is no national cancer registry in Bangladesh even though there is a high prevalence of cancer. They specifically target the effectiveness of communication in cancer interventions in Bangladesh. Their paper picks up on the importance of health literacy to empower individuals and highlights the need for serious investment in providing more-up-to-date technology. Such technology would assist with cancer occurrence data collection to create a national register which would assist with health intervention and information campaigns. The authors note that progress that has been made in some areas of healthcare, but this has not been matched with respect to data collection and active public information dissemination. The authors provide clear directions for improving the Bangladeshi situation and their research signals a way forward that can improve this currently worrying state of affairs. Remaining in the public health domain, Cummings' chapter examines the efficacy of public health campaigns. She investigates the role of cognitive heuristics that are premised on informal fallacies and examines their effect in decision making in the UK and Hong Kong. Cummings found that the public across both countries are subjected to health messages that are flawed in their reasoning and do not assist the public to make informed decisions about what action to take. While she acknowledges some differences between the UK and Hong Kong, Cummings observes that they both fail in their information dissemination. She notes that with more travel and contact with other cultures, there is an increased risk of the spread of disease, ensuring the efficacy of public health messages is now more important than ever. Our final chapter is distinct from all others because it has at its heart methods to develop better natural language processing software for use on untranslated Cantonese data. Yau, Turnbull, Angus and Watson examine the question "can we improve on the interpretation of health professional and patient audio recordings by conducting analysis on Cantonese data rather than relying on translation into English"? Currently, most natural language processing software on low-resource languages (like Cantonese and in contrast to Mandarin Chinese) relies on translation into English or alphabetic languages. These authors have taken data visualisation software and developed workstreams and guidelines so that Cantonese transcripts can be directly uploaded and analysed. Analysing logographic transcripts rather than English translations means that the linguistic subtleties will be retained. This is a positive move towards integrating data from an Asian culture using an analytic tool that has only been used on alphabetic data sets.

In summary, our goal for this edited book is to present a sharing of the knowledge process that informs researchers and practitioners about the work currently occurring in Asian countries. Some of this work is informed by Western medicine and some by traditional Chinese medicine and in a few cases, they are combined. We feel that a more concerted effort to promote an intellectual exchange between these two cultures can serve to inform and improve health communication practice. Importantly, this book is a contact point for researchers to find out what is happening in Asian countries and what can be learned from East and West. We further want this book to breakdown national cultural barriers and promote research collaboration. It is only when researchers and clinicians from these different cultures communicate and share, that meaningful progress can be made.

Contents

Part I
Health Communication and Mental Well-being in Asia

Talking About Trauma in Migrant Worker Returnee Narratives: Mental Health Issues

Hans J. Ladegaard

Abstract This chapter reports on a research project about Indonesian and Filipina migrant worker returnees. Shortly after their return, they were invited to participate in a sharing session with other migrant workers and a researcher about their experiences as migrant workers and about their homecoming. 107 women participated in 30 sharing sessions and all the stories were transcribed and (for some) translated. A large number of the women were (sexually) assaulted while they worked overseas and return to their home countries deeply traumatised. First, the chapter analyses some narrative excerpts in which the women talk about (sexual) assault and other traumatic experiences. The stories are notably incoherent and disconnected, characterised by voids in the narrative flow. This is typical of trauma storytelling but is sometimes used against the women to discredit their stories. Then the chapter discusses the mental health issues involved in these women's stories and what scholars can do to address them. The findings from the current dataset suggest that hundreds of traumatised women return to Indonesia every year with no access to proper healthcare or professional therapy, and the chapter discusses what can be done to meet these women's needs.

Keywords Domestic workers · Trauma · Narrative · Mental health

1 Introduction

Increased migration has become one of the characteristics of globalisation in the twenty-first century. Globalisation has offered augmented opportunities to professionals and skilled workers who can choose to utilise their resources in other parts of the world for longer or shorter periods of time. However, for people at the bottom of the globalisation market, as Blommaert (2010) puts it, globalisation has seriously constrained their lives and opportunities. For refugees, asylum seekers and

H. J. Ladegaard (✉)
The Hong Kong Polytechnic University, Hong Kong, China
e-mail: hans.ladegaard@polyu.edu.hk

© Springer Nature Singapore Pte Ltd. 2020
B. Watson and J. Krieger (eds.), *Expanding Horizons in Health Communication*,
The Humanities in Asia 6, https://doi.org/10.1007/978-981-15-4389-0_1

unskilled migrant workers, migration is not a choice but a necessity. Thus, many people in developing countries are faced with a dilemma: either they stay at home to raise their children who are then kept in poverty with no prospects of a better future, or they go overseas to work, which means more or less permanent separation from their children and other loved ones (Ladegaard, 2017).

The Philippines is one of the world's largest exporters of migrant labour with close to 10 million Filipino migrant workers living and working overseas. Another major supplier of migrant labour is Indonesia with an estimated 6.5 million migrants working overseas and the number is sharply increasing with more than 400,000 new migrant workers leaving Indonesia every year through official channels. Significant numbers also leave the country through illegal channels so the actual number is hard to determine, but 2–4 times the number of documented workers has been suggested (Paul, 2017). Documented migration has dropped significantly in recent years, largely due to a government ban because of widespread reports of abuse of particularly female migrant workers in the Middle East. However, it is still a huge, largely unaddressed problem that so many young women leave their families and communities in rural Indonesia every year without being prepared for the trials and tribulations that await them.

Young Indonesian women, particularly in East and Central Java, are recruited by local agents who work for recruitment agencies in receiving countries/regions in Asia (predominantly Malaysia, Hong Kong, Taiwan and Singapore) and the Middle East (predominantly Saudi Arabia, United Arab Emirates and Kuwait). The women are often recruited through male family members who receive money from the recruiter for signing up their wives or daughters for migrant labour. The women are transferred to a training centre to learn basic cleaning and cooking skills, as well as receive a crash course in the language of the country to which they are going. After 3–6 weeks of training, they are recruited by an overseas agent who negotiates the terms with an employer in a receiving country. They work on 2-year contracts and usually have to live with their employers.

The women are often unprepared for the hardships they experience in many of the receiving countries, particularly in the Middle East where there are virtually no migrant labour laws to protect their rights. While Filipina domestic workers tend to be mature, relatively well educated and speak good English, the Indonesian women tend to be young, have received little formal education and speak little or no English. These factors appear to be important in the widespread abuse of Indonesian domestic migrant workers (DMWs). Several of the women whose narratives were recorded for this study confirmed that they were 16 or 17 years old when they left home and therefore the recruitment agency issued them with fake identity papers so they could pass the Indonesian government's minimum age requirement of 21. They also confided that they knew no English and could not read the employment contract they signed, let alone talk to their employer when they arrived at the final destination. DMWs going to Hong Kong usually receive a 3-week crash course in Cantonese but that does not mean they can speak the language (Ladegaard, 2019).

This chapter analyses DMW returnee narratives. It draws on a sample of 112 narratives recorded during field trips to Indonesia and the Philippines. Overall, the Filipina women's migratory experiences were fairly positive: they took pride in the work they had done and the income they had provided for their families, and they recalled mostly positive experiences. The Indonesian women, on the other hand, recounted mostly negative experiences: they reported widespread exploitation and abuse, including physical and sexual assault, and, despite their poverty, they had no desire to go overseas again (Ladegaard, 2019). This chapter focuses on the Indonesian women's stories of the abuse and exploitation they were subjected to as DMWs. It outlines the characteristics of trauma storytelling, and it presents a discourse analytic study of selected excerpts in which the women talk about their traumatic experiences and their ensuing emotions. The chapter also discusses the mental health issues identified through these women's stories. Presumably hundreds of migrant workers return to Indonesia every year with untreated trauma, and the final part of the chapter explores the likely consequences and discusses what can be done to address their problems.

2 Trauma Storytelling

No matter the content, form and circumstances, trauma narratives are always difficult to tell because "tellability ... is compromised by the unacceptability of the events. They are stories about things that *shouldn't* happen rather than about things that *didn't* happen" (emphasis added) (Shuman, 2005: 19–20). Thus, trauma storytelling is unsettling; it poses a challenge, first and foremost for the storyteller who needs to recall traumatic experiences and the emotional impact they had on her, but also for the audience and the analyst who need to make sense of stories that may appear piecemeal, incoherent and sometimes even contradictory. Hydén and Brockmeier (2008: 10) have coined the term "broken narrative" to explain the essence of trauma storytelling. They define it as "an open and fluid concept, emphasizing problematic, precarious, and damaged narratives told by people who in one way or another have trouble telling their story." Another challenge of trauma, for the teller, the audience and the analyst, is that it may "shatter the established ways in which we have previously understood our self, life, and the world" (McTighe, 2018, p. 46). Trauma storytelling violates listeners' expectations and therefore, it becomes difficult to propose fixed interpretive frameworks (Harvey, 2000).

In terms of structure, trauma narratives are often characterised by voids in the narrative flow (Brockmeier, 2008). The problem is that "ordinary" language cannot capture the experience and this may lead to a "traumatic gap" between the experience on the one hand and the language available to describe it on the other. Thus, as Langer (1980) argues in his discussion of the dilemma of choice in the Holocaust death-camps, because there is no vocabulary of annihilation, trauma victims have to rely on what Levi has called "free words created and used by free men" (Langer, 1980: 224). This means, Langer (p. 224) continues, that in the interpretation of trauma, "we must bring to every 'reading' of the [Holocaust] experience a wary consciousness of the way in which 'free words' and their associations may distort the facts or alter them into more manageable events."

An important question that is often neglected in the literature is how we define trauma narrative. Most of the existing trauma narrative research has been done by health professionals who tend to pay little or no attention to language. Most studies use interviews or written accounts of traumatic events and the focus is usually on post-traumatic stress disorder and other health-related issues (O'Kerney & Perrott, 2006). In a discourse analytic study of trauma narratives, the emphasis must be on language and what it signifies emotionally and psychologically. In previous research drawing on a large corpus of more than 300 narratives recorded at a Hong Kong church shelter for DMWs, I have argued that we should understand trauma narrative in terms of what the traumatic experience does to the teller, rather than using the seriousness of the offence to determine whether it should be classified as traumatic (Ladegaard, 2015). Thus, I propose that the women's *response* to their experiences should impact whether and to what extent the event should be defined as traumatic. However, other scholars have argued that stories may fall short of the listener's stereotypical expectations of what trauma storytelling sounds like and yet, constitute a traumatic experience for the teller. In her analysis of narratives by rape victims, Trinch (2013: 289) rightly points out that analysts may inadvertently focus their attention on "women's pain, suffering, and victimization at the expense of understanding rape when it is reported in the absence of any perceived psychological damage." Based on an in-depth analysis of 175 narratives, 41 of which were defined as trauma narratives, I have previously proposed that the four criteria listed below could function as an indicator of trauma storytelling but by no means exclude other narratives that do not show all of these characteristics[1] (derived from Ladegaard, 2015: 194–195).

(1) There is continuous crying, either throughout the telling of a narrative, or repeatedly during the storytelling.
(2) The trauma leads to some form of existential crisis. At some point during the storytelling, the women would question the meaning of life, their faith in God or their very existence. Even suicide is mentioned in some cases as the only way out.
(3) Traumatic experiences are narrated repeatedly. The narrator returns to her traumatic experiences at least twice during the course of the telling, which suggests that it is experienced as an emotionally unfinished event which requires repeated attention.
(4) The overriding emotion in trauma storytelling is fear. The women would testify repeatedly that they were always afraid while working for an abusive employer.

We might also add, as mentioned above, that trauma storytelling is often characterised by voids in the narrative flow (cf. Brockmeier, 2008): disfluencies, pauses and hesitations as well as incoherence, or even contradictions, in the storyline

(Ladegaard, 2017). Health professionals tend to use physiological and psychological symptoms as an indicator that a patient is traumatised, and they have mentioned that trauma victims often suffer from post-traumatic stress disorder including insomnia, anxiety and intractable depression (Herman, 1998), and/or depression-related symptoms like traumatic grief, extreme sadness, suicidability, weight loss and fatigue (Briere, Scott, & Jones, 2015). As the analyses will show, some of these symptoms are also visible in the narratives that will be analysed in this chapter, but because this study is trying to make a contribution to the language of trauma storytelling, it is befitting that the focus should be on the linguistic, paralinguistic and structural characteristics of the narratives rather than on the women's physiological symptoms.

Before we turn to the analysis of narratives, I shall briefly outline the characteristics of the data and the data collection, and the theoretical and analytical frameworks that were used to analyse it.

3 The Data

3.1 The Field Trips

The two field trips were organised in close collaboration with local migrant worker NGOs in East and Central Java, Indonesia and in Bohol in the Philippines. Through the Hong Kong branch of these NGOs, I received invitations to visit villages with large numbers of migrant worker returnees, and I also visited former clients and residents of a Hong Kong migrant worker NGO that I worked with. I spent 3–4 weeks in each country travelling around the countryside with a driver and an interpreter. The women had been contacted prior to my arrival by the local NGOs and asked if they wanted to meet with me and share their stories.

Most of the women shared their stories in groups of 4–8 people but some preferred to talk to me and/or the interpreter without their friends present. Each sharing session lasted 1–2 h; it was recorded and transcribed by a bi- or multilingual speaker of Bahasa, Javanese and English (for the Indonesian data) and Tagalog and English (for the Filipino data). Prior to each recording, the purpose of the study was explained to the women (in their mother tongue), and they all gave their consent for their anonymised stories to be used for research and publicity purposes. A total of 107 migrant worker returnees participated in the sharing sessions: 67 in Java and 34 in Bohol, in addition to a pre-departure sharing session with six Indonesian women who had been deported from Hong Kong.

In most of the migrant villages we visited, I stayed with a local family and this gave me the opportunity to observe and participate in life as it is lived in migrant worker communities. A striking feature of all the communities I visited was a lack of employment opportunities. All sending migrant worker communities in Java and Bohol are characterised by extremely high unemployment, and only in one of the

19 villages I visited was there an employment opportunity for DMW returnees: a palm oil factory that provided contract work which paid IDR20,000 (US$1.5) per day. However, what these villages did seem to provide for many of the women was a sense of community with close-knit social networks and a sharing of migratory experiences as well as goods and commodities.

3.2 Theoretical and Analytical Frameworks

The research was informed by an inductive approach to data: no hypotheses or preconceived ideas about findings were proposed. The study was exploratory and data were used to generate new theory and applications adopting qualitative methodologies and analytical concepts from anthropology, sociolinguistics and social psychology. A key concept was the use of sharing sessions (as opposed to interviews) where the idea of *sharing* life stories and experiences was in focus. There was no interview guide or pre-defined research questions; rather, the aim was to get the women to tell stories that were important to them. Only three general questions were used to introduce the sharing sessions (with occasional follow-up questions): (1) What was it like to be a migrant worker; (2) What was it like to come home? (3) What are you thinking about the future? While some groups focused more on the coming-home narratives, other groups never got past the first question because they had so many painful stories to share; these stories will be the focus of this chapter. The stories were collected using the ethnography-of-communication approach (Saville-Troike, 2003), which emphasises the need to observe the research site and include as much contextual information as possible in the interpretation of data. Staying with and talking to migrant worker families was important in terms of understanding their stories, and four years of voluntary work/research at shelters in Hong Kong also proved to be invaluable with respect to analysing the narratives and contextualising the women's experiences.

In terms of understanding how narratives are conceptualised, social constructionism provided the framework (Burr, 2015). Social constructionism claims that narratives are situated and dynamic discursive constructions. Thus, when people talk (and tell stories), they also present and negotiate their identities. A social constructionist approach to narratives would question the assumption that stories are given, and that they represent underlying psychological states. Rather, stories and the identity positions they communicate are constructed in discourse, and the construction involves not just the narrator but also the audience. It would see storytelling as constitutive of context and the people who narrate as social actors (Augoustinos, Walker, & Donaghue, 2014).

The stories were analysed using a combination of Toolan's (2001) linguistic approach to narrative, focusing on identity construction, and White & Epston's (1990) therapeutic approach to storytelling. Toolan argues that analysts should pay equal attention to narrative structure and function, and by closely analysing the linguistic components of narratives, important information about the narratives themselves and about the identity of their narrators is revealed. Any aspect of language can be indexical of the storyteller's identity from phonological features to individual words and complex discourse structures (De Fina, Schiffrin, & Bamberg, 2006). However, this does not mean that everything we do in storytelling should be interpreted as identity construction. We do much more than "speak our identities" (Mishler, 1999) when we narrate. Thus, indexical relationships are not given but created and negotiated in context as the narrative progresses. According to narrative therapy, we live storied lives and people should, therefore, be encouraged to tell their stories in order to make sense of past (traumatic) experiences. A key assumption in narrative therapy is that "our stories do not simply represent us or mirror lived events—they constitute us, shaping our lives and our relationships" (Brown & Augusta-Scott, 2007: ix). Thus, the main idea behind narrative therapy is that helping people to change the stories about their lives will also help them change their actual lives.

4 Data Analysis

The first example is from Rika's story. She is a 33-year old DMW from a small village in Central Java who worked eight years in Hong Kong and two years in Singapore. I met Rika through the Hong Kong NGO that provided her with temporary accommodation and medical aid after she had become pregnant and lost her job. Rika's story is typical of Indonesian first-timers: she worked from 7am until 9 pm every day, she got very little food and she only received 2/3 of her stipulated salary, but she was too scared to complain because "I really needed the job." After four years in Hong Kong, she met her Nepalese boyfriend and when she became pregnant, she lost her job but decided to stay illegally in order to be close to her "husband"[2]. After another child and serious problems with her husband, she turned herself in to the authorities and was eventually deported. When I met her in Indonesia, she had given into pressure from family and neighbours and engaged in a marriage of convenience to a cousin to avoid the shame of being a single mother. A female interpreter (Int) and a male fieldworker (FW) were in all the sessions quoted in this paper; original in English (see transcription conventions in the appendix).

Excerpt 1

1. FW: so you overstayed in Hong Kong? You didn't have a regular employer?

2. Rika: I feel so scared, so scared, so scared that (2.0) also the life of his father is

3.   (2.0) very difficult and also xx thinking of the children (4.0) and I want to

4.   go back but also so scared because when I go, maybe they'll catch me

5.   with the kids, if (1.0) if I go to er: prison that's my (1.0) my (3.0) I cannot

6.   think how (1.0) how to separate from the kids if (1.0) if I go to prison, then

7.   when my children go, they say, some people said they cannot bring the kids

8.   they will separate us, then I feel like, so scared [10 turns left out]

9. FW: you said you were able to leave your husband?

10. Rika: yeah, when the (1.0) when the first time is (1.0) I don't (1.0) I'm (1.0)

11.   I'm so scared when I leave him, then when he needs something then we're

12.   not with that (1.0) I'm so scared because later he tried suicide and yeah

13.   I'm so scared about that and then (2.0) I have something like trauma and

14.   I, you know I feel like so stressed

15. FW: yes

16. Rika: when I separate from him, my pain is all coming, before I (1.0) I put all

17.   inside my heart (1.0) my (1.0) heart that xx and many people give me

18.   support there, they said 'you must be strong for your kids' [sobs] because I

19.   (1.0) I'm so (2.0) and so xx when he need (1.0) that one the, I cannot, also he

20.   don't have money to buy and then what he feel like (2.0) and then I also feel

21.   (1.0) feel, what, **pain**, I also feel pain, he's also [in] pain [sobs]

22. FW: yeah

23. Rika: then I'm thinking I go back to Indonesia xx **for my kids**, for their future [sobs]

Rika is a woman in great distress. She has left the man she loves in Hong Kong because she could not deal with his drug abuse, and because she was terrified of being caught by the police and imprisoned for overstaying (lines 4–5). Being imprisoned meant separation from her children and that is her ultimate fear (lines 7–8). Note how she talks about her fear repeatedly throughout the excerpt. The compound "so scared" is used eight times in this part of her narrative (lines 2, 4, 8, 11, 12 and 13), and in line 2, she repeats it three times for emphasis. Her emotional turmoil is further emphasised by repeated references to the pain she feels (line 16 and 21); she even says that she is traumatised (line 13). Her crying also signifies emotional distress (lines 21 and 23) and could be conceptualised as "a language through which individuals communicate their suffering and also as a curative process" (Labott, 2001: 219). Labott (2001: 222) analysed the use and functions of crying in authentic psychotherapy and she notes that crying occurred when the patient had a great deal of unexpressed or unfinished emotion from earlier events in her life, a great deal of stress and upset in her current life, when she felt safe in the situation, and when she accessed earlier painful memories through storytelling. All of these conditions seem to apply to Rika's story: the repeated references to the fear she experienced while living illegally in Hong Kong suggest unfinished emotions; the stress in her current situation is evident in earlier parts of her story where she talks about being ostracised from the local community, and her constant financial worries and the repeated crying suggests that she is accessing painful memories but also that she feels safe in the context in which she tells her story.

Another feature suggesting that Rika is traumatised is that her story is broken and, at times, has voids in the narrative flow (Brockmeier, 2008). There are several pauses, some of them lengthy (e.g., lines 2, 3, 5, 19), and incomplete utterances: "that's my (1.0) my (3.0) I cannot think how" (line 5), and "I'm so (2.0) and so xx when he need (1.0) that one the, I cannot" (line 19). Rika is a perfectly fluent speaker of English so the disfluency she displays in this excerpt is not due to her inability to speak English, but more likely because she is unable to tell a coherent story due to her emotional distress. While incomplete utterances and (lengthy) pauses are not unusual in casual conversation and "natural" storytelling, their cognitive and emotional manifestations are different in trauma narratives (Ladegaard, 2015). The point is the mismatch between the personal experience of events and the language available to describe them. In his analysis of personal accounts of 9/11, Brockmeier (2008: 21) argues that the more everyday the language of trauma narratives is, the more ordinary or familiar it sounds, "the more it loses the horror of what it attempts to capture." Thus, trauma storytelling often appears incoherent, not so much because the teller is searching for the right words but because a vocabulary that adequately captures the events and their emotional impact is not available (Ladegaard, 2015).

The next example is from a sharing session with six migrant worker returnees in Central Java. Harum, a 44-year old former domestic worker who spent 10 years overseas (in Singapore, Malaysia, Taiwan and Hong Kong), is still struggling with the aftermaths of working for an abusive employer one year after her return. The interpreter has just asked if anybody would share her story about being a migrant worker, and line 1 is the beginning of Harum's story. Original in Bahasa (B) and English (E).

Excerpt 2

1.   Har: I often feel sad when sharing my story, when I'm remembering this (1.0)

2.   imagine it was heavy rain and I was kicked out from the house (B)

3.   Int: okay so she// (E)

4.   Har: //there was no evidence that I steal [sobs] (B)

5.   Int: no evidence (B)

6.   Har: have no evidence, until the police (1.0) examined me twice and the one

7.   who was in the house, in the house, also examined me, but I knew that

8.   was only her reason to kick me out (2.0) did not find any evidence (B)

9.   [12 turns left out during which the interpreter asks for clarification]

10. Int: did you get your compensation? (B)

11. Har: yes (B) but only, did not get one month's salary and ticket (E)

12. FW: very common story unfortunately, yeah, sorry to hear that, yeah (E)

13. Har: that's mhm: I'm working to take care of the baby, cleaning the house is

14.   (1.0) must be very very clean (E)

15. FW: mhm

16. Har: eh: 12 o'clock midnight, still washing cars in the car park (1.0) I'm

17.   sleeping sometimes 1 o'clock 2 o'clock and I wake up 5:30 (E)

18. FW: mhm

19. Har: and then [they do] not give me enough food like that, so I'm always

20.   hungry there [sobs] (E)

21. FW: yeah, yeah (E)

Prior to Harum's story, Mawar told the group how she was accused of stealing a necklace from her Hong Kong employer who reported her to the police. A police officer searched her belongings and eventually took her to the bathroom and ordered her to strip naked. To accuse a DMW of stealing is a way for the employer to terminate the contract without having to pay the compulsory compensation (one month's salary and airfare back to the home country), and sadly, it is quite a frequent practice in Hong Kong (Ladegaard, 2017). Part of the sadness and frustration Harum is going through as she recollects what happened to her is being falsely accused of committing a crime she did not commit. She cries as she remembers how she was searched by the police (line 4) and eventually kicked out of the house while it was pouring down with rain (line 2).

She then recollects what it was like for her to work for almost a year under gruelling conditions. She cleaned every inch of the big house repeatedly every day (line 13–14), she took care of a baby while doing all her other chores (line 13), she had to wash the cars late at night (line 16), and still be ready for work every morning at 5:30 (line 17). Like other DMWs seeking help at shelters in Hong Kong, Harum was worn out from hard labour and extremely long workdays and constantly suffering from hunger (Ladegaard, 2017). She cries when she remembers, as she later testifies, how she was always hungry and always thinking about food (line 19–20). Hunger is a terrible all-encompassing experience but equally traumatising is the fact that DMWs are being positioned by their employers as less than human (Tileaga, 2005). They are treated like expendable household commodities, not like human beings who have a right to eat, rest and relax, and the consequence is a gradual reduction of self. Brison (1999: 41) argues that "victims of human-inflicted trauma are reduced to mere objects by their tormenters"—a process which she refers to as "the undoing of the self by trauma" (bid). Trauma victims are reduced to mere objects, physically weakened by lack of food, rest and sleep, and mentally weakened by lack of recognition and respect.

An important part of this undoing of the self is subjecting somebody to lack of sleep and constant hunger. In a sharing session at a Hong Kong church shelter, Marinol, a 38-year old Filipina DMW, says "I'm desperate [from hunger], I could not sleep well at night because I was **so** very hungry", and when she asked her employer for food, she was told: "you did not come here to eat, you come here to work" (Ladegaard, 2015: 198). Thus, DMWs' experience of food and sleep deprivation can be compared to Levi's account of life in Auschwitz, which, he says, cannot be encompassed by ordinary language, or "free words":

Just as our hunger is not that feeling of missing a meal, so our way of being cold has need of a new word. We say "hunger", we say "tiredness", "fear", "pain", we say "winter" and they are different things. They are free words created by men who lived in comfort and suffering in their homes. If the Lagers (camps) had lasted longer a new harsh language would have been born, and only this language could express what it means to toil the whole day […] and in one's body [feel] nothing but weakness, hunger and knowledge of the end drawing near (cited in Langer, 1980: 223–224).

Some of Levi's accounts of life in Auschwitz are comparable to DMWs' experiences. Like Levi's, their hunger is not that of missing a meal but a constant all-encompassing feeling of never having enough to eat and living off food scraps. It becomes an obsession, a horrifying traumatising experience that "ordinary" language cannot describe. Levi's account again captures an essential aspect of trauma storytelling: the gap between the experience and the language available to describe it.

The codeswitching also deserves a comment. In a sharing session where Bahasa is the dominant language, Harum switches to English in line 11. It might be motivated by the reference to "one month's salary/notice and return ticket", which is very much part of migrant workers' register, and therefore it might be more convenient to borrow these lexical items from English. Speech/communication accommodation (Gallois & Giles, 2015) may also be important. Studies have shown that speakers accommodate to their interlocutors' (perceived) linguistic and communicative behaviour, and in this example, it is possible that Harum is focusing her attention on the English-speaking fieldworker and appeals for his sympathy (Ladegaard, 2018).

The next example is from Sari's narrative. She worked four years in the United Arab Emirates (UAE); like Harum in Excerpt 2, she worked extremely long hours on little food and was eventually accused of stealing a necklace from her employer. She was subsequently arrested by the police, put in jail and deported from the country with a criminal record. Utama (Uta) and three other participants were also in the sharing session. Original in Bahasa (B) and English (E).

Excerpt 3

1. Sari: when I go back [from hospital] they say there's a necklace missing, they say

2.   I took it but I never took it (B)

3. Uta: what was taken? (B)

4. Sari: I continued to stay there to prove that I didn't take it [sobs] then later on

5.   I heard a story while she was talking to her relative, she said that the

6.   necklace was missing before I came (B)

7. Int: mhm

8. Sari: then I said [to the employer] 'the necklace was missing when I came back from

9.   hospital but actually before I came here, before I worked here, it was already

10.   missing, perhaps you used the money for your mother's surgery' I said (1.0)

11.   I was there trying to be loyal and patient, to prove that I'm innocent [sobs]

12.   but thank God there were consequences, there was punishment from

13.   God [sobs]

14.   [15 short turns left out during which the interpreter asks clarifying questions]

15. FW: has anybody helped you talk about this after you came back? (E)

16. Int: okay when//

17. Sari: //yes [sobs] I've talked but I also sometimes have difficulties

18.   expressing [myself], difficult like that (B)

19. Int: okay, it's not easy for her to share her story, she's tried but it's kind of

20.   not easy (E) [quietly to FW]

21. Sari: the trauma is so deep [sobs] (E)

22. FW: yeah, how many years now? (E)

23. Sari: three years (E)

24. FW: three years ago okay (1.0) yeah okay, how do you feel now? (E)

25. Sari: I think everything is the same, what, what I feel is, until now is the same

26.   [sobs] (E)

27. FW: just take your time right (E) (6.0)

Sari is arguably the most visibly distraught of all the DMWs in the sample. She cried continuously throughout her entire story, which lasted approximately 15 min, and even three years after her return to Indonesia, she is still struggling with the aftermath of trauma (line 21). Sari is required to stay with the employer's mother while she undergoes surgery in hospital. She looks after her for 10 days and sleeps on the floor next to her bed, and when she comes back from hospital, she is accused of theft (lines 1–2). Her female employer concocted a story and got another Indonesian helper in the household to support her, and together they framed Sari as the culprit despite the fact that the employer admitted to a relative that the necklace went missing before Sari joined the household (lines 4–6). It is this ultimate betrayal from two women who claim to be her Muslim sisters that plunges Sari into depression.

A noticeable feature of the turn-taking in this excerpt is that Sari ignores a question (line 3) and interrupts a comment (line 17) from one of the other participants. This is not because she is an inconsiderate speaker but more likely because she is so engulfed in her storytelling that the story takes over and tells itself as it were (Ladegaard, 2017). This could be a consequence of her emotional turmoil which is also evident in the lines immediately following Excerpt 3: "it's always like this when I raise it [the trauma], also I cannot, I cannot, right? (1.0) the pain is the same, I go home I'm sick (2.0) I cannot xx [sobs]". Thus, at times during the storytelling, Sari's narrative becomes "like a raging river sucking up everything in its path; a stream of consciousness out of control" (Medved & Brockmeier, 2008: 61).

The first part of Sari's story is narrated in Bahasa but in line 21, she switches to English. The reason could be speech accommodation, as we saw it in Excerpt 2, since the fieldworker has just asked a question in English (line 15) and the interpreter has translated into English (lines 19–20). But it might also have to do with the emotional impact of the storytelling. Scholars have argued that switching to a less emotionally charged language (usually the L2) might lessen the emotional impact of trauma storytelling (Tehrani & Vaughan, 2009). Thus, using an L2 is believed to bring about some form of psychological detachment so that the teller is able to talk about the events without being overwhelmed by grief. However, Sari's forceful emotional response in lines 17, 21 and 26 suggests that the switch to English did not lessen the emotional impact. What Sari's story as well as several other examples in the data suggest is that codeswitching and emotionality are aligned. When the women recall particularly difficult, emotionally charged experiences, they tend to switch from Bahasa into English, but we do not know whether the issue is emotional detachment, or an attempt to increase the quality of the emotional content of the experience by narrating it in the language in which the incident was encoded (Tehrani & Vaughan, 2009; Ladegaard, 2018).

However, what is arguably more important in Sari's case is that three years after her return to Indonesia, she is still overwhelmed by grief and unable to come to terms with what happened to her. The trauma is "so deep" (line 21) and nothing has changed or improved regarding her emotional state since she came back (line 25). The next example is from a pre-departure sharing session with five Indonesian DMWs in Hong Kong. All the women have had babies out of wedlock; therefore, they have overstayed and eventually been deported. Ratu, a 29-year old domestic helper who worked for seven years in Singapore, Malaysia and Hong Kong, is telling the group that she got pregnant by her boyfriend, an African asylum-seeker who left her before the baby was born to marry a Chinese woman. Like the other women in this group, Ratu's father is adamant that "until I see the baby's father, don't bring him [the baby] to Indonesia", so she has no idea where to go when she leaves Hong Kong. Notions of shame and guilt, particularly if related to women's sexual behaviour, are very strong in Indonesian sending communities (Chan, 2018), and the women's sense of failure is very real. About 5 min into her story, Ratu tells the group that she is traumatised (original in English).

Excerpt 4

1. Ratu: me, traumatised already as domestic helper because uhm (1.0)

2.   the first time I'm working in Singapore, I have, my employer is

3.   really very bad

4. FW: yeah

5. Ratu: and then after that I worked here [Hong Kong], it's also very bad

6. FW: uhm

7. Ratu: so I, I'm scared to be a domestic helper

8. FW: okay, yeah

9. Ratu: yeah, in Singapore before my boss want to kill me with a knife

10. FW: oh my goodness

11. Ratu: yeah, and then uhm (2.0) the second one here [Hong Kong] the boss,

12.   the (1.0) sir (2.0) and then always, I don't know, he's maybe not

13.   working, and then like (1.0) stressed

14. FW   uhm

15. Ratu: and then sometimes he ask me more (2.0) something like that, ask me

16.   to do this one (1.0) it's not my job but he ask me to do it

17. FW: okay

18. Ratu: so (1.0) if I work, if I go back to Indonesia and then I want to uhm (1.0)

19.   I don't want to become a domestic helper (1.0) I will find another job

20.   but it's not domestic helper

21. FW: yeah, yeah, right

22. Ratu: because I'm really scared already

Like we saw it with Rika (Excerpt 1) and Sari (Excerpt 3), Ratu also testifies to being traumatised (line 1), and it is caused by bad experiences during her previous employments. Her Singapore employer threatened to kill her with a knife (line 9), and there is reason to suspect that her Hong Kong employer took advantage of her sexually. Although she never says explicitly that she was sexually assaulted, there are several linguistic and paralinguistic cues suggesting that she was. First, she hesitates and pauses repeatedly (lines 11–13, 15–16), she uses false beginnings (lines 11–12) and hedges (lines 12–13) and she mitigates the employer's actions in advance by saying that he was unemployed and stressed (lines 12–13). Then she testifies that he sometimes asked for more (line 15), and she eventually uses a euphemism ("to do this one", line 16) followed by a mitigating statement: "it's not my job but he ask me to do it" (line 16), which serves as a form of self-defence. Sadly, some young DMWs are asked to provide sexual services to male family members, and the experience is associated with embarrassment, shame and guilt (Ladegaard, 2013). As in Ratu's case, the "confession" is usually presented piecemeal and gradually and more often than not, never explicitly mentions sex[3], presumably due to the shameful nature of the experience. The overarching emotion derived from her overseas work experiences is fear (lines 7, 22), which has scarred her and made her vow that she will never be a domestic helper again.

The final example is from Riana's story. She is a 45-year old former DMW who spent 10 months in Kuwait. Due to a mistake made by her Indonesian recruiter, she was brought to Kuwait on a tourist visa, which does not allow her to work. She is discovered because she eventually runs away from her abusive employers (original in Bahasa, except for the quote in lines 5–6).

Excerpt 5

1. Riana: I was not paid for three months, for three months I was not paid, I

2.   called the agent, and the agent said 'yes later I will ask your employer'

3.   [3 turns left out] I was not paid for three months, I was asking for my salary,

4.   it was not given (1.0) then my employer said 'when your employer is

5.   away, there is no need for you to go out' [English] even the garbage

6.   could not be thrown out [3 turns left out] if the employer went out the door

7.   must be locked, if there are people knocking on the door, I couldn't open,

8.   just like that (1.0) after three times I doubted it, then I called the agent, I

9.   was not allowed to go out, even to throw the garbage was not allowed, the

10.   employer said [they were] afraid there are police (1.0) then the agent said

11.   'don't be afraid, the most important thing is you must do what your

12.   employer has told you' [4 turns left out] after three months I was [still] not

13.   paid I called the embassy and [they] said 'just come here but use a taxi', just

14.   like that [3 turns left out during which Riana explains that her employer had

15.   taken her passport] before they [the embassy] could make a temporary

16.   passport, I had already been caught by the police (1.0) then I was brought

17.   to the police station, for 3 months and 13 days I was in prison in the police

18.   station

19. Int: you were imprisoned?

20. Riana: because according to the police, 'you're not guilty, the mistake was made

21.   by the office in Indonesia', they said it like that, but I was stripped naked

22.   and beaten with a rattan

23. Int: why were you stripped naked ma'am?

24. Riana: [they were] afraid I was hiding weapons, or something like that

Riana spent only 10 months overseas and she has been back in Indonesia for seven years at the time of the recording. However, she is still visibly distraught when she tells her story and later confides that she is traumatised by the experiences she had in Kuwait. Note how she keeps repeating that she was not paid any salary for three months (twice in line 1, line 3, lines 12–13), which underlines the importance of the issue. Money is the reason DMWs leave their families to earn a living overseas. It was brought up repeatedly in sharing sessions at the shelter that they came to Hong Kong for the sake of their family, and as long as they are paid, they will endure almost any humiliation (Ladegaard, 2017). Sadly, underpayment or non-payment is shockingly common, particularly among Indonesian domestic helpers. In his survey of 2,500 DMWs in Hong Kong, Chiu (2005) found that 50% of the Indonesian workers in his sample were underpaid. Underpayment/ non-payment is a means to effectively belittle domestic workers and deprive them of the recognition their work deserves. Taylor (1994: 25) argues that non-recognition can function as "a form of oppression, imprisoning someone in a false, distorted, and reduced mode of being." Thus, non-payment has serious consequences for DMWs' lives, first and foremost financially but it may also contribute to the "reduction of self" (Brison, 1999).

There are several other examples of blatant abuse and dehumanisation in Riana's story. She is kept inside the house and not allowed to open the door (line 7), her employer keeps her passport to prevent her from leaving (lines 14–15), and she is eventually arrested and imprisoned for not having a valid employment visa (lines 17–18), and while in prison, she is stripped naked and beaten (line 21–22). Although she does not say so, it is possible that she was sexually assaulted, or at least, extremely humiliated for appearing naked in front of male police officers. During her ordeal, she calls her local agency to which she has paid extortionate fees and asks for help only to be told that she needs to be obedient and do what her employer tells her to do (lines 11–12). This again is a typical reply to DMWs who seek help from their employment agencies no matter the issue and, like employers' control of their domestic workers, it signifies "an attempt to reduce them to docile social bodies, to deprive them of full personhood, and to craft for them a less morally ambivalent—but sufficiently subordinate—position within the household" (Constable, 1997: 553). Thus, controlling domestic helpers and restricting their freedom is one way of exerting authority and ensure that they would never take up any position of authority in the family, or in the societies in which they live.

However, as Riana testifies later in her story, the ultimate humiliation for her is coming home to her village with nothing. Despite the sacrifices she has made, and despite her personal suffering, the ultimate defeat is coming home with her clothes wrapped in an ugly piece of cloth from prison, not even a suitcase. And when her son asks, "mom, where's the money", she says, "I took the money from my pocket, just coins (1.0) this is my money [sobs]." In her research in sending communities in Central Java, Chan (2018) found that villagers perceive labour migration positively, but only to the extent that return migrants bring back money so that the family can buy land and build a house. If they don't, they are considered failures and tend to be subjected to gendered and moral blame: the implication is that they did something wrong which is why their migratory journey failed.

5 Discussion and Conclusion

Among 101 recorded and transcribed DMW returnee narratives and 6 pre-departure narratives, this chapter has analysed five excerpts, which are prototypical examples of the migratory experiences of the Indonesian migrant women in my data. All five women admitted to being traumatised, and they displayed all or most of the recognisable features identified earlier as signs of trauma: repeated crying, existential crisis or disillusionment about life, repetition of the traumatic experience and expressions of fear as the overriding emotion. In this final part of the chapter, I shall discuss the wider mental health issues that this research has uncovered.

Out of a corpus of narratives by 73 Indonesian DMWs (67 returnees and 6 pre-departure narratives), as many as 1/3 of the women displayed signs of being traumatised if we use the criteria stated above. Thus, we may assume that hundreds (possibly thousands) of traumatised migrant workers return to Indonesia every year with no prospects of receiving professional counselling, or any kind of medical support to put their horrific experiences behind them and move on with their lives[4] (Prusinski, 2016). An equally valid concern is the fact that the perpetrators are not brought to justice. The DMWs in this study suffered because of human-inflicted trauma. Herman (2003) argues that although victims of a human-inflicted crime who decide to seek justice may initially experience their role in the legal system as "revictimization", there is potential that legal system intervention will have positive effects on the victim's mental health. One factor in the healing process would be that the perpetrator is brought to justice. Although the victim's healing process may still be long and painful, she may acquire a sense of closure that is likely to advance her healing if the perpetrator is punished (Brison, 2002). However, for none of the women who participated in this research was there any closure; not in one single case (known to me) was the perpetrator brought to justice and the women have to rely on their own resources for healing. Thus, the decision to take (or not to take) a rape case to court that Herman alludes to does not exist for these Indonesian women, just like trauma counselling does not exist.

The only potential for help that exists in these communities is at grass-roots level. During their storytelling, some of the women did share heart-warming stories of support and compassion in the community. In some cases, friends and neighbours would support a storyteller and help her through a particularly difficult part of her narrative; or stories of abuse would spread from one community to the next and serve as warnings for other women. Such stories would deter some women from going (back), or they would help prepare other women for the problems they may face, and inform them of NGOs they could turn to for help. However, there were also stories of women who felt condemned by neighbours and family and who became the objects of gossip and slander (e.g., Rika in Excerpt 1). This happened in particular if they had violated social norms, such as becoming pregnant out of wedlock, or if their migratory journey had failed and they did not bring back any monetary gains (see Chan, 2018).

At the personal level, stories have the potential to initiate a process of healing. The stories we tell are rich sources of identity, both in terms of who we are and what we would like to be. As Cortazzi (2001: 388) argues, "Through life stories individuals and groups make sense of themselves; they tell what they are or what they wish to be, and as they tell so they become, they *are* their stories." Thus, as narrative therapy posits, storytelling has the capacity to change our lives, but help is usually required in order for the storyteller to construct more helpful stories for him/herself. The fact that some of the women whose stories were analysed in this chapter have been back in Indonesia for years but still not been able to come to terms with their traumatic experiences suggests that they have not received the help they needed. However, this reflects reality in rural Indonesia: there are few doctors and virtually no professional counselling. Therefore, as scholars in health communication and related disciplines, who feel a responsibility to not only disseminate our research findings but also to engage in some form of social activism, we have to think about other means that may assist these women in their healing. This chapter proposes three possible avenues that may be considered.

First, we must insist with Brison (1999: 48) that "*saying* something about traumatic memory *does* something to it" and therefore, we should keep encouraging trauma victims to talk about their experiences. There is no miracle cure and the healing process will most likely be lengthy, but, as narrative therapy argues, by telling and retelling trauma narratives, dominant repressive discourses may be questioned (or even silenced) and the victim may receive the help she needs to rewrite her story from victimhood to survival and beyond (Duvall & Béres, 2007). This does not necessarily require professional counsellors but can happen with the support from migrant worker NGOs, or even in conversations among neighbours and friends. Scholars have argued that empathy is essential (and arguably more important than psychological training) and will go a long way towards facilitating healing (Shuman, 2005; Ladegaard, 2017).

Second, we need to reject the idea that traumatic experiences can and should be converted to coherent stories. Apparently, as several studies have found, life-threatening and all-inclusive traumatic experiences cannot be transformed into a traditional temporal framework of storytelling with a before and after but will always, as Langer (1991) agues, stand outside of time: "frozen, static, ever-present and not forgotten" (in Harvey, 2000: 294). The problem is that most audiences do not want to listen to survivors' accounts of atrocities; they want coherent stories, stories that make sense and which move from "a state of suffering and pain to one of wholeness and recovery" (ibid. p. 294). But, as this chapter has demonstrated, this is not the story Indonesian migrant workers tell. Trauma narratives will always be unsettling and we must learn to hear what they have to tell us, even when these stories are not what we want to hear, and when they do not match the theories we prefer and the cultural plots we are familiar with.

Finally, we may need to consider alternative ways of engaging in trauma storytelling. In their work among traumatised African refugees in Australia, Puvimanasinghe, Denson, Augoustinos, and Somasundaram (2014) found a tendency for the participants to suppress thoughts and actions related to the trauma because sharing the experiences had negative impact on their self-identity and self-worth. Therefore, the researchers found a need "to move beyond words to listen to the silence and blank spaces of the stories untold" (ibid. p. 70). They found that "non-verbal techniques such as visualization, progressive relaxation, mindfulness, and religious rituals facilitated psychological healing" (ibid. p. 88). The non-verbal techniques could take many forms and include innovative therapeutic means such as "theatre of the oppressed" and "art therapy". The point about these non-verbal techniques is that they "could be more culturally familiar and hence more acceptable; or they circumvent[ed] the need to be exposed to emotional turmoil in order to heal" (ibid. p. 88).

Dealing with traumatised migrant worker returnees in rural Indonesia may require alternative approaches and interpretations. This chapter has provided further evidence of the rampant abuse and exploitation of DMWs that happens all over the world, not least in the Middle East (Jureidini, 2005). The findings in this chapter have wide-reaching ramifications. Cheung, Tsoi, Wong, and Chung (2019) found that Filipina DMWs in Hong Kong had more than a 25% depression level, as opposed to 2.9% in Hong Kong's general population, and they explain the significantly increased levels of depression by reference to the victimisation of domestic helpers which increases their vulnerability to depression, leads to low self-esteem and makes them less likely to be able to escape violence and abuse. Given that Indonesian DMWs are more likely to be exploited an abused than Filipinas (Ladegaard, 2017), we may assume the problem also applies to Indonesians, and possibly to an even greater extent.

This chapter concludes by making two recommendations. First, that future research on trauma should include more discourse analytic work. It is arguably harder to cover up linguistic "leaks" in trauma storytelling than psychological "leaks", which may be revealed through traditional clinical instruments[5]. Therefore, discourse analytic research also has the potential to introduce other forms of "treatment", including compassionate responses to trauma: to suffer *with* the storyteller rather than just showing empathy. Second, this study insists, perhaps even more explicitly than the scientific rationale behind the project, that telling untold stories of human suffering is a moral obligation (Shuman, 2005). Herman (1998: S149) argues that a natural response to trauma is repression but she also issues a warning that those who forget the past are likely to repeat it. Therefore, she argues, "that public truth-telling is the common denominator of all social action."

Notes

(1) These characteristics are similar to the features mentioned in a more comprehensive list of utterance categories in rape narratives by patients receiving therapy for post-traumatic stress disorder. Foa, Molnar, & Cashman (1995, p. 682) noted that repetitions, desperate thoughts/disorganised thoughts, unfinished thoughts and negative feelings frequently appear in trauma storytelling.

(2) DMWs sometimes form relationships with other non-local residents, such as refugees and asylum seekers or illegal migrant workers, and because they do not have legal status in the city, it is not possible for them to marry legally. Therefore, they may go to a mosque or church to pray for God's blessing on their relationship and then consider their partners their husband. However, this does not constitute a legal marriage so the women are still considered single and therefore looked down upon if they have a child.

(3) Sadly, as revealed in a sharing session at a church shelter in Hong Kong, some young domestic workers are being asked to provide sexual services to male family member. The services are usually not intercourse but intimate massage followed by masturbation, and it is often the grandfather in the family who requests these "services" (Ladegaard, 2013).

(4) This estimation is supported by an article in *The Jakarta Post* ("Returning migrant workers dogged by mental problems" by Burhaini Faizal, 26 June 2012), which claims that the continuous psychological pressure migrant women experience while working overseas leads to depression, psychosis and suicidal tendencies. The article also claims that the number of returning migrant women suffering from mental disorders is increasing.

(5) I am grateful to an anonymous reviewer for making this important point.

Acknowledgements The research reported in the chapter was supported by a General Research Grant from the University Grants Committee of Hong Kong [grant number PolyU-2444/13H]. Staff and volunteers at Pathfinders organised my field trip to Indonesia and I'm very grateful for their support. My gratitude also goes to the Indonesian migrant worker NGOs who helped me, and to all the migrant workers who willingly shared their stories with me—many of them personal and painful. I'll never forget the moments we shared and the stories I heard!

Appendix

Transcription Conventions
   Bold = pronounced with stress/emphasis
   [it's a] = word(s) inserted by the transcriber to ease comprehension
   , = short pause, less than 0.5 s
   (2.0) = pause in seconds
   'give me that' = reporting direct speech
   : (as in ah:) = the vowel sound is prolonged
   xx = incomprehensible
   // = interruption;//as I said// = overlapping speech
   ? = question/rising intonation
   […] turn(s) left out

References

Augoustinos, M., Walker, I., & Donaghue, N. (2014). *Social cognition: An integrated introduction*. Thousand Oaks, CA: Sage.

Blommaert, J. (2010). *The sociolinguistics of globalization*. Cambridge: Cambridge University Press.

Briere, J. N., Scott, C., & Jones, J. (2015). The effects of trauma. In J. N. Briere & J. Jones (Eds.), *Principles of trauma therapy* (2nd ed., pp. 25–61). Thousand Oak, CA: Sage.

Brison, S. J. (1999). Trauma narratives and the remaking of the self. In M. Bal, J. V. Crewe, & L. Spitzer (Eds.), *Acts of memory: Cultural recall in the present* (pp. 39–54). Hanover, NH: Dartmouth College Press.

Brison, S. J. (2002). *Aftermath: Violence and the remaking of a self*. Princeton, NJ: Princeton University Press.

Brockmeier, J. (2008). Language, experience and the 'traumatic gap': How to talk about 9/11? In L. Hydén & J. Brockmeier (Eds.), *Health, illness and culture: Broken narratives* (pp. 16–35). New York: Routledge.

Brown, C., & Augusta-Scott, T. (2007). Introduction: Postmodernism, reflexivity, and narrative therapy. In C. Brown & T. Augusta-Scott (Eds.), *Narrative therapy: Making meaning, making lives (ix-xlii)*. Thousand Oaks, CA: Sage.

Burr, V. (2015). *Social constructionism* (3rd ed.). London: Routledge.

Chan, C. (2018). *In sickness and in wealth: Migration, gendered morality, and central Java*. Bloomington, IN: Indiana University Press.

Cheung, J. K. T., Tsoi, V. W. Y., Wong, K. H. K., & Chung, R. Y. (2019). Abuse and depression among foreign domestic helpers. A cross-sectional survey in Hong Kong. *Public Health, 166,* 121–127.

Chiu, S. W. K. (2005). *A stranger in the house. Foreign domestic helpers in Hong Kong*. Hong Kong: Hong Kong Institute of Asia-Pacific Studies and the Chinese University of Hong Kong.

Constable, N. (1997). Sexuality and discipline among Filipina domestic workers in Hong Kong. *American Ethnologist, 24*(3), 539–558.

Cortazzi, M. (2001). Narrative analysis in ethnography. In P. Atkinson, A. Coffey, S. Delamont, J. Lofland, & L. Lofland (Eds.), *Handbook of ethnography* (pp. 384–394). London: Sage.

De Fina, A., Schiffrin, D., & Bamberg, M. (2006). Introduction. In A. De Fina, D. Schiffrin, & M. Bamberg (Eds.), *Discourse and identity* (pp. 1–23). Cambridge: Cambridge University Press.

Duvall, J., & Béres, L. (2007). Movement of identities: A map for therapeutic conversations about trauma. In C. Brown & T. Augusta-Scott (Eds.), *Narrative therapy: Making meaning, making lives* (pp. 229–250). Thousand Oaks, CA: Sage.

Foa, E. B., Molnar, C., & Cashman, L. (1995). Change in rape narratives during exposure therapy for posttraumatic stress disorder. *Journal of Traumatic Stress, 8*(4), 675–690.

Gallois, C., & Giles, H. (2015). Communication accommodation theory. In K. Tracy (Ed.), *The international encyclopedia of language and social interaction* (pp. 159–176). Oxford: Wiley-Blackwell.

Harvey, M. R. (2000). In the aftermath of sexual abuse: Making and remaking meaning in narratives of trauma recovery. *Narrative Inquiry, 10*(2), 291–311.

Herman, J. L. (1998). Recovery from psychological trauma. *Psychiatry and Clinical Neuroscience, 52*(S1), S145–S150.

Herman, J. L. (2003). The mental health of crime victims: Impact of legal intervention. *Journal of Traumatic Stress, 16*(2), 159–166.

Hydén, L., & Brockmeier, J. (Eds.). (2008). *Health, illness and culture: Broken narratives*. New York: Routledge.

Jureidini, R. (2005). Migrant workers and xenophobia in the Middle East. In Y. Bangura & R. Stavenhagen (Eds.), *Racism and public policy* (pp. 48–71). London: Palgrave Macmillan.

Labott, S. (2001). Crying is psychotherapy. In J. J. M. Vingerhoets & R. R. Cornelius (Eds.), *Adult Crying: A Biopsychosocial Approach* (pp. 213–226). Hove, UK: Brunner-Routledge.

Ladegaard, H. J. (2013). Laughing at adversity: Laughter as communication in domestic helper narratives. *Journal of Language and Social Psychology, 32*(4), 390–411.

Ladegaard, H. J. (2015). Coping with trauma in domestic migrant worker narratives: Linguistic, emotional and psychological perspectives. *Journal of Sociolinguistics, 19*(2), 189–221.

Ladegaard, H. J. (2017). *The discourse of powerlessness and repression: Life stories of domestic migrant workers in Hong Kong.* London: Routledge.

Ladegaard, H. J. (2018). Codeswitching and emotional alignment: Talking about abuse in domestic migrant-worker returnee narratives. *Language in Society, 47*(5), 693–714.

Ladegaard, H. J. (2019). Reconceptualising 'home', 'family' and 'self': Identity struggles in domestic migrant worker returnee narratives. *Language and Intercultural Communication, 19* (3), 289–303.

Langer, L. L. (1980). The dilemma of choice in the deathcamps. *Centerpoint, 4,* 222–231.

Langer, L. L. (1991). *Holocaust testimonies: The ruins of memory.* New Haven: Yale University Press.

McTighe, J. P. (2018). *Narrative theory in clinical and social work practice.* Cham, Switzerland: Springer.

Medved, M., & Brockmeier, J. (2008). Talking about the unthinkable: Neurotrauma and the catastrophic reaction. In L. Hydén & J. Brockmeier (Ed.), *Health, illness and culture. Broken narratives* (pp. 54–72). New York: Routledge.

Mishler, E. G. (1999). *Storylines: Craftartists' narratives of identity.* Cambridge, MA: Harvard University Press.

O'Kerney, R., & Perrott, K. (2006). Trauma narratives in posttraumatic stress disorder: A review. *Journal of Traumatic Stress, 19*(1), 81–93.

Paul, A. M. (2017). *Multinational maids: Stepwise migration in the global labor market.* Cambridge: Cambridge University Press.

Prusinski, E. (2016). 'Because it is our fate': Migration narratives and coping strategies among Indonesian migrant women workers. *Asian Journal of Social Science, 44,* 485–515.

Puvimanasinghe, T., Denson, L. A., Augoustinos, M., & Somasundaram, D. (2014). Narrative of silence: How former refugees talk about loss and past trauma. *Journal of Refugee Studies, 28* (1), 69–92.

Saville-Troike, M. (2003). *The ethnography of communication* (3rd ed.). Oxford: Blackwell.

Shuman, A. (2005). *Other people's stories: Entitlement claims and the critique of empathy.* Urbana and Chicago, Illinois: University of Illinois Press.

Taylor, C. (1994). The politics of recognition. In A. Gutman (Ed.), *Multiculturalism: examining the politics of recognition* (pp. 25–73). Princeton, NJ: Princeton University Press.

Tehrani, N., & Vaughan, S. (2009). Lost in translation: Using bilingual differences to increase emotional mastery following bullying. *Counselling and Psychotherapy Research, 9*(1), 11–17.

Tileaga, C. (2005). Accounting for extreme prejudice and legitimating blame in talk about Romanis. *Discourse and Society, 16*(5), 603–624.

Toolan, M. (2001). *Narrative: A critical linguistic introduction* (2nd ed.). London: Routledge.

Trinch, S. (2013). Recalling rape. Moving beyond what we know. In C. Heffer, F. Rock, & J. Conley (Ed.), *Legal-lay communication. Textual travels in the law* (pp. 288–306). Oxford: Oxford University Press.

White, M., & Epston, D. (1990). *Narrative means to therapeutic ends.* New York: Norton.

Prompting Strategies and Outcomes in Picture-Based Counseling

Dennis Tay, Jin Huang, and Huiheng Zeng

Abstract Pictures are an innovative resource in the verbal activity of psychological counseling (Ginicola, Smith, & Trzaska, 2012; Malchiodi, 2011). Counselors often guide clients to interpret and explore them as figurative representations of their situation (Stevens & Spears, 2009). Picture-based counseling is, however, under-explored from both clinical and discourse perspectives, with few published guidelines and analyses of the nature of counselor prompts and client interpretations. Informed by metaphor theory, this paper examines 34 counterbalanced matched-pairs of elicited picture interpretations responding to either a topic-present or topic-absent prompt in Mandarin Chinese. Topic-present metaphor prompts indicate a specific topic to be connected to the picture, while topic-absent metaphor prompts do not. The resulting transcripts were coded for five variables reflecting key aspects of metaphor construction—sources, topics, source–topic connections, uncertainty markers, and metaphor signals. Spearman correlations were calculated and compared across the two prompt conditions, supported by qualitative analysis of examples. Results show stronger correlations and by implication greater integration among the variables in the topic-present condition. This suggests that people are better able to contextualize pictorial elements to a specified target topic of discussion. The present findings motivate follow-up research incorporating more direct counseling outcome measures.

Keywords Pictures · Counselling · Metaphor theory · Mandarin chinese

1 Introduction

In psychological counseling, counselors apply mental health principles to assist clients to modify problematic behaviors, cognitions, and emotions (Norcross, 1990) by "talking through" them. Picture-based counseling (PBC) is an innovation

D. Tay (✉) · J. Huang · H. Zeng
Hong Kong Polytechnic University, Hong Kong, People's Republic of China
e-mail: dennis.tay@polyu.edu.hk

© Springer Nature Singapore Pte Ltd. 2020
B. Watson and J. Krieger (eds.), *Expanding Horizons in Health Communication*,
The Humanities in Asia 6, https://doi.org/10.1007/978-981-15-4389-0_2

29

practiced across different counseling paradigms, supplementing their traditional conversational delivery. Counselors show clients a picture at some point in the session and prompt them to explore its meaning and potential relevance to their situation. The central rationale is that pictures allow clients to "discuss an issue and express emotions in a creative way" (Ginicola et al., 2012: 311), while maintaining some distance from things they might not be ready to directly confront. The communicative task faced by clients in PBC could be described as drawing symbolic connections between two typically unrelated things—the picture, and the issues in their lives.

Various types of symbolic languages can be expected in clients' spontaneous interpretation of pictures. Among them, metaphor—defined as describing and potentially thinking of something in terms of something else (Semino, 2008)—is likely to be predominant and interesting to communication researchers and healthcare practitioners alike. A typical example is an expression "life is a journey", where the speaker describes and is potentially thinking about life in terms of a journey. In the terminology of metaphor theory, "life" is the target concept, or the thing to be described, and "journey" is the source concept, or the thing used to describe it. It would seem intuitive for clients to use pictorial elements as "source" concepts whose meanings could be transferred onto the "target" concepts. It has been shown across languages and cultures that metaphors are important to understand abstractions in terms of something more concrete and familiar (Cameron & Maslen, 2010; Kövecses, 2000; Lakoff & Johnson, 1999; Yu, 1998), like our example of depicting life in terms of a journey. In counseling, metaphors are believed to help clients express difficult-to-describe feelings (McMullen, 1996), appreciate alternative perspectives (Kopp & Craw, 1998; Lyddon, Clay, & Sparks, 2001), and enhance their sense of participation (Gelo & Mergenthaler, 2012; Rasmussen & Angus, 1996). Lyddon et al. (2001: 270–271) suggest that "metaphors may be useful tools for helping clients access (and) symbolize emotions that may have been previously unexpressed, unexplored, or even unrecognized".

Counselors have, therefore, asked how best to use metaphors (Stott, Mansell, Salkovskis, Lavender, & Cartwright-Hatton, 2010), manage client metaphors (Kopp & Craw, 1998), and/or "co-construct" them with clients (Tay, 2016). It has been suggested that counselors should use metaphors or help to develop client metaphors in a systematic fashion; i.e., ensure that source and target concepts are clearly mapped onto each other (Kopp & Craw, 1998; Sims & Whynot, 1997). For example, if a client describes his HIV-positive condition as a "large dark cloud hanging over me that will rain AIDS down upon me" (Kopp & Craw, 1998), the counselor should explore how various expressed or implied aspects of the source (e.g., the cloud, the rain, whether the shelter is available, and if the rain will stop) relate to the client's perception of his condition. It has also been suggested that counseling-related metaphors should be hedged to maintain awareness that they are ultimately tools for conceptualizing the situation, rather than literal statements of it. There is thus a subtle but important difference between saying "your husband is a tyrant" and "it sounds like your husband is sort of a tyrant for you" (Tay, 2014). Nevertheless, there is a scant opportunity to test these suggestions in a more empirical way due to the difficulties of imposing a controlled design on the spontaneous nature of counseling and metaphor. McMullen (1996), for instance, points out that artificially encouraging and restricting metaphor use in order to compare counseling outcomes would implicate difficult-to-control covariates like counselor/client attitudes and engagement. The nature of PBC, however, presents an opportunity for a more systematic study of discourse outcomes because it begins with a predetermined counselor-initiated prompt followed by uninterrupted client elaboration. This facilitates controlled elicitation and contrastive analyses of different prompting strategies and their outcomes, while largely preserving the authentic PBC process even in a (quasi)-experimental context. Such analyses are exigent given that there are currently no standardized PBC procedures, and very little empirical research into optimal ways of prompting clients to interpret the picture (Goessling & Doyle, 2009; Rampton et al., 2007; Stevens & Spears, 2009). This may be particularly true in cultural contexts like Hong Kong and mainland China. Mental health services have only gradually gained acceptance in Chinese societies in recent decades, due to conflicts between psychotherapeutic and traditional cultural values like not revealing "shameful" personal matters to nonfamily members (Zhong, 2011). This chapter is, therefore, well-placed to investigate aspects of PBC in a Mandarin Chinese-speaking context.

2   Topic-Present Versus Topic-Absent Prompting Strategies

To gain an initial sense of how counselors spontaneously prompt clients in PBC, relevant transcripts from a Chinese university counseling center were manually examined. Consider the following two observed prompts. The picture at hand (not reproduced here) shows an angry man standing next to his broken-down car in the middle of a long road.

> 我这里有一张图片, 你看了这张图片之后, 你自己想个小故事, 随意, 你自己发挥想象力 Here is a picture, look at it and think of a small story. Do as you like, use your imagination

> 看这张图, 你生活中有没有这样类似的一些经历? 见过的或者是发生在你身上的? Do you have life experiences similar to what you see in this picture? What you've witnessed or experienced?

Both prompts encourage the client to use the picture as a symbolic platform to talk about other things. In metaphor theoretic terminology again, the subtle difference between them is that the first prompt does not specify an intended target topic ("a small story", "do as you like", "use your imagination"), whereas the second prompt fixes the target topic as "life experiences". We may accordingly call the first a topic-absent prompt and the second a topic-present prompt. This is an example of a (potentially) systematic and observable difference in practice that can be hypothesized to lead to different outcomes. For instance, to what extent would the subsequent spontaneous metaphor construction (or other types of symbolic language) by clients show the "ideal" characteristics described earlier, and how does this vary across the prompting strategies? How might these differences inform prompting strategies in return, given the scarcity of relevant guidelines?

We report findings from a mixed-methods discourse analytic study comparing metaphor-related characteristics and their correlational structures across elicited picture interpretations, following topic-absent versus topic-present prompts. The findings are part of a larger experimental study which also compared how different prompts are associated with affective arousal levels using skin conductance measures. This chapter will only report the discourse analytic component. Interested readers may refer to Tay, Huang, & Zeng (2019) for a fuller account of both methodological components and how they inter-relate.

3 Methodology

3.1 Participants and Stimuli Selection

34 native Mandarin Chinese-speaking university students (10 male, 24 female) were recruited by convenience sampling through advertisements posted on the campus of the Hong Kong Polytechnic University. They participated in this study with informed consent. While they were not actual counseling clients, it is acceptable to employ suitable role-played subjects in counseling research (e.g., Van Parys & Rober, 2013). The study was approved by the university's Human Subjects Ethics subcommittee.

The PBC literature advocates flexible use of different types of pictures ranging from photographs to abstract art (Malchiodi, 2003). For present research purposes, however, the following selection criteria were imposed: i) the pictures should have structures and elements that are reasonably familiar and easy to describe; ii) they should not evoke strong emotional responses like disgust and fear. This is to avoid ceiling effects for the skin conductance measures (not reported here). The left picture in Fig. 1 shows an acceptable example. The right picture, common in stimuli sets to investigate a wide range of emotional assessments (e.g., the International Affective Picture System Lang, Bradley, & Cuthbert, 2008), is deemed unacceptable for present purposes. From a random pool of internet images, two pictures were eventually determined by all three authors as fulfilling both criteria, and used for the study.

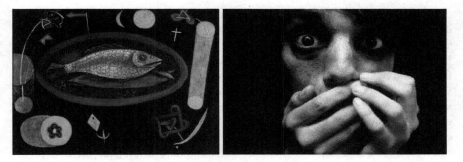

Fig. 1 Acceptable and unacceptable picture stimuli

3.2 Elicitation of Spontaneous Interpretations

Each participant was randomly assigned one of the two pictures and prompted to interpret it three times in randomized sequence—once per prompting strategy, including a nonfigurative control prompt that is more relevant for comparing the electrodermal activity measures. The experiment was conducted in a face-to-face setting in a quiet room to facilitate the explanation and clarification of the procedures. This paper will focus on a comparative analysis of the interpretation following the topic-present and topic-absent prompts only.

> Topic-present prompt: This picture symbolizes what you think about life. Can you interpret what it means?

> Topic-absent prompt: This picture can symbolize anything you like. Can you interpret what it means?

Participants responded for as long as needed following each prompt, after which a one-minute rest was given before the next prompt. The main purpose was to allow electrodermal activity to return to baseline levels and give participants time to reorient themselves.

3.3 Coding and Analysis

The present mixed-methods approach comprises two main steps: (i) inductive coding of metaphor-related variables, which is a qualitative process, followed by (ii) comparative and correlational analyses of variable frequencies, which is a quantitative process supported by qualitative exemplification.

Audio recordings of all interpretations were transcribed and examined by two native Mandarin-speaking raters with postgraduate degrees in metaphor and discourse analysis for a general understanding of their content. This was followed by identifying and counting the frequencies of discourse elements related to the content, co-text, and structure of metaphors. Five variables were identified: source units, target units, metaphor signals, uncertainty markers, and domain switches, all illustrated in the following subsections. Following established guidelines for inductive metaphor analysis (Cameron & Maslen, 2010), inter-rater reliability was maximized by regular discussion and cross-checking rather than quantification. The five variables collectively comprise the basic "building blocks" of spontaneous metaphor construction, and allow us to see if metaphors produced under different conditions reflect characteristics espoused in the counseling literature; e.g., clear co-occurrence of and correspondence between sources and targets (Sims & Whynot, 1997), and suitable "hedging" of metaphors to indicate their subjective character (Prince, Frader, & Bosk, 1982; Tay, 2014).

3.4   Source and Target Units

Source and target meanings are often conflated in a single unit (e.g., *I struggle to convince him*), and the identification of metaphors rests upon the idea that some aspect of the unit's "basic meaning" is used to understand its "contextual meaning" (Pragglejaz Group, 2007; Steen et al., 2010). In the above example, the basic physical meaning of "struggle" is used to understand its more abstract contextual meaning of difficulty. Basic meanings are, therefore, the source, and contextual meanings of the target. In the present data, sources and targets turn out to be relatively easy to identify because they are not often conflated, but instead appear as juxtaposed units. Furthermore, source units are mostly picture elements and their anaphoric pronominal forms. Target units mostly relate to the prescribed target topic in the topic-present condition, and other counseling-related issues in the topic-absent condition. A translated example is given below. "Thing", "arrow", and "it" are source units while "the things we need in life" and "process" are target units.

> 这个东西是一些人生需要的要素.　然后这个箭头其实我也不是很了解。我觉得会把它理解成代表了一个过程 This thing represents the things we need in life. And then this arrow, I don't really understand. I think I can see it as representing a process.

3.5   Metaphor Signals

Variously known as signaling devices (Goatly, 1997), tuning devices (Cameron & Deignan, 2003), and metaphor flags (Steen et al., 2010), metaphor signals refer to linguistic units which draw attention to the use of metaphor, such as the prototypical English example *like* in *my dog is like a cat*. Many researchers also include in this category elements which convey the speaker's stance towards the metaphor. For example, *in a way* in *I was in a way a child again* not only signals metaphor use, but also suggests a hedged comparison. In the present study, however, these stance-marking elements are separately coded (see next variable) because they are often expressed apart from core markers of metaphoricity. Metaphor signals, therefore, refer only to stance-neutral elements whose primary function is to indicate a metaphorical comparison, not how the speaker feels toward it. The following examples illustrate the use of "represents" and "like" in this regard.

我觉得这代表着男女之间的关系 I think this represents the relationship between men and women

那个深蓝色的东西像一个海，要自己去面对很多风浪 That dark blue thing is like the sea, to face many waves alone

3.6 Uncertainty Expressions

Uncertainty expressions, which express tentativeness toward the metaphor (Cameron & Deignan, 2003; Goatly, 1997), are technically only part of a larger category of stance-marking elements. Their conceptual opposite would be expressions which enhance the degree of metaphoricity, such as *very much* in *life is very much like a journey*. Not unlike spontaneous psychotherapy and counseling talk (Tay, 2014), however, tentativeness constitutes the predominant stance expressed by participants when describing the source, target, and/or relationship between them. Such tentativeness also tends to be expressed in addition to core metaphor signals such as *like*. The following examples are illustrative.

这里有一个类似是，远看像一匹马，近看也不知道是什么，代表着 。。。Here is something like a, looks like a horse from far, but I don't know what it is up close, representing…

像有月亮有太阳，就是类似于可以说用星河大海这样的东西去形容旁边来围绕它这些东西 There is the moon and the sun, so we can sort of say we are using stars, rivers, seas, and such to describe these things surrounding it

3.7 Domain Switches

A "domain switch" is not a tangible linguistic form, but the boundary between a source and target unit. The number of domain switches thus provides a measure of how extensively participants juxtapose a source with a corresponding target when constructing an interpretation. Constant source-target juxtaposition has been observed to characterize more systematic, "correspondent type" explication of target topics, and vice versa for more impressionistic, "class inclusive" type descriptions (Wee, 2005a). In the following example, the two domain switches are indicated by slashes. The speaker describes the source picture, relates it to the target of life, and then switches to the source once more.

那他应该也是可以翻越过这些障碍，可以走到他想去的地方。那我觉得这幅画的意思就是，表达，比如说/像人生中有很多种选择，另外就是/自己想走的那条路总归都不会太容易也不会太轻松，但是他也还是有很多渠道的 So he should be able to overcome these obstacles and walk where he wants to. So, I think this picture is trying to show that life has many choices, and also, the road you want choose will not be easy and relaxing, but there are still many possible channels.

The variable frequencies were then analyzed in three ways: (i) pairwise comparisons of each variable between the topic-present and absent conditions; (ii) comparison of the variable correlational structure between the two conditions; (iii) qualitative analysis of the selected illustrative examples.

4   Results and Discussion

Table 1 shows the mean frequencies, standard deviations, and normalized means of the five variables following each prompting strategy. Normalization is done by dividing each variable frequency by the number of words in that interpretation.

Nonparametric tests were used in the following comparative and correlational analyses as not all variables met parametric testing assumptions (e.g., normality of distribution). Firstly, paired comparisons across the topic-present and topic-absent prompts with Wilcoxon signed-rank tests reveal no statistically significant differences in the normalized means for all five variables: source units ($Z = -0.686$, $p = 0.493$), target units ($Z = 1.195$, $p = 0.232$), metaphor signals ($Z = 1.07$, $p = 0.285$), uncertainty expressions ($Z = -0.333$, $p = 0.739$), and domain switches ($Z = 0.588$, $p = 0.557$). This implies that participants employ these key building blocks of metaphor construction to similar extents regardless of the type of prompt received.

Next, the correlational structure of these metaphor building blocks was examined, as potential relationships between any two variables might have distinct meanings and implications. Figures 2 and 3 show the Spearman's correlational

Table 1 Variable frequencies in topic-present and topic-present conditions

Variable	Prompt	Mean ($N = 34$)	SD	Normalized mean
Source units	Topic-present	9.129	7.49	0.03
	Topic-absent	7.032	4.99	0.034
Target units	Topic-present	13.323	12.08	0.041
	Topic-absent	8.194	6.65	0.039
Metaphor signals	Topic-present	3.258	2.54	0.011
	Topic-absent	2.032	2.27	0.009
Uncertainty expressions	Topic-present	5.097	3.53	0.018
	Topic-absent	4.097	2.86	0.019
Domain switches	Topic-present	11.774	10.66	0.037
	Topic-absent	8.194	7.35	0.035

Variable	domain switch	source	target	signal	uncertainty
domain switch	1	0.786***	0.771***	0.567***	0.515**
source	0.786***	1	0.499**	0.461**	0.382*
target	0.771***	0.499**	1	0.591***	0.518**
signal	0.567***	0.461**	0.591***	1	0.173
uncertainty	0.515**	0.382*	0.518**	0.173	1

* p < .05, ** p < .01, *** p < .001

Fig. 2 Correlational heatmap of variables in the topic-absent condition

Variable	domain switch	source	target	signal	uncertainty
domain switch	1	0.861***	0.762***	0.609***	0.647***
source	0.861***	1	0.613***	0.436**	0.528**
target	0.762***	0.613***	1	0.604***	0.679***
signal	0.609***	0.436**	0.604***	1	0.529**
uncertainty	0.647***	0.528**	0.679***	0.529**	1

* p < .05, ** p < .01, *** p < .001

Fig. 3 Correlational heatmap of variables in the topic-present condition

heatmaps for the five variables in the topic-absent and topic-present conditions, respectively. The cells show the value of Spearman's ρ, the number of asterisks indicates the corresponding p-value, and darker colors indicate stronger correlations.

The first general observation is that all variables are positively correlated in every situation regardless of statistical significance. This is unsurprising and reflects the fact that all five variables are co-constitutive in the process of spontaneous metaphor construction. However, the correlations are generally stronger in the topic-present than topic-absent condition, suggesting nuanced differences in the construction of interpretations. The scatterplots in Figs. 4 and 5 provide a clearer visualization of variable relationships in the topic-absent and topic-present conditions, respectively (with histograms, regression lines, and 95% confidence intervals). The following discussion focuses on and exemplifies cases, where the correlation is higher by at least one α-level (e.g., $p < 0.05$ vs. $p < 0.01$).

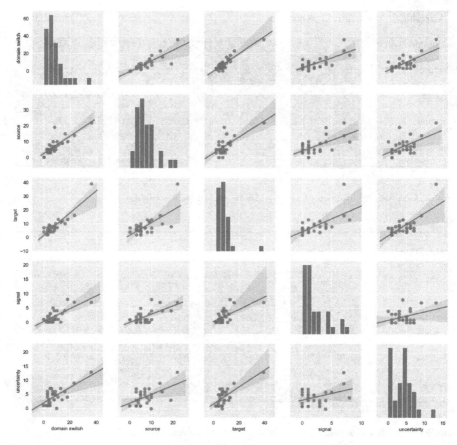

Fig. 4 Scatterplots of variables in the topic-absent condition

4.1 Source–Target Correlation

Source–target correlation here does not refer to connections between substantive source and target concepts (i.e., conceptual metaphors), but the extent to which source units mentioned in discourse are accompanied by target units. It is substantially stronger in the topic-present ($r_s = 0.613$, $p < 0.001$) than topic-absent condition ($r_s = 0.499$, $p = 0.004$), suggesting two distinct discourse strategies in constructing a metaphor-oriented interpretation. Consider the two examples below from the same participant, following a topic-present and topic-absent prompt, respectively.

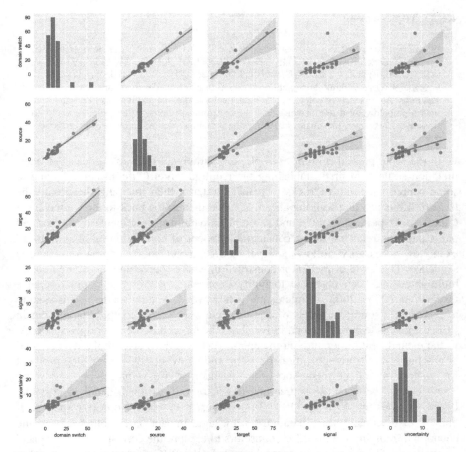

Fig. 5 Scatterplots of variables in the topic-present condition

4.1.1 Topic-Present

如果要从人生的角度来看的话，就是那可能这些石头，就是圆圈的这种，就是我们要走的路。因为他用的这个蓝色，就是给我的感觉就是水嘛。就是，就像人生就是在，人生本来就是在深渊中前进，然后这些石头就是可以供我们走向自己想去的路 If I were to see this from the perspective of "life", maybe these rocks, these circular rocks, are the path we walk on. Because the blue color feels like water to me. That is, life is like, life is just like walking ahead in an abyss, and these rocks pave the way for us to walk the path we want

4.1.2 Topic-Absent

我觉得这张图片很复杂。就因为有很多含义在吧。但是它用的颜色就是，上面是比较, 颜色比较浅, 下面像水, 水蓝色一样。然后画的这个人的腿又特别的长, 就感觉是他想要, 就是跨过这个, 就是这些水就像深渊吧, 就是可能说他生活中有一些烦吧, 然后他想跨越过去 I think this picture is complicated, because there are many hidden meanings. But in terms of color, it has a lighter color at the top, and it looks like water, like aqua blue below. And this person's legs are exceptionally long, it feels like he wants to cross over, this water, like an abyss. Perhaps he is feeling troubled and wishes to cross over them.

In the topic-present prompt example, the participant follows a consistent interpretation strategy of first establishing the required target ("life"), then referring to some source element(s) ("rocks", "path", "water"), then mapping these onto the target ("life is just like walking ahead…"), and then going back to the source again ("these rocks pave the way"), and so on. This pattern is quite consistent across all participants as reflected in the considerable extent of correlation, although not all examples necessarily follow a strict source–target–source domain switching sequence. This style of metaphor construction where source and target are equally highlighted has been observed to typify explicatory genres like popular science texts (Wee, 2005a, 2005b)—interestingly, however, in such texts the task is usually to construct a source in order to account for a structurally complex target, but in PBC the task is to construct a narrative about the target based on a pre-given source. In the mental health literature on metaphor, such a style is also implicitly favoured or emphasized by some practitioners. Kopp and Craw's (1998) seven-step protocol for elaborating client metaphors, for instance, advises counselors to develop "connections" between the source and target topic in as much detail as possible. Likewise, Sims and Whynot (1997:343) suggest that "each addition to the development of the image has a parallel, but unstated impact on the other side of the equation", implying the need for counselors to explore the corresponding "impact" on the target for every new source element. In the PBC context, where such theoretical ideas on metaphor construction have not been discussed, topic-present prompts combined with a structurally rich picture could be ideal in cases where the counselor wants the client to arrive at a structurally coherent narrative about the target topic at hand. Conversely, in the topic-absent prompt example, the participant's interpretation strategy is less focused on a balanced account of source and target units. There is instead an extended, detailed description of the source ("color", "water", "person's legs", "cross over", "abyss"), followed by a tentative comment on what these elements could symbolize ("feeling troubled and wishes to cross over them"). This appears to be a less explicatory but more exploratory style, where the client does not feel compelled to match perceived sources with target counterparts, but is instead prompted toward a more comprehensive, thematic understanding of the source first. This style of prompting and interpretation in the PBC context might then be suitable for counseling objectives centered around initial exploration of feelings, attitudes, and even rapport building (George, Iveson, & Ratner, 1999).

4.1.3 Relative Co-occurrence of Signals with Sources Versus Targets

Metaphor signals are defined in this paper as elements that draw attention to metaphor use, which is in turn often expressed in terms of both a source and target unit. It, therefore, seems intuitive to expect these signals to co-occur equally with both source and target. However, in the present data the target–signal correlation is stronger than the source–signal correlation in both the topic-absent ($r_s = 0.591$, $p < 0.001$ vs. $r_s = 0.461$, $p = 0.009$) and topic-present conditions ($r_s = 0.604$, $p < 0.001$ vs. $r_s = 0.436$, $p = 0.014$). This is surprising because even though the source picture is by definition more palpable in both conditions, and the target topic is undefined in the free condition, the signaling of metaphor still tends to be more closely tied to statements of the target topic at hand rather than the source. The following two examples from a topic-present and topic-absent interpretation respectively are illustrative.

4.1.4 Topic-Present

当然这一条鱼放在中间就可以象征着一个人。因为所有的旁边，像有月亮有太阳，就是类似于有可以说用星河大海这样的东西去形容让旁边来围绕它这些东西。围绕他这些东西有可能代表这一生经历的挫折，有可能是这一生经历的欢乐，或者其他的一些东西吧 Of course, this fish in the middle can symbolize a person. Because everything beside it, the moon and the sun, we can sort of say we are using stars, rivers, seas, and such to describe these things surrounding it. These surrounding things might represent the setbacks in life, happiness in life, or something else.

4.1.5 Topic-Absent

首先中间有一条鱼，放在一个类似盘子一样的地方。然后上面它的周围围了一些东西，有什么月亮，太阳，或是一个蓝色的管子还是什么的，可能表示一个周期，一个循环之类的 Firstly, there is a fish in the middle, in something like a plate. Then there are things surrounding it like the moon, the sun, or something like a blue tube, perhaps they indicate a period or a cycle of sorts

In the first example, the target topic was fixed as "life". The participant begins expectedly with a statement juxtaposing the source ("fish"), target ("person"), and signal ("symbolize"), and then proceeds to elaborate the picture elements in some detail, producing a series of source units along the way. These source units are then collectively linked to several aspects of the fixed target ("setbacks", "happiness"). Similarly, in the second example, the interpretation begins with an extended description of the source picture before a collective linking of the many source units to the tentatively signaled target topic of a "period" or "cycle of sorts". Both these examples suggest that in the PBC context, even when no specific target topic is provided in the counselor's prompt, people are likely to regard metaphor as a target-oriented rather than source-oriented interpretation strategy; i.e., their elaboration of source elements is diverse but eventually aimed toward producing a description for a more concisely stated target topic. On the one hand, the willingness and ability of participants to expand upon the source image affirms the general efficacy of PBC. On the other hand, it is important for PBC practitioners to critically reflect on when the converse situation might be ideal, and how it could be encouraged; i.e., where clients present a concise description of the source, signal it accordingly, and offer a diverse elaboration of the target topic instead. As the present findings suggest, it may well be the case that PBC provides an initial step toward this. Although source elaboration appears more forthcoming in the narrow context of this counselor-prompted activity, the outcomes and insights can be subsequently followed up with other techniques outside the context of the picture.

4.1.6 Co-occurrence of Uncertainty Expressions with Other Variables

The final aspect to be discussed is the expression of uncertainty vis-à-vis other variables. It reflects the greatest contrast between the two conditions, as the correlation between uncertainty expressions and every other variable is stronger in the topic-present than topic-absent condition by at least one α-level. Recall that this does not mean more uncertainty in topic-present interpretations, but a more synchronized expression of uncertainty with source units, target units, signals, and domain switches. Four examples are provided below, the first two from topic-present and the latter two from topic-absent interpretations.

4.1.7 Topic-Present

他是站在海平面上的，就可能代表他已经在人生当中寻找到一个自己如何去适应社会的一个方法，就是去站的更高，就把自己的某些技能发挥一下，加强一下某些技能，起码是他去适应了整个社会的潮流吧，而不是被社会的洪波冲掉吧。他的衣服是黑色的，就可能说明其实还是，就在社会实践中可能他还是需要掩盖一下自己的内心想法，就不能把太多内心的东西说出来吧 He is standing at sea level, maybe it represents that he has found a way to fit into society in life, which is to stand higher and show off his skills, strengthen his skills. At least he has adopted to societal trends and has not been washed away by the wave of society. His shirt is black, maybe it represents that in actual society he still needs to conceal his thoughts, and not fully speak his mind

自己暂时无法逃离这个状态，需要外界的一个帮助的一个感觉。就是这种感觉。嗯。还是不知道这四个圈圈是什么意思。但是我不是很理解为什么作者画这么长的腿，走过很多的路吗?嗯，就应该还是刚才说的就他应该经历的事情挺多 I cannot escape this situation for the time being, and need some external help. Yes, this is my feeling. I still don't know what these four circles mean. But I don't quite understand why the author drew such long legs, does it mean walking a long distance? Yes, it is probably what I said just now, he has experienced a lot

The first example has two expressions of uncertainty with "maybe". Both occur at the juncture of prior source picture elaboration and subsequent inferencing about what this implies for the fixed target topic of "life". Therefore, they also co-occur with a domain switch from source to target, as well as a metaphor signal ("it represents"). The second example is structurally similar except that it starts with a target topic elaboration, before expressing uncertainty about the source ("I still don't know what these four circles mean"). The sequence is then reversed to resemble the first example, with a source unit ("such long legs"), followed by an uncertainty expression ("does it mean"), and then an inference about the target ("walking a long distance"). Contrast this with the following examples from the topic-absent condition.

4.1.8 Topic-Absent

应该是一个人他想要走出一个困境, 但是没有什么具体的办法, 所以他把这个腿拉的很长很长, 想要看一看, 这个包围住他的东西外面是什么。可是他拉长之后看见外面的这个, 外面困境, 就是包围住他这个东西外面好像也并没有什么具体的, 也没有什么具体的实物, 就很, 有点忧郁的, 一幅画。嗯, 这个这个地方明明有梯子啊, 有梯子他却没有选择, 就是爬上这个梯子去看远方 It probably is someone who wants to walk out of a difficult situation, but has no clear solution, so he stretches his legs a lot, he wants to see what is surrounding him. But after he stretches his legs to see what is outside, surrounding him, there seems to be nothing concrete as well. It is like, a very melancholic picture. Yes, there is clearly a ladder here, but he does not choose to climb it and look far

我觉得这个人像是在渴望一些什么吧, 可能, 所以需要独自去, 思考一下自己到底, 就是内心世界会比较丰富一点吧, 可能在这个, 这样一个环境里, 他这样孤独地站着。然后, 对, 就没有别的想法。就可能周围这个环境是他曾经, 或者是经历过什么的一个地方。我感觉。这是一个有故事的人, 然后这个环境是一个提供给他一定回忆的地方, 可能是这样。然后他在思考什么或者盼望什么 I feel this person desires something, maybe he needs to be alone and think deeply, so he has a rich mental world. Maybe, in this environment, he stands in loneliness, and thinks of nothing else. Maybe he once experienced these surroundings. I think this is a person with a story, and this environment is bringing back memories, maybe it's like that. And he is contemplating or hoping for something

In the first example, the uncertainty expression occurs at the beginning ("it probably is"), after which there is an extensive elaboration of the source picture. The second example is similar except that the source elaboration has three uncertainty expressions ("maybe") within. Both examples differ from the topic-present interpretations above in that there is no systematic relationship between these expressions and the rest of the metaphoric inferencing process; i.e., reference and switching to the target topic, which accounts for the weaker correlations. Regarding implications for PBC and metaphor use in counseling in general, the expression of uncertainty in healthcare communication contexts remains underexplored (Prince et al., 1982; Tay, 2014). Previous accounts argue that uncertainty in counselor talk is strategic. It conveys recognition that while metaphors are useful because sources are inferentially productive and targets are relevant to the client, source-to-target inferences are ultimately nonfactual or approximate. The present findings suggest that spontaneous client discourse also shares these characteristics, but more so when counselors offer a clearly defined target topic. Uncertainty expressions have a higher chance of occurring in a structured ensemble with sources, targets, and signals following topic-present prompts, but tend to focus on source elaboration when no obvious target is in sight.

5 Conclusion

PBC is a promising healthcare communicative resource that remains under-researched both in terms of efficacy and discourse outcomes. The present study reported one aspect of this much-needed research in the Chinese context. A comparative discourse analysis of metaphorical interpretations following topic-present and topic-absent prompting strategies revealed nuanced differences with implications for PBC practice. Participants who were given a target topic tended to produce metaphorical expressions in a more systematic ensemble consisting of a source unit, target unit, metaphor signal, and uncertainty expression. On the other hand, although participants who freely decided on the target topic demonstrated less systematicity, they still had little trouble orienting their use of metaphor toward a useful conceptualization of the target. Finding the optimal prompting strategy, therefore, requires the counselor to judge what style of metaphor elaboration best fulfills the context-specific objectives at hand, since it is premature to conclude that systematicity is an inherently superior style.

There are several limitations to this study. Firstly, the analysis of metaphors was exclusively focused on their structural make-up, and overlooked their contents such as the actual sources and targets used. Future research could explore whether, and how, structural make-up might vary with content-related variables like sources and targets. Secondly, the frequencies-based correlational analysis could not specifically pinpoint exactly where, or how near/far apart, the features were from one another. Doing so would require a detailed qualitative examination of each transcript that is beyond the present scope. Another direction to be considered for follow-up research is to incorporate nonlinguistic outcome measures such as counselor and client perceptions of PBC, thus investigating not only intra-linguistic relationships, but more direct interfaces between discourse strategies and clinical outcomes.

Funding Acknowledgement This research is supported by a General Research Fund from the Research Grants Council, University Grants Committee, Hong Kong SAR (Funding no. PolyU 156033/18H), and Departmental Research Grants from the Department of English, The Hong Kong Polytechnic University (G-UAEH, G-YBMA), awarded to the first author.

References

Cameron, L., & Deignan, A. (2003). Combining large and small corpora to investigate tuning devices around metaphor in spoken discourse. *Metaphor and Symbol, 18*(3), 149–160.
Cameron, L., & Maslen, R. (Eds.). (2010). *Metaphor Analysis*. London, UK: Equinox.

Gelo, O. C. G., & Mergenthaler, E. (2012). Unconventional metaphors and emotional-cognitive regulation in a metacognitive interpersonal therapy. *Psychotherapy Research, 22*(2), 159–175.

George, E., Iveson, C., & Ratner, H. (1999). *Problem to Solution: Brief Therapy with Individuals and Families*. London, UK: BT Press.

Ginicola, M. M., Smith, C., & Trzaska, J. (2012). Counseling Through Images: Using Photography to Guide the Counseling Process and Achieve Treatment Goals. *Journal of Creativity in Mental Health, 7*(4), 310–329.

Goatly, A. (1997). *The Language of Metaphors*. London, UK: Routledge.

Goessling, K., & Doyle, C. (2009). Thru the lenz: Participatory action research, photography, and creative process in an urban high school. *Journal of Creativity in Mental Health, 4*(4), 343–365.

Kopp, R. R., & Craw, M. J. (1998). Metaphoric language, metaphoric cognition, and cognitive therapy. *Psychotherapy, 35*(3), 306–311.

Kövecses, Z. (2000). *Metaphor and Emotion. Language, Culture and Body in Human Feeling*. Cambridge: Cambridge University Press.

Lakoff, G., & Johnson, M. (1999). *Philosophy in the Flesh: The Embodied Mind and its Challenges to Western Thought*. New York: Basic Books.

Lang, P. J., Bradley, M. M., & Cuthbert, B. N. (2008). *International affective picture system (IAPS): Affective ratings of pictures and instruction manual. Technical Report A-8*. Gainsville, FL.

Lyddon, W. J., Clay, A. L., & Sparks, C. L. (2001). Metaphor and change in counselling. *Journal of Counseling & Development, 79*(3), 269–274.

Malchiodi, C. A. (2003). *Expressive Therapies*. New York: Guilford Press.

Malchiodi, C. A. (Ed.). (2011). *Handbook of Art Therapy* (2nd ed.). New York: Guilford Press.

McMullen, L. M. (1996). Studying the use of figurative language in psychotherapy: the search for researchable questions. *Metaphor and Symbolic Activity, 11*(4), 241–255.

Norcross, J. C. (1990). An eclectic definition of psychotherapy. In J. K. Zeig & W. M. Munion (Eds.), *What is Psychotherapy? Contemporary Perspectives* (pp. 218–220). San Francisco, CA: Jossey-Bass.

Pragglejaz Group. (2007). MIP: A Method for Identifying Metaphorically Used Words in Discourse. *Metaphor and Symbol, 22*(1), 1–39.

Prince, E., Frader, J., & Bosk, C. (1982). On hedging in physician-physician discourse. In R. J. di Pietro (Ed.), *Linguistics and the Professions* (pp. 83–97). Norwood, NJ: Ablex.

Rampton, T. B., Rosemann, J. L., Latta, A. L., Mandleco, B. L., Roper, S., & Dyches, T. T. (2007). Images of life: Siblings of children with Down syndrome. *Journal of Family Nursing, 13*(4), 420–442.

Rasmussen, B. M., & Angus, L. E. (1996). Metaphor in psychodynamic psychotherapy with borderline and non-borderline clients: A qualitative analysis. *Psychotherapy, 33*(4), 521–530.

Semino, E. (2008). *Metaphor in Discourse*. Cambridge and New York: Cambridge University Press.

Sims, P. A., & Whynot, C. A. (1997). Hearing metaphor: An approach to working with family-generated metaphor. *Family Process, 36*, 341–355.

Steen, G. J., Dorst, A. G., Herrmann, J. B., Kaal, A. A., Krennmayr, T., & Pasma, T. (2010). *A Method for Linguistic Metaphor Identification: From MIP to MIPVU*. Amsterdam and Philadelphia: John Benjamins.

Stevens, R., & Spears, E. H. (2009). Incorporating photography as a therapeutic tool in counseling. *Journal of Creativity in Mental Health, 4*(1), 3–16.

Stott, R., Mansell, W., Salkovskis, P., Lavender, A., & Cartwright-Hatton, S. (2010). *Oxford Guide to Metaphors in CBT. Building Cognitive Bridges*. Oxford and New York: Oxford University Press.

Tay, D. (2014). An analysis of metaphor hedging in psychotherapeutic talk. In M. Yamaguchi, D. Tay, & B. Blount (Eds.), *Approaches to Language, Culture, and Cognition* (pp. 251–267). Basingstoke, UK: Palgrave MacMillan.

Tay, D. (2016). Finding the Middle Ground between Therapist-Centred and Client-Centred Metaphor Research in Psychotherapy. In M. O'Reilly & J. N. Lester (Eds.), *The Palgrave Handbook of Adult Mental Health* (pp. 558–576). London: Palgrave Macmillan.

Tay, D., Huang, J., & Zeng, H. (2019). Affective and discursive outcomes of symbolic interpretations in picture-based counseling: A skin conductance and discourse analytic study. *Metaphor & Symbol, 34*(2), 96–110.

Van Parys, H., & Rober, P. (2013). Micro-analysis of a therapist-generated metaphor referring to the position of a parentified child in the family. *Journal of Family Therapy, 35*(1), 89–113.

Wee, L. (2005a). Class-inclusion and correspondence models as discourse types: A framework for approaching metaphorical discourse. *Language in Society, 34*(2), 219–238.

Wee, L. (2005b). Constructing the source: Metaphor as a discourse strategy. *Discourse Studies, 7*(3), 363–384.

Yu, N. (1998). *The Contemporary Theory of Metaphor: A Perspective from Chinese*. Amsterdam and Philadelphia: John Benjamins.

Zhong, J. (2011). Working with Chinese patients: Are there conflicts between Chinese culture and psychoanalysis? *International Journal of Applied Psychoanalytic Studies, 8*(3), 218–226.

Understanding the Perspectives of Counsellors and Clients in School-Based Counselling in Hong Kong

Mark Harrison and Phoenix Lam

Abstract The growing incidence of mental health problems in adolescents is a significant global concern. School-based counselling, where a student meets with an individual, trained counsellor a number of times in a school setting, is a common component of holistic mental health programmes to support the well-being of students. In Hong Kong, however, professional counselling is in general not well-developed, and school-based counselling has been severely under-researched. Drawing on data from interviews with 8 counsellors and 25 student clients in local secondary schools, the present study aims to investigate the perspectives of counsellors and clients on the practice of school-based counselling in Hong Kong. Following a thematic approach, the study compares the key themes identified in the reflections of counsellors and clients on their experience of counselling. Similarities and differences in the discursive construction and realisation of themes are examined in detail. Representative examples are discussed in context to illustrate the views from both the service providers and users of school-based counselling. Findings from this study will inform and enhance understanding of how school-based counselling can help to promote the mental well-being of students in the local educational setting and in the broader Asian context.

Keywords Mental health · Adolescents · School-based counselling

M. Harrison
Department of Psychology, The Education University of Hong Kong, Hong Kong, People's Republic of China

P. Lam (✉)
Department of English, The Hong Kong Polytechnic University, Hong Kong, People's Republic of China
e-mail: wyplam@polyu.edu.hk

© Springer Nature Singapore Pte Ltd. 2020
B. Watson and J. Krieger (eds.), *Expanding Horizons in Health Communication*, The Humanities in Asia 6, https://doi.org/10.1007/978-981-15-4389-0_3

1 Introduction

The growing incidence of mental health problems in adolescents is a significant global concern, with up to a fifth of children and adolescents worldwide experiencing mental health issues (Kieling et al., 2011). In the US, for instance, the lifetime prevalence of mental disorders has been increasing, with around half of all cases beginning by age 14 (Kessler et al., 2005). Similarly, adolescents in Hong Kong are experiencing serious mental health problems. In a recent survey of secondary school students (Baptist Oi Kwan Social Service, 2017), more than half of the 15,560 respondents showed symptoms of depression, with a quarter showing symptoms of anxiety. Given the severity of mental health problems among secondary school students, it is imperative that prevention and early treatment interventions for mental health conditions focus on adolescents (Kessler et al., 2005).

The importance of schools in supporting the mental well-being of students has been increasingly recognised in recent years. The American School Counselor Association (2012) and the International School Counselor Association (Fezler & Brown, 2011) have developed models to address mental health issues in schools, for example. Previous studies have shown that programmes in schools that address young people's mental well-being are most effective when teachers are supported by trained counsellors who provide responsive services to students (Kourkoutas & Giovazolias, 2015; Kyriacou, 2015). School-based counselling (SBC), where a student meets with an individual, trained counsellor a number of times in a school setting, is one of the most common forms of psychological therapy for secondary school students in the UK and the US.

In Hong Kong, local schools generally adopt a whole-school approach to supporting the mental health of young people (Education Bureau, 2015). This approach highlights the collaborative efforts of teaching staff and supporting personnel such as social workers. Few schools, however, employ trained counsellors to provide responsive services (Harris, 2014). In both the US and the UK, training and accreditation are required for counsellors to practise in schools (American Counseling Association, 2012; Stein & DeBerard, 2010) whereas in Hong Kong, counselling in secondary schools is usually carried out by social workers, teachers and other paraprofessional staff. This lack of professional counselling provision in secondary schools reflects the low status of the counselling profession in Hong Kong, where many local people have little or no experience of counselling and are unwilling to see a counsellor (Yu et al., 2010). The dismissal of counselling as a viable means to address the mental health issues of young people is also evident in the attitude of the local educational authorities. In the Education Bureau's (2016) recent report on student suicide prevention, for example, counselling was only briefly mentioned for helping 'needy parents' and post-secondary students. Together, these are telling signs that counselling, in particular SBC for adolescents, is not supported widely in Hong Kong society.

Despite recent research providing convincing evidence for the effectiveness of counselling in tackling mental health problems among adolescents in Western countries (Hanley & Noble, 2017), there remains a severe dearth of research in this area locally. More research into counselling with Hong Kong adolescents is needed to assess its effectiveness and the extent to which findings from Western contexts may be transferable. Importantly, understanding the perspectives of the key stakeholders in SBC in Hong Kong will contribute to the evidence-base for SBC implemented in the local setting. This constitutes the focus of the present study.

2 Literature Review

2.1 The Effectiveness of Counselling with Adolescents

A large body of research strongly indicates that counselling is effective in addressing adolescents' mental health problems. Several different counselling approaches have been found to be effective for a large number of issues, and young people have reported a range of positive outcomes as a result of attending counselling, including increased self-esteem, self-efficacy and confidence, better emotional regulation, improved concentration and engagement at school, better relationships, greater empathy, better listening skills, greater insight, and increased feelings of happiness (see, for example, Crocket et al., 2015; Fedewa et al., 2016; Gibson & Cartwright, 2014; McArthur et al., 2016; McLaughlin et al., 2013).

Despite the research consensus into the effectiveness and benefits of adolescent counselling, however, little is understood about the processes taking place which lead to therapeutic change. While some work has tentatively proposed mechanisms to explain the ways in which positive change comes about in counselling, the nature of such change processes remains largely unexplored (Fedewa et al., 2016).

2.2 Processes in Counselling with Adolescents

Process in counselling can be thought of as a series of phases through which an individual passes as the counselling relationship develops. Such phases or stages may be conceptualised chronologically. Mearns and Thorne (2007), for example, divide counselling simply into 'beginnings,' 'middles' and 'ends'. Egan (2013) offers a three-stage process: identifying problems, developing ideas for constructive change and planning action. McLeod (2013) identifies several stages of counselling including: negotiating expectations, establishing a working alliance, assimilation of problematic experiences and ending counselling.

Some research explores adolescents' experiences as they move through the different phases of the counselling process. Young people are often apprehensive and nervous about attending counselling and find their first experiences unfamiliar and strange (Binder et al., 2011). These feelings of insecurity are associated with young people being unsure about whether they can trust the counsellor. Prior (2012) found that developing trust is essential for engagement in counselling, and that trust is more easily established when the counsellor is perceived as being accepting, non-judgemental and capable of assuring confidentiality. Once a counselling relationship has been established, young people have described their counsellors as being 'genuinely caring' and showing 'sensitivity' and a 'welcoming attitude' (Binder et al., 2011). They value not being judged (McArthur et al., 2016), 'being treated like an equal' (Prior, 2012), 'feeling understood' (Cooper, 2009; Crocket et al., 2015) and 'feeling valued and accepted' (Cooper, 2009). Self-disclosure in limited amounts by the counsellor seems to be appreciated by young people, though professionalism and the maintenance of proper boundaries is expected (Binder et al., 2011). The relationship formed between the counsellor and the client, as well as the characteristics of the client and the counsellor, are thought to have a significant impact on therapeutic outcomes (Cooper, 2009).

Some of the most common change processes by adolescents identified in previous research include 'getting things off my chest,' 'talking about emotions leading to relief,' 'exploring alternative ways of behaving,' 'finding answers for themselves,' 'increasing self-worth,' 'developing insight,' 'enhancing coping strategies,' 'improving relational skills' and 'releasing tension' (Cooper, 2009; Griffiths, 2013; McArthur et al., 2016). Change processes are generally understood to be overlapping and not mutually exclusive. Importantly, they may be influenced by contextual factors, including socio-cultural ones.

2.3 The Influence of Socio-Cultural Factors

Cultural beliefs about the self in relation to wider society may influence the individual's experience of psychological distress (refer to chapters by Chan and Jin in this edition for discussion of cultural differences in communication). Such beliefs will also affect help-seeking behaviour and the way counselling is perceived.

As a city in China with a primarily ethnic Chinese population, Hong Kong society has been heavily influenced by Confucianism, where the identity of the individual is defined by his/her place in the wider social network, particularly the family, and where 'collectivism and conformity' are central (Hofstede, 2018). Hong Kong Chinese society has thus been described as 'low trust', meaning that individuals are less willing or able to form strong relationships with individuals outside the family (Fukuyama, 1996). As such, Hong Kong adolescents may be more reluctant to seek help for mental health problems since disclosing personal information outside the family may be considered shameful and disruptive to family harmony (Kim et al., 2009). Asymmetrical relationships and hierarchical social structures are also key features of Confucianism, which may lead individuals to see counsellors as authority figures. This appears to be reflected in the language used to describe counselling and counsellors. In Hong Kong, 'counselling' is usually rendered as '輔導', which connotes the giving of advice or guidance. People often refer to their counsellor as '老師', meaning 'teacher'. Chinese clients may, therefore, prefer a counsellor who is directive in style and oriented towards problem-solving (Ng & James, 2013). Given that Confucianism has influenced school guidance in Hong Kong (Hue, 2008), any study which investigates SBC in the territory should take socio-cultural factors, particularly the influence of Confucianism, into account.

2.4 Linguistic and Discourse Studies on Counselling

Most linguistic and discourse studies on counselling focus on the actual interactions taking place within a counselling session, typically through conversation analysis, rather than investigating separately the reflections of stakeholders outside a counselling session. Specifically, they focus on the discursive strategies or linguistic features employed by either counsellors or clients, but not a comparison of both groups. Some studies have examined how counsellors responded to students' advice requests (Vehviläinen, 2003), managed students' negative emotions and trouble-telling (Svinhufvud, Voutilainen & Weiste, 2017) or displayed empathy (Stommel & Te Molder, 2018). Others have investigated how clients resisted collaborating with counsellors (Hutchby, 2002), or ended e-counselling chats based on their level of satisfaction (Christodoulidou, 2018). While these studies provide useful insights into the internal workings of counselling as it happens, they do not explicitly ask counsellors and clients directly about what counselling means to them and what it encompasses. In this connection, we argue that a reflective genre like an open-structured interview is pivotal to the understanding of counselling practice, as it invites counsellors and clients to take an outsider role to observe and evaluate; encourages them to consider more deeply their own actions and experiences; and offers them the opportunity to communicate explicitly their perspectives on counselling which are often not apparent or feasible in a counselling session. Such direct insights into the stakeholders' reflective cognitive processing can complement the observations found in counselling interactions to provide a more thorough and nuanced view of the practice of counselling.

3   Aim and Research Questions of the Study

The study aims to understand the perspectives of counsellors and clients in SBC in Hong Kong as constructed and realised in discourse with the following research questions:

1. What are the perspectives of counsellors and clients on their experience of SBC?
2. What are the similarities and differences between counsellors' and clients' perspectives on their experience of SBC?
3. How are the reported experiences of clients and counsellors discursively and linguistically constructed and realised?

4   Methods

4.1   Data Collection

The 25 student participants were ethnically Chinese, born and raised in Hong Kong, between 14 and 19 years of age, from families of middle to high socio-economic status (SES), and had attended at least six sessions of counselling at their school within the past 6 months prior to data collection. All were recruited from three fee-paying co-educational schools in Hong Kong, which served a majority of ethnically Chinese students. They were fluent English speakers who were able to effectively articulate their experience through the language. A wide range of mental health issues was involved, the most frequent of which were relationship problems and stress caused by schoolwork. The eight counsellor participants were qualified counsellors trained to at least certificate level or qualified social workers trained to masters' level with additional training and experience in counselling in school settings. Four were native Cantonese speakers, one was a native Mandarin speaker and three were native English speakers.

Ethics approval was granted by the university with which the first author is affiliated. Consent forms were signed by the principals of the participating schools and by the participants, and assent from parents was obtained. Participants were told that all interviews were confidential and would be anonymised and that they could withdraw from the research at any time.

Semi-structured interviews were conducted with all participants in English. The student participants were interviewed using focus questions based on the client change interview developed by Elliott (1996). Counsellors were interviewed using a similar but modified version of the focus questions. In total, 25 interviews with students (mean age 16.7 years; SD 1.0 years) and 8 interviews with counsellors, amounting to approximately 22 hours of recording, were conducted. The mean length of the interviews was 34.4 min (SD 6.9 min) for students and 55.9 min (SD 6.0 min) for counsellors. The interviews were then orthographically transcribed and resulted in transcripts of over 100,000 words of data for analysis.

4.2   Data Analysis

4.2.1   Thematic Analysis

Analysis of the data was first carried out thematically using the method outlined by Braun and Clarke (2006) within a philosophical paradigm of critical realism (Maxwell, 2012), in which psychological experiences such as thoughts and emotions are regarded as ontologically real. These experiences may be modified by social interactions, and the way in which they are understood and communicated is also socially constructed. The use of Braun and Clarke's (2006) method allowed us to develop themes that captured shared meanings across many participants.

Transcripts were read several times to develop familiarity with the content of the interviews, and the transcripts were coded using a computer programme (NVivo 11). Codes were clustered into themes characterised by a central organising concept (Clarke et al., 2015). Initial data analysis was carried out at a descriptive level in order to capture the participants' experience of counselling as accurately as possible.

In line with the Standards for Reporting Qualitative Research recommendations (O'Brien, Harris, Beckman, Reed, & Cook, 2014), several steps were taken to ensure the credibility and trustworthiness of the data analysis and subsequent findings. Ongoing discussion took place with colleagues as data were analysed and themes were developed; an audit of the method was carried out; and participants were given the opportunity to comment on preliminary findings. Triangulation of data by including the perspectives of both counsellors and students in analysis also contributed to the credibility of the study's findings.

4.2.2 Discourse Analysis

Once the themes were identified in the thematic analysis, the text samples instantiating the themes were subject to discourse analysis. This involved examining each text sample in question in context to observe the strategies and features used in relation to the text producer's role in the counselling process. Then all the text samples realising each main theme were analysed together to identify any common patterns of prominent strategies and features employed in the discursive construction and realisation of the main themes. In the analytic process, we explored the similarities and differences between counsellors and student clients. We then reviewed and synthesised the findings with our interpretation. We also specifically compared findings from the present study on SBC in the local context with those found in relevant studies in other geographical areas, especially in Western contexts, to identify any distinct observations pertinent to the present setting, and to discuss how socio-cultural factors might account for such observations.

5 Findings

Three themes were developed from the interviews regarding the perspectives of counsellors and clients on their experience of SBC. In their narration of these themes, participants often described how the themes were associated with the chronological stages of a counselling relationship in SBC. These three themes are thus organised here in relation to four interlocking and partially overlapping stages of SBC and are visually summarised in Fig. 3.1.

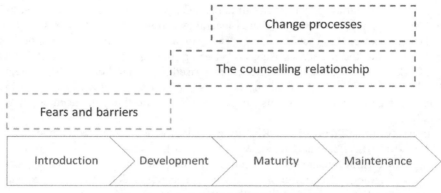

Fig. 3.1 Relationship between Themes Developed from the Data and Stages of School-based Counselling

5.1 Fears and Barriers

The first theme identified concerns the negative emotions that clients experience which inhibit them from participating in counselling. This theme is particularly relevant to respondents in the introduction and development stages, i.e. the period before counselling begins and when they start to engage with counselling initially.

5.1.1 The Clients' Perspective—Approaching Counselling with Doubt and Hesitation

Most students experienced considerable doubt and hesitation before they began counselling. These fears and barriers mainly concerned confidentiality, other people's perceptions and the effectiveness of counselling. In Example 1, a student explained her fear of the breach of confidentiality if the counsellor talked to her parents:

Example 1

I thought she was going to maybe talk to my parents. That was a really big thing because—I don't know. I thought she was going to call my parents and talk to them about it, and that was something that scared me (Student C).

The use of a number of hedges, and expressions of uncertainty and vagueness (*I thought, maybe, I don't know, something*) in Example 1 presented the student's fear as speculative and hypothetical. She further used an intensifier (*really*) to amplify the scale of her fear, portraying the counsellor talking to her parents as 'a really big thing'. At the same time, she used an emotion verb (*scared*) to explicitly describe her negative personal feeling. In describing how their parents, classmates and friends characterise those receiving counselling, clients commonly employed negative labelling by such terms as 'an attention seeker', 'a lunatic', 'losers', 'the bad students', 'messed up people' and 'weak people'. The usefulness of counselling was also often dismissed by the frequent use of the negator *not* and negative emotive words, as in '*I didn't feel like it was going to be that effective*' and '*I did feel suspicious and feel like, doubt the effectiveness of it*'.

Such negativity, suspicion and doubt surrounding the clients' assumptions of counselling could also be seen in the ways in which counsellors were referred to by clients. In these preliminary stages of counselling, clients distanced themselves from counsellors by using expressions which highlighted the unfamiliarity between them, as shown in Example 2.

Example 2

For the first time it was difficult, and I hesitated a little bit because you're telling your feelings to someone that you don't know, a complete stranger (Student Q).

5.1.2 The Counsellors' Perspective—Approaching Counselling with a Balanced View

While counsellors also reported the initial fears and barriers that clients experienced, their views were more balanced in that they acknowledged such feelings as normal and they presented positive as well as negative impressions of clients on their initial encounters of counselling. Example 3 shows how a counsellor normalised the negative feelings that some students had at the beginning.

Example 3

Any young person who is sitting in a room with a vaguely strange adult... I think they have a natural apprehension and a natural reluctance to talk to anybody because they're teenagers (Counsellor A).

Instead of highlighting the undesirable emotions that students went through, the counsellor in Example 3 normalised such feelings by using the indefinite 'any' and 'anybody', thus suggesting that these feelings were common and applied to everyone. The use and repetition of the adjective 'natural' with positive connotation before the nouns 'apprehension' and 'reluctance' also presented the feelings as legitimate, unsurprising and acceptable. Interestingly, when counsellors described clients' initial positive views towards counselling, they tended to generalise these views to a wider population, as in Example 4 with the use of the pronoun 'most', associated with the positive feelings of being 'open' and 'okay' with counselling that students quickly experienced, after they knew what counselling was from the counsellor.

Example 4

Most of the student they are open to it. They don't quite actually know what counselling is, but once I explain it to them, "This is about talking about your problem and trying to resolve the issue together", most of them they are okay with this (Counsellor F).

Conversely, when counsellors described clients' initial negative views, they tended to hedge more and hence suggested that such views only partially applied, as in Example 5 with the use of the pronoun 'some' associated with the feeling of being 'very weird'.

Example 5

Obviously, some of them think that it is very weird because "I don't know this person and I have to sit here and talk to her" (Counsellor B).

The strategic choice of pronouns denoting the number of clients concerned, therefore, allowed counsellors to present clients' positive perceptions as widespread and negative perceptions as occasional, thereby highlighting the positive aspects of such first impressions. In either case, while presenting collective views of clients, counsellors avoided over-generalisation with the omission of such quantifiers as 'all' and 'every' to give a less lopsided and more measured assessment of their clients' feelings.

5.2   The Counselling Relationship

The second theme identified concerns how clients and counsellors characterise the nature of their relationship at different stages of counselling. The building of this relationship starts at the development stage, after clients have overcome their initial fears and barriers in the first few encounters with their counsellor. The relationship then continues to grow through the maturity stage, when counsellors and clients have engaged in counselling for some time. In the maintenance stage, clients derive ongoing support from their counsellor, often seeing them irregularly or simply keeping in touch without meeting.

5.2.1   The Clients' Perspective—Highlighting Benefits to Self

Once students got over their anxieties and qualms about counselling, they came to see its benefits and embraced the experience of being counselled. Example 6 details the way in which a client perceived the change of his relationship with the counsellor over time:

Example 6

It was quite formal at first, I was not relaxed at all. It was just like talking to a deputy principal. His face looks quite serious, like he doesn't smile. It wasn't like that afterwards. Things become less formal, and soft. I don't need to sit up straight to talk to him anymore. I can just relax and have a casual conversation (Student F).

A number of negative words were used to describe the stress and rigidity perceived in the early counselling experience and relationship: the meeting was 'quite formal', the client was 'not relaxed at all', and the counsellor was an authoritative and intimidating figure who 'looks serious' and 'doesn't smile'. As the relationship proceeds, it was described with more positive words (*less formal, soft, relax* and *casual*) and actions (*I don't need to sit up straight*) associated with comfort and ease. Similar to the ways in which initial fears and barriers tended to be dramatised, clients often used intensifiers to amplify their subsequent positive experience of counselling with the use of words such as 'very' and 'so'. In Example 7, the dramatisation was achieved through intensifiers together with the contradiction of the expectation set up at the beginning of the extract.

Example 7

I was expecting questions and writing down stuff and being very specific on targets. I didn't know that it would be so conversational, and something that's very natural for me so that it would actually lead me to talk more. It was very pleasant (Student A).

Other students also characterised the counselling relationship with such intensification as 'very casual', 'a lot more effective' and 'a lot more useful'. This dramatic change in clients' perceptions of counselling could be seen further in the ways in which they referred to their counsellors. Many clients referred to their counsellor as 'a friend'. Some emphasised the solidarity and emotional support in the relationship through such expressions as 'someone who was on my side every time', 'someone who was like an older brother to me', 'someone to talk to', 'someone that can listen to me' and 'someone to share about my feelings and experience'. Counsellors were no longer strangers whom clients did not know or powerful professional figures who they did not relate to personally. As the relationship matured, many students considered counselling a long-term relationship and an ongoing source of support. They felt that they could seek help from counsellors when needed without the arrangement of regular meetings. This perception of counselling as a long-term relationship is evident in Example 8 where the client emphasised the closeness of the relationship (*really close*) and the extent of the counsellor's knowledge about the client (*they know so much about you*).

Example 8

I feel like this is a long-term thing, really, because you build this connection with the counsellor that's really close. They know so much about you (Student A).

5.2.2 The Counsellors' Perspective—Taking Wider Issues into Account

Like clients, counsellors conceptualised the counselling relationship in positive terms. Instead of highlighting such attributes as informality and comfort, however, counsellors focused more on creating a safe and non-judgemental counselling environment, both physically and emotionally. Making students feel safe and not judged was thus a central and recurring topic in the counsellors' perspective, as shown in Example 9 where these qualities were highlighted through the connection of three adjectives in asyndetic coordination, the quantifier 'all' and the intensifier 'really' before 'important'.

Example 9

We don't judge. Not judgemental, calm, safe space, I think all of that's really important (Counsellor A).

Counsellors, at the same time, acknowledged the challenges and practical constraints involved in building a relationship with clients and the factors that might affect a counselling relationship. In other words, counsellors took into account a number of wider issues in articulating this theme, rather than simply focusing on expressing their own perception on the nature of one single relationship. Their construction of the theme, therefore, entailed the consideration of individual differences and variation in SBC. Example 10 describes a difficult situation that a counsellor faced, the options he had and the possible effects of the options.

Example 10

So I do struggle sometimes when I do get referrals to- How do I approach this in a very- to make them feel safe, they're not being- or to call them in, because being called to the counselling office can be quite daunting I think (Counsellor C).

This internal struggle could be seen structurally through the use of incomplete sentence fragments and false starts, with the dilemma presented in contrast through near-antonyms (*safe* and *daunting*). In addition to having a more macro, multidimensional view which took into account other aspects of the counselling relationship, counsellors also differed from clients in their understanding of the length of SBC. Counsellors regarded counselling in the school setting to be temporary, with many pointing out the possible negative effects of long-term counselling, using such negative metaphorical terms as 'a crutch' and 'somewhere to hide' to describe their role when the counselling relationship remained for longer than necessary. Example 11 illustrates a counsellor's rejection of long-term SBC, indicating her reluctance of being a 'shelter' metaphorically.

Example 11

Usually, I keep a distance from them because I don't want to still be the shelter (Counsellor B).

This emotional distancing from the clients was also evident in the ways in which counsellors referred to the clients. Terms marking the clients' age and institutional role (*kids, children, students*) were commonly used. While more emotional vocabulary (*a mommy figure, a big sister*) was sometimes used to refer to their own role for clients, these terms nonetheless showed a strongly hierarchical relationship. No counsellors in the interviews described their relationship with the clients as an equal one such as friendship, as perceived by many clients.

5.3 Change Processes

The third and last theme identified concerns how clients experience the processes of change, often brought about or facilitated by counsellors, in SBC. Since such changes take place over time, clients often go through such change processes only after their relationship with the counsellors becomes more stable, i.e. the maturity stage. Such change processes continue well into the maintenance stage when clients do not receive regular counselling. Three change processes are commonly discussed by both clients and counsellors: fostering new ways of thinking; developing better relationships; and experiencing positive emotions.

5.3.1 The Clients' Perspective—Effecting Changes as an Active Agent

Students conceptualised change processes as self-directed, underlining their own responsibility in effecting changes, with the counsellors only in an assisting but not a leading role. Instead of giving the clients a solution or answer, counsellors often assisted by listening, asking questions or suggesting alternative scenarios. In Example 12, a client explained how counselling prompted her to think differently:

Example 12

It helped me think in a different mindset compared to what I've always been thinking it (Student C).

In describing the change processes that she was undergoing, the student in Example 12 used the structure 'helped me think' with SBC as the subject and the client as the object of the first verb 'helped' but also the subject of the second verb 'think'. Similar structures with the second verb expressing a mental or existential state (*helped/made me see/think/realise/understand/feel/get over/change/become*) were found repeatedly. This suggests that while counselling promotes the change processes, it is the client who is the agent responsible for a number of cognitive and transformative activities.

Another common structure clients used to highlight change processes was the juxtaposition of the present with the past. In Example 12, there is an explicit comparison between the new way of thinking brought about by counselling and the old way of thinking in the past. This structure contrasting the present and the past was often combined with positive words associated with the present and after counselling, and negative words associated with the past and before counselling. This linguistic realisation is illustrated in Example 13, when a client explained how counselling helped her feel more positively, expressed her emotions more easily, and in turn develop a better relationship with her parents.

Example 13

After counselling, I feel I'm more open to my parents.... I wasn't able to tell my parents anything, like my feelings and emotions. But after I went through counselling, it was more easier for me to tell my parents (Student Q).

The juxtaposition of the present situation filled with positive adjectives in the comparative form (*more open, more easier*) with the past depicted in negative terms (*wasn't able to tell my parents anything*) accentuated the transformation experienced by the client and in turn amplified the benefits of SBC.

5.3.2 The Counsellors' Perspective—Facilitating and Assessing Cautiously

Similar to their clients, counsellors considered their role as a facilitator in promoting change processes. Further, they gave credit to students for finding their own solutions, as in Example 14:

Example 14

They're seeking somebody to discuss things with and think them through, you know, the guided question, the have you thought about-? what about-? and letting them express really what their own solutions are. Most of our students have their own solutions (Counsellor A).

By strategically asking guiding questions, counsellors indirectly acknowledged students' abilities to change on their own, with solutions already in place in them which only required expressing, or verbalising clearly, as some counsellors described their clients' thoughts as 'all jumbled up' and their task as 'unpacking the jumbled mess of thoughts, feelings, emotions'.

Compared with the clients' portrayed contrast between the present and the past, however, counsellors focused more on the here-and-now positive aspects of change processes without an explicit comparison with the past. In consequence, there were also fewer words with negative meanings specifically associated with the time before counselling. In particular, counsellors highlighted the different positive dimensions of self-improvement that students experienced after counselling, as discussed in Example 15.

Example 15

They may gain some confidence about themselves, their self-esteem enhanced, and for some of them, they may find it easier to deal with the challenges and their struggles (Counsellor B).

While positive words concerning self-improvement (*gain, confidence, self-esteem, enhanced, easier*) abound in Example 15, the extract is also highly mitigated. As with the construction of the other two themes, counsellors explained the possible change processes experienced by clients in a cautious tone by using the weak modal 'may' twice, the indefinite pronoun 'some' and the comparative form 'easier' to avoid over-generalisation of the impact of SBC on students and to highlight individual differences.

6 Discussion

Three main themes were found to be central in the discursive construction and realisation of the experience of SBC by both clients and counsellors. These three common denominators documented the emotional and developmental ups and downs in our four-stage conceptualisation of SBC. At the early introduction and development stages, the negative feelings of fears and barriers by clients surrounding SBC were emphasised by both groups of stakeholders. This sense of insecurity in young clients associated with the pre- and initial-counselling period is consistent with findings from previous research (Binder et al., 2011). At the later maturity and maintenance stages, by contrast, the positive emotions experienced through the establishment of a counselling relationship, and the emotional and developmental benefits from change processes, were common in the portrayal by both groups. This supports the effectiveness of SBC in promoting mental health among adolescents in Hong Kong, a finding also reported in other cultural contexts (Hanley & Noble, 2017). Again, many of the desirable qualities reported in the present study regarding the nature of the counselling relationship are similar to those in previous studies, where not being judged (McArthur et al., 2016) and mutuality (Prior, 2012) are found to be valued by teenage clients.

In relation to change processes, both clients and counsellors highlighted the importance of self-directedness, or 'finding answers for themselves', echoing what has been found in counselling studies conducted both in Western contexts (Cooper, 2009; Griffiths, 2013; McArthur et al., 2016) and also locally (Hue, 2008). In discourse studies, the same notion of self-directedness and the avoidance of giving direct advice by counsellors have been much discussed (Vehviläinen, 2003). The three change processes as observed in the findings earlier, namely fostering new ways of thinking; developing better relationships; and experiencing positive emotions, also bear a close resemblance to those experienced by adolescents reported in earlier research, particularly 'exploring alternative ways of behaving', 'talking about emotions leading to relief' and 'improving relational skills' (Cooper, 2009; Griffiths, 2013; McArthur et al., 2016). These similarities suggest that the three main themes shared by counsellors and clients in SBC in Hong Kong in the present study may be universal and central to young peoples' experience of counselling globally.

It is, however, also important to note the differences between counsellors and clients in their perspectives of SBC in Hong Kong, how such perspectives are constructed and realised differently, and how such perspectives may differ from those in Western contexts. One important difference observed in the findings between the counsellors and clients lies in the scope and intensity of the construction and realisation of the themes. On the one hand, clients' perspectives on the themes were more localised in scope and extreme in intensity, focusing largely on their own personal feelings and experiences without extending them to other individuals through the use of a large number of positive and negative evaluative words peppered with intensifiers. The deep anxiety reported by clients, in particular, may be compounded by the highly collectivist culture in which they are embedded. In the past, the social stigma associated with counselling has been found to positively correlate with Asian cultural values (Miville & Constantine, 2007). Given that such social stigma associated with counselling not only applies to the student receiving the service but also to the entire social network (Kim et al., 2009), the pressure imposed on young clients to conform, rather than to differ by going to counselling, may be greater than in Western contexts, where more individualistic cultures are observed. The contrast between pre- and post-counselling was further dramatised by clients through the employment of comparative expressions, parallel structure juxtaposing the present and the past, and the selection of opposite terms used to refer to the counsellor at different stages. While intensifiers have been well-documented as characteristic in teenage talk (Stenström, Andersen & Hasund, 2002), other features seem to be unique in the current context. As the most directly engaged stakeholder group in SBC, student clients may feel the need to employ particular strategies and features to express the high intensity and polarised sentiments of their first-hand experience.

On the other hand, counsellors' perspectives on the themes were broader in scope and more moderate in intensity, covering a wider range of issues and presenting more balanced views through more strongly mitigated language. While counsellors commended the benefits of SBC, they also explicitly and realistically acknowledged its limits and challenges. At the same time, they highlighted the variation in SBC by avoiding over-generalisation. To balance clients' negative portrayal of their fears and barriers, counsellors employed the strategy of normalising to legitimise and naturalise clients' feelings as normal and common (cf. Svinhufvud, Voutilainen & Weiste, 2017). Linguistically, the use of mitigators and hedges allowed counsellors to present their perspectives in a more measured, neutral tone, which in turn helped them build a professional and practical image.

In relation to the discursive and linguistic construction and realisation of the counselling relationship, counsellors and clients differ in their perception of how hierarchical it is and how long it should last. Counsellors tended to perceive the relationship to be hierarchical and temporary, as reflected in their choice of reference terms marking the level of seniority and their use of metaphors with a negative meaning in warning against longer term counselling. In this respect, their perspective seems to be more attuned to the value of Confucianism, whereby counsellors are typically seen as figures of authority rather than as equals. Since deference to authority figures as an Asian cultural value has been found to foster stronger alliances between counsellors and clients (Kim et al., 2002), this view by the counsellors may actually enrich the experience and outcome of counselling. In the local context, the hierarchy in the counselling relationship seems particularly relevant, as counsellors often also serve as teachers in schools (cf. Hue, 2008). Clients, in comparison, characterised the relationship as a long-lasting friendship with more equal status, as reflected by their choice of reference terms marking solidarity and comradeship and by their more positive portrayal of the benefits of long-term counselling. This mismatch in the perception of the counselling relationship between stakeholders coming from the same culture suggests that the ways in which cultural values may affect the experience of SBC are varied, intricate and complex, awaiting further investigation (see, for example, Miville & Constantine, 2007).

7   Limitations

The students participating in the study were of middle socio-economic status, and so the present study's findings may not be more broadly transferrable to other Chinese adolescents in Hong Kong or those from other ethnic groups. Although fluent in English, the student participants did not use their first language in the interviews and so there may have been limitations on the extent to which they were able to express themselves in a clear and nuanced way. Participants came from three fee-paying schools, a category of secondary day schools only making up about one-fifth of the total, which may indicate an SES bias and thus may not be representative of most schools in Hong Kong.

8   Conclusions

This study has identified and analysed three common main themes from interviews regarding the perspectives of counsellors and clients on their SBC experience in Hong Kong. The similarities and differences between counsellors and clients in their perspectives on these common main themes have been discussed, with an examination and comparison of how such themes have been discursively and linguistically constructed and realised. Given the scarcity of research conducted in SBC in Asian contexts in general, and the dearth of linguistic and discourse studies examining critical self-reflections of counselling experience rather than counselling sessions in action, the present study is a timely attempt to address an important yet much under-researched area in mental health communication. Specifically, the examination of the first-hand reflections of the two key stakeholder groups in the study allows us to understand better the obstacles and rewards involved at different stages of SBC in Hong Kong, and to provide policymakers and mental health professionals with a window into the views of those directly engaged in local educational counselling.

Future research can investigate the themes which are unique to different stakeholder groups, compare the reflections of counselling experience with the actual interactions in counselling sessions, and directly study the impact of different cultural factors on SBC, especially in Asian contexts. It is hoped that this study will inform and enhance our understanding of the benefits of SBC, and the challenges to its successful implementation in Hong Kong, which will in turn improve the practice of SBC and promote the mental well-being of students in the local educational setting and beyond.

References

American School Counseling Association. (2012). *The ASCA national model: A framework for school counseling programs*. Herndon, VA: American School Counseling Association.
Baptist Oi Kwan Social Service. (2017). Secondary school students' depression and anxiety survey 2017. Retrieved from https://www.bokss.org.hk/content/press/27/MHI_PressRelease2017_final2.pdf.
Binder, P. E., Moltu, C., Hummelsund, D., Sagen, S. H., & Holgersen, H. (2011). Meeting an adult ally on the way out into the world: Adolescent patients' experiences of useful psychotherapeutic ways of working at an age when independence really matters. *Psychotherapy Research, 21*(5), 554–566.
Braun, V., & Clarke, V. (2006). Using thematic analysis in psychology. *Qualitative Research in Psychology, 3*(2), 77–101.
Christodoulidou, M. (2018). Consultee satisfaction in ending chats of an e-counseling service. *Discourse Studies, 20*(4), 461–487.
Cooper, M. (2009). Counselling in UK secondary schools: A comprehensive review of audit and evaluation data. *Counselling and Psychotherapy Research, 9*(3), 137–150.
Crocket, K., Kotzé, E., & Peter, M. (2015). Young people's perspectives on school counselling: A survey study. *New Zealand Journal of Counselling, 35*(1), 22–43.
Education Bureau, Hong Kong Government. (2015). *Guide on comprehensive student guidance service (revised version August 2015)*. Hong Kong: Education Bureau.
Education Bureau, Hong Kong Government. (2016). Committee on prevention of student suicides final report (November 2016). Retrieved from https://www.edb.gov.hk/attachment/en/student-parents/crisis-management/about-crisis-management/CPSS_final_report_en.pdf.
Egan, G. (2013). *The skilled helper: A problem-management and opportunity-development approach to helping*. Belmont, CA: Cengage Learning.
Elliott, R. (1996). *Client change interview schedule*. Unpublished research instrument. Toledo, OH: Department of Psychology, University of Toledo.
Fedewa, A. L., Ahn, S., Reese, R. J., Suarez, M. M., Macquoid, A., Davis, M. C., et al. (2016). Does psychotherapy work with school-aged youth? A meta-analytic examination of moderator variables that influence therapeutic outcomes. *Journal of School Psychology, 56*, 59–87.

Fezler, B., & Brown, C. (2011). The international model for school counseling programs. *Association of American Schools in South America*, 36–49.

Fukuyama, F. (1996). *Trust: The social virtues and creation of prosperity*. London: Free Press.

Gibson, K., & Cartwright, C. (2014). Agency in young clients' narratives of counseling: "It's whatever you want to make of it". *Journal of Counseling Psychology, 60*(3), 340.

Griffiths, G. (2013). *Scoping report for MindEd: helpful and unhelpful factors in schoolbased counselling: Clients' perspectives*. Lutterworth: BACP.

Hanley, T., & Noble, J. (2017). Therapy outcomes: Is child therapy effective? In N. Midgley, J. Hayes, & M. Cooper (Eds.), *Essential research findings in child and adolescent counselling and psychotherapy* (pp. 59–78). London: Sage.

Harris, B. (2014). Locating school counseling in the Asian-Pacific region in a global context. Brief reflections on a scoping review of school counseling internationally. *Journal of Asia Pacific Counseling, 4*(2), 217–245.

Hofstede, G. (2018). Hofstede Insights—What about China? Retrieved from https://www.hofstede-insights.com/country/china/.

Hue, M. T. (2008). The influence of Confucianism: A narrative study of Hong Kong teachers' understanding and practices of school guidance and counselling. *British Journal of Guidance and Counselling, 36*(3), 303–316.

Hutchby, I. (2002). Resisting the incitement to talk in child counselling: Aspects of the utterance 'I don't know'. *Discourse Studies, 4*(2), 147–168.

Kessler, R. C., Berglund, P., Demler, O., Jin, R., Merikangas, K. R., & Walters, E. E. (2005). Lifetime prevalence and age-of-onset distributions of DSM-IV disorders in the National Comorbidity Survey Replication. *Archives of General Psychiatry, 62*(6), 593–602.

Kieling, C., Baker-Henningham, H., Belfer, M., Conti, G., Ertem, I., et al. (2011). Child and adolescent mental health worldwide: Evidence for action. *The Lancet, 378*(9801), 1515–1525.

Kim, B. S. K., Li, L. C., & Liang, C. T. H. (2002). Effects of Asian American client adherence to Asian cultural values, session goal, and counselor emphasis of client expression on career counseling process. *Journal of Counseling Psychology, 49*, 342–354.

Kim, B. S., Ng, G. F., & Ahn, A. J. (2009). Client adherence to Asian cultural values, common factors in counseling, and session outcome with Asian American clients at a university counseling center. *Journal of Counseling and Development, 87*(2), 131–142.

Kourkoutas, E., & Giovazolias, T. (2015). School-based counselling work with teachers: An integrative model. *The European Journal of Counselling Psychology, 3*(2), 137–158.

Kyriacou, C. (2015). Social pedagogy and pastoral care in schools. *British Journal of Guidance and Counselling, 43*(4), 429–437.

Maxwell, J. A. (2012). *A realist approach for qualitative research*. London: Sage.

McArthur, K., Cooper, M., & Berdondini, L. (2016). Change processes in school-based humanistic counselling. *Counselling and Psychotherapy Research, 16*(2), 88–99.

McLaughlin, C., Holliday, C., Clarke, B., & Ilie, S. (2013). *Research on counselling and psychotherapy with children and young people: A systematic scoping review of the evidence for its effectiveness from 2003–2011*. British Association for Counselling and Psychotherapy: Lutterworth, UK.

McLeod, J. (2013). *An introduction to counselling*. New York: Open University Press.

Mearns, D., & Thorne, B. (2007). *Person-centred counselling in action*. London: Sage.

Miville, M. L., & Constantine, M. G. (2007). Cultural values, counseling stigma, and intentions to seek counseling among Asian American college women. *Counseling and values, 52*, 2–11.

Ng, C. T. C., & James, S. (2013). "Directive approach" for Chinese clients receiving psychotherapy: is that really a priority? *Frontiers in Psychology, 4*, 49.

O'Brien, B. C., Harris, I. B., Beckman, T. J., Reed, D. A., & Cook, D. A. (2014). Standards for reporting qualitative research: A synthesis of recommendations. *Academic Medicine, 89*(9), 1245–1251.

Prior, S. (2012). Young people's process of engagement in school counselling. *Counselling and Psychotherapy Research, 12*(3), 233–240.

Stein, D. M., & DeBerard, S. (2010). Does holding a teacher education degree make a difference in school counselors' job performance? *Journal of School Counseling, 8*(25), 25.

Stenström, A.-B., Andersen, G., & Hasund, I. K. (2002). *Trends in teenage talk. Corpus compilation, analysis and findings.* Amsterdam: John Benjamins.

Stommel, W. & Te Molder, H. (2018). Empathically designed responses as a gateway to advice in Dutch counseling calls. *Discourse Studies,* 20(4), 523–543.

Svinhufvud, K., Voutilainen, L., & Weiste, E. (2017). Normalizing in student counseling: Counselors' responses to students' problem descriptions. *Discourse Studies, 19*(2), 196–215.

Vehviläinen, S. (2003). Avoiding providing solutions: Orienting to the ideal of students' self-directedness in counselling interaction. *Discourse Studies, 5*(3), 389–414.

Yu, C., Fu, W., Zhao, X., & Davey, G. (2010). Public understanding of counsellors and counselling in Hong Kong. *Asia Pacific Journal of Counselling and Psychotherapy, 1*(1), 47–54.

What Happens to the Holistic Care of Patients in Busy Oncology Settings?

E. Angela Chan

Abstract Cancer patients suffer from emotional issues and/or distress, for which they require appropriate care. However, effective communication that translates into recognition of patients' cues/concerns remains an issue. Barriers to effective communication include nurse shortages, time constraints and limited healthcare communication training for cancer nurses. Exploring how nurses fare in communicating with patients by responding to their cues/concerns for emotional and/or informational needs is important. This ethnographic study examined a busy cancer ward and its nursing care as a subculture. Content analysis from patient interviews was conducted, and a statistical analysis of the nurses' cue-responding behaviours. Findings revealed that despite no emotional counselling, nurses exhibited positive cue-responding behaviours and patients expressed appreciation for this care. This conclusion is striking at a time when nurses stated there was no time to talk to patients and Hong Kong faces a shortage of nurses, even as the emphasis on holistic care is growing. Findings challenge the cultural expectations of emotional care in oncology wards. The perception that emotional care must be addressed separately from the nurses' everyday physical and technical care is challenged and should be re-assessed with reintegration of the physical with the emotional in the nursing care provided to patients.

Keywords Nursing · Cancer · Ethnography · Descriptive content analysis

1 Background

The phrase 'I don't have the time to talk to patients' is commonly heard in any clinical setting. However, is there a common understanding of what that means? Does it mean that one does not have the time to listen, or that one does not have the

E. A. Chan (✉)
School of Nursing, The Hong Kong Polytechnic University, Hung Hom,
Kowloon, Hong Kong
e-mail: e.angela.chan@polyu.edu.hk

© Springer Nature Singapore Pte Ltd. 2020
B. Watson and J. Krieger (eds.), *Expanding Horizons in Health Communication*,
The Humanities in Asia 6, https://doi.org/10.1007/978-981-15-4389-0_4

skill to communicate effectively under a tight schedule? Or is it simply a common response when healthcare professionals are asked about their relationship with their patients? Among the barriers, a heavy nursing workload and a lack of time are most often mentioned as obstacles to effective nurse–patient communication. Studies have indicated that anxious patients, such as those who suffer from cancer, need the most emotional support, but often express their concerns implicitly.

Given that Chinese patients seldom express their concerns and feelings about their health, the expectation is that their psychological needs will be met by family members, while implicit communication is to be used with outsiders. Health professionals are regarded as people who occupy a space between insiders and outsiders. Since nurses spend the most time with patients, patients were found to express cues more often in conversations with nurses than with physicians (Dunn et al., 2013). An emotional cue is a covert or overt expression that something is or may be important or a cause of concern (Heaven & Green, 2001). Cue-responding refers to the need for healthcare providers to understand and respond to 'the meaning of messages conveyed by cues about the patients' feelings' (Goldberg et al., 1984, p. 574). However, few researchers within the Asian region, including Hong Kong, have explored healthcare interactions that occur in real time and in real contexts between patients and nurses through the cue-responding behaviours of nurses (refer to the chapter by Jin in this edition for a novel contribution to the study of the *opening and closings* of medical consultations in China). In addition, more than a quarter of Asian cancer patients have experienced depression and anxiety (Chen, Chang, & Yeh, 2000). It is hence imperative to gather empirical evidence in Asia about this kind of communication, since such evidence is limited. The aim of this study was to examine the psychosocial care delivered by nurses to the cancer patients of a busy oncology ward.

1.1 Differences Between Psychotherapy and Psychosocial Care

Before advancing the discussion, an overview of the phenomenon is required to establish the context. Situated as they are within the culture of a busy hospital ward, and given the shortage of nurses in Hong Kong, it is common to hear nurses say that they have no time to talk to patients, even as there is an increased emphasis on providing oncology patients with holistic care. The question is, how do nurses fare in communicating with patients by responding to their cues and concerns for emotional or/and informational needs and what are the patients' experiences like? With evidence-based practice being the motto for nursing practice, and given the importance of psychosocial care in reducing distress and improving the quality of life of cancer patients, nurses have the obligation to attend to the psychosocial aspect of care. However, a general lack of research on the significant levels of distress experienced by patients points to the need to explore the experiences of cancer patients (Jacobsen, 2009). Among those studies that have been conducted, diverse findings have led to inconclusive results. The construct of psychological distress is fundamental to the psychosocial aspect of the experience of the illness. However, the term psychosocial distress has a wide construct at the practical and operational levels (Muzzalti, Bomben, Flaiban, Mella, & Annunziata, 2016). Annunziata, Giovannini, and Mussatti (2012) asserted that psychological distress needs to be differentiated from other psychosocial dimensions of cancer, for instance, issues related to body image, cognitive limitations (Soussain et al., 2009), post-traumatic growth (Sawer, Ayers, & Field, 2010), cancer-related fatigue (Stone & Minton, 2008) and sexual difficulties (Horden, 2008). Psychosocial distress ranges from normal feelings of apprehension about the cancer diagnosis to different intensities/levels of depression and anxiety that may interfere with treatment and daily living.

Since it is important for nurses to communicate effectively by responding to cues if they are to provide psychosocial care to cancer patients, there is a need to clarify the meaning of psychosocial care in cancer nursing and the importance of cue-responding in nurse–patient communication for therapeutic care.

Cancer has become a chronic illness, and the number of patients in both curative and palliative care continues to rise globally (Ferlay et al., 2010). Various psychosocial strategies have been proposed in the field of psycho-oncology for the prevention and early detection of psychosocial distress, and for the provision of psychosocial care for cancer patients (AWMF, 2014). The term 'psychosocial distress' refers to the emotional, cognitive, social and functional problems experienced by patients (Weis, 2015). However, psychosocial distress is understood as a continuum from a normal to a high level of distress and psychiatric conditions. Hence, dealing with psychosocial distress is not simply about the early detection of distress and a subsequent referral of the patient to someone who can provide psychosocial care to improve the patient's quality of life. Rather, what is required is a stepped-care model with the systematic identification of needs and integrated delivery of psychosocial care from counselling to psychoeducation to psychotherapy (Braeken et al., 2013). The emphasis on psychosocial aspects in caring for cancer patients may inadvertently lead to the isolation of these aspects from the holistic view of a biopsychosocial model. Yet, in providing everyday nursing care to cancer patients, nurses still refer to the term 'psychosocial care', which is theoretically embedded in the biopsychosocial model. However, this apparent split in the understanding of the meaning of biopsychosocial care might also be influenced by an understanding of the psychosocial interventions that are available for managing the pain and symptoms of cancer (Novy & Aigner, 2014). Nonetheless, in 1977 Engel (1977) had already argued that the purpose of the biopsychosocial model was to bridge the separation between mind and body, in order to address the complex interactions among all of the determinants that contribute to the well-being of humans. Somehow, nurses worldwide have inadvertently separated the mind from the body in their language when they refer to the lack of time that they have to attend to the psychosocial needs of patients or when they say that they simply 'don't have the time to talk to them'. This would result in the provision of halfistic rather than holistic care (Gordon, 2006).

Abrahamson et al. (2011) asserted that, although common, psychosocial distress is frequently underdiagnosed because its diagnosis often depends on the psychosocial care and subjective judgement of busy clinicians. Muzzalti et al. (2016) conceded that the prevalence of anxiety and depression, which are common forms of psychosocial distress, varies, being generally higher among cancer patients than among the general population (Hinz et al., 2010). Globally, standardized screening and information technology have increased the ease and efficiency of making psychosocial assessments. The issue, however, is that an agreed-upon definition of distress for treatment pathways seems to be lacking. Hence, the mention of nurses having no time to talk or make any psychosocial assessments may refer to the lowest level of the continuum. However, such assessments in cancer care are important, as the patients' level of psychosocial distress can increase if their psychosocial needs are left unattended. The monitoring of psychosocial distress is the monitoring of emotions so that they do not become chronic problems requiring interventions (Muzzalti et al., 2016). The impact of psychological distress on the management of the patients' physical symptoms, and vice versa, merits attention, as it is an important issue in the provision of holistic care.

Psychological distress can easily occur when cancer patients are experiencing poor physical functioning, increased pain and fatigue, difficulties in communicating with healthcare professionals, and a lack of social support (Hill et al., 2011). It is well documented that inadequate attention is paid to the psychosocial needs of oncology patients, and that this often relates to ineffective nurse–patient communication (Hack et al., 2012).

2   Ethical Considerations

Ethical approval was obtained from the Research Ethics Committee of the hospital and the Departmental Research Committee of The Hong Kong Polytechnic University.

3   Method

This study is part of a larger focused ethnographic study investigating the processes of nurse–patient communication through an exploration of the socio-cultural context and practices of providing nursing care in busy oncology wards. Data were collected through participant observations in the field to construct a cultural analysis of the ward. Interviews with patients and the nurse–patient communication that took place during routine care were audiotaped. Transcripts of these conversations were produced and codes were developed by examining the transcripts using the Medical

Interview Aural Rating Scale (MIARS) (Heaven & Green, 2001). The patients' turns of speech (Sandvik et al., 2002) were studied to determine whether they contained any cues. The patients' emotional cues were categorized under three levels. Level 1 cues contain hints of worry or concern; level 2 cues are the direct expression of an emotional state or concern; and level 3 cues contain a clear expression of a strong emotion. The nurses' turns of speech, on the other hand, were separated into positive and negative responses to the patients' cues. Positive responses included (i) acknowledgement and exploration, and (ii) adequate acknowledgement but no exploration; while negative responses contained, (iii) inadequate acknowledgement but no exploration, (iv) acknowledgement and distancing and (v) distancing.

A content analysis was conducted of the interviews with the patients, as well as an analysis of the cue-responding behaviours of the nurses (Uitterhoeve et al., 2009). Using the MIARS, a patient's disclosure and the nurse's response to the patient's cues/concerns were rated and coded independently into two categories: adequate response and inadequate response. The interrater reliability coefficient among two raters was 0.8, indicating consistency in the coding. Interviews were transcribed verbatim for ethnographic analysis, using the approach of Hammersley and Atkinson (2007). A coding framework with different categories was established by two independent researchers. The team further discussed and analysed the codes and reached a consensus on them. The emic–etic synergy of the study (Hammersley & Atkinson, 2007) was revealed through a construction of the experiences of the nurses and patients and a predefined coding system for cue-responding behaviours. The qualitative findings based on interviews with the patients ($n = 93$) and the audiotaped cue-responding behaviours of the nurses in nurse–patient communications, ($n = 200$) during procedural care ($n = 110$) are reported in this chapter.

4   Results

A total of 63 conversations were recorded during the nurses' provision of procedural care. The mean number of patient cues per conversation was 2.92 ± 2.41, with a range of 1–10. The most common emotional cue that patients gave was the level 2 cue, which explicitly revealed the patients' worries or concerns (mean number of cues per conversation = 2.08 ± 1.95), followed by the level 1 cue, which hinted at a worry or concern (mean number of cues per conversation = 0.84 ± 1.13). Level 3 cues, which are the clear expression of emotions, were not observed in the conversations.

Table 1 Examples of nurses' responses to patients' level 1 and level 2 cues using MIARS coding

	Patients' cues and nurses' responses	MIARS coding
Patient (PN37)	It has been a long time. I have been admitted for a week	Cue-Level 1 (Hinted that he was worried about a long hospital stay)
Nurse (NNF11)	Yes, almost a week	Negative response: Acknowledgement but no exploration
Patient (PN07)	Another nurse did not give me Panadol. She asked me to take morphine	Cue-Level 1 (Hinted that he wanted to take Panadol for pain relief instead of morphine)
Nurse (NNM07)	Do you want to take morphine?	Negative response: Acknowledgement and distancing
Patient (PN40)	May I have morphine?	Cue-Level 2 (Directly expressed the need for morphine)
Nurse (NNM08)	It will be given to you later today	Negative response: Acknowledgement but no exploration
Patient (PS01)	I am always scared of injections	Cue-Level 2 (Directly expressed a fear of injections)
Nurse (NSF01)	Don't be scared.... Don't rub the insertion site or it will become bruised	Negative response: Acknowledgement and distancing
Patient (PS04)	I can't move. When I move, I feel a lot of pain	Cue-Level 2 (Directly expressed pain upon moving)
Nurse (NSF03)	Who helped you to clean the wound? If you don't move or turn your body, the wound cannot heal	Negative response: Distancing

4.1   The Cue-Responding of Nurses

The oncology nurses used positive cue-responding behaviours (mean number of cues per conversation = 2.32 ± 2.03) more often than negative cue-responding behaviours (mean number of cues per conversation = 0.60 ± 1.23). Of the 184 cues that the patients sent out, the nurses responded to more than half with acknowledgement and exploration (55.98%), followed by adequate acknowledgement but no exploration (23.37%). The remaining cues were met with negative cue-responding behaviours (20.65%). Examples of the nurses' different responses to the expression of level 1 and level 2 cues by the patients are given in Table 1 using MIARS coding.

In their interviews, the patients gave vivid descriptions of their recognition of the heavy workload shouldered by the nurses. The nurse–patient ratio in Hong Kong is high, averaging 1:10/12 in comparison to the average of 1:4/6 in the West. The following quotations were drawn from the patients' interviews about the nurses' communication with them on psychosocial issues. The patients commented on the inability of the nurses to attend to their psychosocial needs since the majority of them did not expect to receive explicit emotional support as psychosocial care from the nurses.

> *I believe that clinical psychologists and doctors are trained in counselling skills, and have lots of tools and medications to help [patients] psychologically.... It is difficult to become familiar with [the nurses] during a one- to two-day [hospital stay].*(PN 25, interview)

> *[Nurses] don't have the ability to help me. Asking the doctor to make a referral to a convalescent sanatorium is the only thing that they can do for me.* (PN38, interview)

The patients thought that it was more feasible and realistic for nurses in busy cancer wards to provide physical rather than psychosocial care, in terms of emotional counselling. However, while some patients were not familiar with the busy nurses, others were frequently admitted to the hospital. As these patients became more familiar with the nurses, this familiarity, and the relationship established through the nurses' physical and technical work, caused the patients to develop an appreciation of the heavy demands on the nurses, and hence of their care. Their familiarity with the nurses also made the patients more willing to ask the nurses for help, although mostly with regard to physical rather than emotional aspects.

> *... [I] haven't talked about my worries ... [the nurses] can't solve the problems; actually, they can't help because they have their own responsibilities. They have already done a lot [physically] for [the patients]. If they were social workers or chaplains, then I would talk [about my concerns] because they would be specialists in counselling, that is, in helping [patients] gain relief. PN35*

While the patients did not think that the nurses could help them with emotional counselling given the time constraints and the roles that they expected nurses to play, their concerns about physical care would prompt them to seek help, even if the nurses were busy.

> *I vomited something like blood before. I told [a nurse] about it, even though she looked very busy. It is important. [Nurses] need to make a record of it and let the doctor know.* (PS06, interview)

> *Today, there is nothing wrong with the blood vessel. If it is swollen and painful, I'll ring the call bell to find the nurses ... no worries ... [the nurses] will try their best to help us.... [Patients] should be considerate of them. Their work is very hard ... [their performance is] already satisfactory enough. [A nurse] has no time to talk with [patients]. He/she has a lot of work to do.* (PS14, interview)

> *If I have missed any medications [from my previous prescriptions], I'll tell the nurse directly and let him/her inform the doctor.* (PS01, interview)

The following also shows the dialogue that took place between the nurse and the patient, which involved the nurse giving positive responses to cues from the patient. The nurse reassured the patient and explored the weakness in the patient's legs. The nurse then provided care during the procedure of administering medications, which reduced the patient's worries.

> *NSF06: After taking [the analgesic] tonight, please let us know if you're unwell, or whether it is ineffective and you have more pain at night.*

PS17: Don't you mind?

Patient's cue: asking to clarify with the nurse if it will be indeed fine for her to raise the issue of the effect and side-effects of taking the medication for pain at night.

NSF06: No, I don't. By the way, about the analgesic that was given to you before phys-iotherapy – was it useful?

Nurse's response: good acknowledgement + exploration (the nurse responded to the patient's query and further explored the effects on the patient of taking the analgesic).

PS17: Yes ... but my legs are weak ... floating.

Patient's cue: directly indicating her weak legs.

NSF06: Yes, because you have been resting in bed these few days. You have to build up your strength. That's why I give you morphine before physiotherapy every time.... If you don't feel well, please tell us using the call bell. We can give you [an analgesic] any time.

PS17: Thanks, that is helpful to know and I felt less worried. (PS17, audiotaped routine care)

The nurse's response reveals good acknowledgement plus exploration. The nurse acknowledged the patient's concern and tried to relate the issues with the legs and bed rest to the need for physiotherapy. The explanation helped the patient to better understand the reason for her weakness and eased her concern. The nurse also clarified the need for the patient to take morphine before undergoing physiotherapy, and further reassured the patient about feeling free to request more analgesics if necessary.

When nurses respond to cancer patients' queries about their physical symptoms by caring for the patients' condition and giving them information by teaching them, this clearly benefits the patients' mental well-being. More examples are given below.

> *The nurse would check on me to see whether or not my nausea and vomiting had improved after the treatment of the target therapy, or she would clear up my uncertainties about the removal of the gastric tube upon discharge, so that I felt my anxiety was reduced.* (PS36, interview)

> *The nurse has taught me and helped me to better understand how I can give myself injections. Having the knowledge helped to minimize my fears.* (PS42, interview)

> *The nurse (NNM08) administered the mouthwash to alleviate my pain from the mouth ulcer. I felt much better after rinsing my mouth, and was able to eat better. I was worried about not being able to eat, and became weak because of the mouth sores. I am grateful to the nurse for giving me physical help, which made me feel less worried.* (PN31, interview)

Accordingly, it appears that the patients considered physical care to be more important than psychosocial care in terms of emotional counselling, and more feasible and realistic to provide in a busy cancer ward. This was mostly because the patients did not think that it was the role of nurses to deal with their emotional needs, nor did they think that the nurses could help, given the constraints on their time. The qualitative findings from the interviews were very much supported by the quantitative measures of nurses' cue-responding behaviours during their provision of routine care. The findings from the descriptive statistics in this study indicate that the nurses displayed a higher percentage of positive cue-responding behaviours (75%) and a lower percentage of negative cue-responding behaviours (25%), which is different from the often lower percentage of positive cue-responding behaviours (45%) and a higher percentage of negative cue-responding behaviours (55%) of nurses in the West (Sheldon, Blonquist, Hilaire, Hong, & Berry, 2015). The level of the nurses' cue-responding behaviours was 0.61, which represents a high level of competence in communication. Given that there was little in the way of responses to the patients' direct emotional needs, the higher percentage of positive cue-responding from the nurses can be attributed to responses to the informational needs of the patients.

5   Discussion

Attending to the negative emotions of oncology patients is essential for patient-centred care. However, any discussion of the subject requires an exploration of the issue of what most nurses do in a busy oncology setting and what most patients actually want. Most importantly, nurse–patient communications are influenced by specific cultural norms and values (Liu, Mok, & Wong, 2005). For example, Asian and Western patients tend to process socio-emotional cues in very different ways (Liu, Rigoulot, & Pell, 2015). Given the embedded understanding of culture in health (Helman, 2007), a knowledge of Chinese cultural norms and values is essential to promoting patient-centred care (Hsu, O'Connor, & Lee, 2009; Lau, Mok, Lai, & Chung, 2013; Zheng, Johnson, Wang, & Hu, 2014). This, in turn, could lead to cross-cultural comparisons of cultural beliefs and environments. Lin, Lee, Chou, Liu, and Tang's (2017) work examining the competence of nurses in Taiwan in responding to simulated emotional cues from standardized patients with cancer revealed that the nurses' cue-responding behaviours were less adequate than those of nurses in other countries. However, this also prompts the important question of what is adequate within the context of Chinese culture in providing psychosocial care?

In fact, we found in our study in Hong Kong that a high percentage of responses to patients' cues seemed to involve responses by nurses to informational rather than emotional cues. Similarly, Zhang, Wong, You and Zheng (2012), who analysed the content of telephone follow-ups by nurses of Chinese cancer patients, reported that psychosocial concerns only accounted for 3.8% of the total content. It seems that patients have no expectations of receiving emotional counselling from nurses, given their perception of the time constraints on nurses and of the roles of the nurses. Perhaps a partial explanation for this result can be found in the strong influence of Confucianism on the Chinese culture, which does not encourage the verbalizing of emotional concerns, especially to outsiders (Cheng et al., 2013; Lai, 2006). In addition, Chinese patients are reluctant to disclose their emotional concerns to healthcare professionals in the belief that patients should control their own emotions and avoid disturbing the nurses (Zheng, Zhang, Qin, Fang, & Wu, 2013). Instead, they prefer to seek psychosocial support from close family members (Lam, Fabrizio, Ho, Chan, & Fielding, 2009; Liu, Mok, & Wong, 2005; Wong, Fielding, Wong, & Hedley, 2009; Wu, Koo, Tseng, Liao, & Chen, 2015). Such support is often expressed in tangible ways, such as in the preparation of food or performance of domestic tasks for the patient (Chan, Molassiotis, Yam, Chan, & Lam, 2001).

As the role played by nurses in providing psychosocial care could go beyond the delivering of emotional care to include assessing the needs of the patients, managing their symptoms of distress, and providing education, this study shows that nurses can respond positively to patients' cues by providing physical attention and information, especially in the Chinese healthcare setting. Indeed, Chinese patients tend to place more emphasis on informational needs related to their disease than on psychosocial support (Lam et al., 2009; Tang et al., 2006; Zheng et al., 2014). In a cross-cultural comparison, Lam et al. (2011) found that Hong Kong Chinese patients prioritized informational needs, while German patients focused on psychosocial support. In our study, we also found that Hong Kong Chinese patients valued the support that the nurses provided to their physiological needs, particularly in a busy oncology setting.

There is also a taken-for-granted perception that emotional care, which is a cultural expectation of nurses working in oncology settings, is a separate matter from the everyday physical and technical care that nurses provide, giving rise to Gordon's (2006) point about the provision of halfistic rather than holistic care. Perhaps this perception of a divide stems from the emphasis on the psychosocial distress that may arise when patients have psychosocial needs that are not attended to. While there is merit in the debate that physical care and psychosocial care could be two separate realms of holistic care, nurses should not overlook the argument that the physical and the psychosocial are inter-related dimensions of holistic care, and that there is a cultural aspect to the understanding of psychosocial care. Another possible explanation for the emphasis on the reference to psychosocial care may relate to the recognized lack of such care within severe time constraints and the clinical environment often faced by nurses in Hong Kong. The crowded and noisy environment in the wards also does not make it easy for nurses to talk to patients (Chan, Wong, Cheung, & Lam, 2018). Yet another possible reason relates to the fact that nurses in Hong Kong are trained predominantly in the Western model (Chen, 2001), which advocates providing not only physical but emotional care to patients. This, in turn, has prompted nurse educators in Hong Kong to reconsider the broader social and cultural context of nursing in their curriculums. As nursing students are socialized in their profession to be caring nurses expected to render holistic care to patients, there is a need to re-emphasize the importance of learning about caring communication to respond to the often subtle cues expressed by Chinese patients and to introduce mindfulness training to address the demands of a busy work environment. More practice of reflection is vital if nursing students and graduates are to deepen their understanding of the meaning of nursing, and of themselves in a busy and complex healthcare environment. The importance of having nursing students and graduates translate their theoretical understanding of holistic care into practice through mentoring is essential to developing value-based nursing.

Overall, our findings also indicate that the stress felt by nurses could be alleviated somewhat if, rather than using a deficit model to examine how nurses are not paying enough attention to the psychosocial needs of patients, we instead take the appreciative stance of defining psychosocial needs from the patients' understanding of how busy the nurses are. It is perhaps time to revisit and highlight what nurses are doing in a busy cancer ward to promote the emotional/psychosocial aspects of care through the provision of quality physical attention.

When effective nurse–patient communication in cancer care is examined in the literature (de Leeuw et al., 2014; Dong et al., 2016; Song et al., 2016; Uitterhoeve, Bensing, Grol, Demulder, & van Achterberg, 2010; Welton, 2016), and the role of nurses in psychosocial care is raised, one sees not only discussions about letting patients vent their emotions and meeting their affective needs, but also about meeting their cognitive needs and ensuring that they receive psychosocial comfort from nurses. In fact, to Chinese patients the extension of emotional support is less important than meeting informational or physiological needs related to the management of their disease (Ding, Hu, & Hallberg, 2015; Lee, Francis, Walker, & Lee, 2004). They tend to view medical professionals as service providers instead of as comforters (Ding et al., 2015; Lam et al., 2009). The National Comprehensive Cancer Network (2017) describes the roles played by nurses in psychosocial care as being not only about managing symptoms of distress and offering individual/family counselling, but also about clarifying treatment options, providing education, assessing needs, and building trust in patients.

Our findings are consistent with the results of previous studies (Bracher, Corner, & Wagland, 2016; Song et al., 2016) that examined psychosocial care from the perspectives of patients, which revealed the importance of communicating with patients and providing them with medical information. Indeed, informed patients are often less distressed than uninformed patients (Echlin & Rees, 2002; Matthews, Sellergren, Manfredi, & Williams, 2002). On the other hand, unmet informational needs are associated with anxiety and depression (Li et al., 2013), and with an overall poor quality of life (So, Chan, Choi, Wan, & Mak, 2013). It is important for nurses to be aware that, for oncology patients, the meaning of psychosocial needs goes beyond emotional counselling. The psychosocial support that nurses have been rendering to patients when they give them information and take care of their physiological functioning in busy oncology settings should not be taken for granted.

6 Conclusion

Given the consistent, positive qualitative findings from the interviews with patients about their perspectives of nurse–patient communication during their procedural care and the quantitative statistical analysis of the nurses' cue-responding behaviours, it seems clear that, unlike in many countries, it is not common for patients in Hong Kong to solicit emotional care. While the talk is of patient-centred care, cancer patients' perspectives of the physical care provided by the nurses, which involves the exchange of information and the provision of everyday nursing care, has an impact on the patients' psychosocial needs. This aspect is equally important to the patients and should not be undervalued. As it is difficult for nurses to work in such a complex and busy environment, the patients' perspectives reinforce the value of the interactions that take place between the two parties during taken-for-granted routines, and highlight the importance for nursing of reintegrating the physical and the emotional in the care that they provide to cancer patients.

Acknowledgements This study was funded by the General Research Fund, PolyU 156003/15H.

References

Abrahamson, K., Durham, M., Norton, K., Doebbeling, B. N., Doebbeling, C. C., & Anderson, J. G. (2011). Provision of psychosocial care for cancer patients: Service delivery in urban and rural settings. *Journal of Primary Care & Community Health, 2*(4), 220–224.

Annunziata, M., Giovannini, L., & Mussatti, B. (2012). Assessing the body image: Relevance, application and instruments for oncological settings. *Supportive Care in Cancer, 20,* 901–907.

AWMF. (2014). Leitlinienprogramm Onkologie (Deutsche Krebsgesellschaft, Deutsche Krebshilfe, AWMF): Psychoonkologische Diagnostik, Beratung und Behandlung von erwachsenen Krebspatienten. AWMF Registernummer: 032/051OL. Retrieved from www.awmf.org/uploads/tx_szleitlinien/032-051OLl_S3_Psychoonkologische_Beratung_Behandlung_2014-01_1.1.pdf.

Bracher, M., Corner, D. J., & Wagland, R. (2016). Exploring experiences of cancer care in Wales: A thematic analysis of free-text responses to the 2013 Wales Cancer Patient Experience Survey (WCPES). *British Medical Journal Open, 6*(9), e011830.

Braeken, A. P., Kempen, G. I., Eekers, D. B. P., Houben, R. M., van Gils, F. C., Ambergen, T., et al. (2013). Psychosocial screening effects on health-related outcomes in patients receiving radiotherapy. A cluster randomised controlled trial. *Psycho-Oncology, 22*(12), 2736–2746.

Chan, C. W., Molassiotis, A., Yam, B. M., Chan, S. J., & Lam, C. S. (2001). Traveling through the cancer trajectory: Social support perceived by women with gynecological cancer in Hong Kong. *Cancer Nursing, 24*(5), 387–394.

Chan, E. A., Wong, F., Cheung, M. Y., & Lam, W. (2018). Patients' perceptions of their experiences with nurse-patient communication in oncology settings: A focused ethnographic study. *PLoS ONE, 13*(6), 1–17.

Chen, M. L., Chang, H. K., & Yeh, C. H. (2000). Anxiety and depression in Taiwanese cancer patients with and without pain. *Journal of Advanced Nursing, 32*(4), 944–951.

Chen, Y. C. (2001). Chinese values, health and nursing. *Journal of Advanced Nursing, 36*(2), 270–273.

Cheng, H., Sit, J. W., Chan, C. W., So, W. K., Choi, K. C., & Cheng, K. K. (2013). Social support and quality of life among Chinese breast cancer survivors: Findings from a mixed methods study. *European Journal of Oncology Nursing, 17*(6), 788–796.

de Leeuw, J., Prins, J. B., Uitterhoeve, R., Merkx, M. A., Marres, H. A., & van Achterberg, T. (2014). Nurse-patient communication in follow-up consultations after head and neck cancer treatment. *Cancer Nursing, 37*(2), E1–E9.

Ding, Y., Hu, Y., & Hallberg, I. R. (2015). Chinese women living with cervical cancer in the first 3 months after diagnosis: A qualitative study. *Cancer Nursing, 38*(1), 71–80.

Dong, S. T., Butow, P. N., Tong, A., Agar, M., Boyle, F., Forster, B. C., ... Lovell, M. R. (2016). Patients' experiences and perspectives of multiple concurrent symptoms in advanced cancer: A semi-structured interview study. *Supportive Care in Cancer, 24*(3), 1373–1386.

Dunn, J., Ng, S. K., Holland, J., Aitken, J., Youl, P., Baade, P. D., et al. (2013). Trajectories of psychological distress after colorectal cancer. *Psycho-Oncology, 22*(8), 1759–1765.

Echlin, K. N., & Rees, C. E. (2002). Information needs and information-seeking behaviors of men with prostate cancer and their partners: A review of the literature. *Cancer Nursing, 25*(1), 35–41.

Engel, G. L. (1977). The need for a new medical model: A challenge for biomedicine. *Science, 196*, 129–136.

Ferlay, J., Shin, H. R., Bray, F., Forman, D., Mathers, C., & Parkin, D. M. (2010). Estimates of worldwide burden of cancer in 2008: GLOBOCAN 2008. *International Journal of Cancer, 127*(12), 2893–2917.

Goldberg, D. P., Hobson, R. F., Maguire, G. P., Margison, F. R., O'Dowd, T., Osborn, M., et al. (1984). The clarification and assessment of a method of psychotherapy. *British Journal of Psychiatry, 144*, 567–575.

Gordon, S. (2006). The new Cartesianism: Dividing mind and body and thus disembodying care. In S. Nelso & S. Gordo (Eds.), *The complexities of caring: Nursing reconsidered.* Ithaca, NY: Cornell University Press.

Hack, T. F., Ruether, J. D., Pickles, T., Bultz, B. D., Chateau, D., & Degner, L. F. (2012). Behind closed doors II: Systematic analysis of prostate cancer patients' primary treatment consultations with radiation oncologists and predictors of satisfaction with communication. *Psycho-Oncology, 21*(8), 809–817.

Hammersley, M., & Atkinson, P. (2007). The process of analysis. In M. Hammersley & P. Atkinson (Eds.), *Ethnography: Principles in practice* (3rd ed., pp. 158–190). London: Routledge.

Heaven, C. M., & Green, C. (2001). *Medical Interview Aural Rating Scale.* Manchester, England: Psychological Medical Group, Christie Hospital, Stanley House.

Helman, C. G. (2007). *Culture, health and illness: An introduction for health professionals* (2nd ed.). London: CRC Press.

Hill, J., Holcombe, C., Clark, L., Boothby, M. R. K., Hincks, A., Fisher, J., ... Salmon, P. (2011). Predictors of onset of depression and anxiety in the year after diagnosis of breast cancer. *Psychological Medicine, 41*(7), 1429–1436.

Hinz, A., Krauss, O., Hauss, J. P., Höckel, M., Kortmann, R. D., Stolzenburg, J. U., et al. (2010). Anxiety and depression in cancer patients compared with the general population. *European Journal of Cancer Care, 19*(4), 522–529.

Horden, A. (2008). Intimacy and sexuality after cancer: A critical review of the literature. *Cancer Nursing, 31*, E9–17.

Hsu, C. Y., O'Connor, M., & Lee, S. (2009). Understandings of death and dying for people of Chinese origin. *Death Studies, 33*(2), 153–174.

Jacobsen, P. B. (2009). Clinical practice guidelines for the psychosocial care of cancer survivors: Current status and future prospects. *Cancer, 115*(S18), 4419–4429.

Lai, A. (2006). Eye on religion: Cultural signs and caring for Chinese patients. *Southern Medical Journal, 99*(6), 688–689.

Lam, W. W., Au, A. H., Wong, J. H., Lehmann, C., Koch, U., Fielding, R., et al. (2011). Unmet supportive care needs: A cross-cultural comparison between Hong Kong Chinese and German Caucasian women with breast cancer. *Breast Cancer Research and Treatment, 130*(2), 531–541.

Lam, W. W., Fabrizio, C., Ho, E., Chan, L., & Fielding, R. (2009). Perceived importance of evidence-based psychosocial clinical guidelines for Hong Kong Chinese women with breast cancer: Opinions of patients and health care providers. *Supportive Care in Cancer, 17*(3), 219–229.

Lau, L. K. P., Mok, E., Lai, T., & Chung, B. (2013). Quality-of-life concerns of Chinese patients with advanced cancer. *Social Work in Health Care, 52*(1), 59–77.

Lee, Y. M., Francis, K., Walker, J., & Lee, S. M. (2004). What are the information needs of Chinese breast cancer patients receiving chemotherapy? *European Journal of Oncology Nursing, 8*(3), 224–233.

Li, W. W., Lam, W. W., Au, A. H., Ye, M., Law, W. L., Poon, J., … Fielding, R. (2013). Interpreting differences in patterns of supportive care needs between patients with breast cancer and patients with colorectal cancer. *Psycho-Oncology, 22*(4), 792–798.

Lin, M. F., Lee, A. Y., Chou, C. C., Liu, T. Y., & Tang, C. C. (2017). Factors predicting emotional cue-responding behaviors of nurses in Taiwan: An observational study. *Psycho-Oncology, 26* (10), 1548–1554.

Liu, J. E., Mok, E., & Wong, T. (2005). Perceptions of supportive communication in Chinese patients with cancer: Experiences and expectations. *Journal of Advanced Nursing, 52*(3), 262–270.

Liu, P., Rigoulot, S., & Pell, M. D. (2015). Culture modulates the brain response to human expressions of emotion: Electrophysiological evidence. *Neuropsychologia, 67*, 1–13.

Matthews, A. K., Sellergren, S. A., Manfredi, C., & Williams, M. (2002). Factors influencing medical information seeking among African American cancer patients. *Journal of Health Communication, 7*(3), 205–219.

Muzzalti, B., Bomben, F., Flaiban, C., Mella, S., & Annunziata, M. A. (2016). Psychological distress in cancer patients: From recognition to management. In A. Compare, C. Elia, & A. G. Simonelli (Eds.), *Psychological distress*. Hauppauge, NY: Nova Science Publishers Inc.

National Comprehensive Cancer Network. (2017). NCCN clinical practice guidelines in oncology. Retrieved from https://www.nccn.org/professionals/physician_gls/f_guidelines.asp#supportive.

Novy, D. M., & Aigner, C. J. (2014). The biopsychosocial model in cancer pain. *Current Opinion in Supportive and Palliative Care, 8*(2), 117–123.

Sandvik, M., Eide, H., Lind, M., Graugaard, P. K., Torper, J., & Finset, A. (2002). Analyzing medical dialogues: Strength and weakness of Roter's Interaction Analysis System (RIAS). *Patient Education and Counseling, 46*(4), 235–241.

Sawer, A., Ayers, S., & Field, A. (2010). Posttraumatic growth and adjustment among individuals with cancer or HIV/AIDS: A meta-analysis. *Clinical Psychology Review, 30*, 436–447.

Sheldon, L. J., Blonquist, T. M., Hilaire, D. M., Hong, F., & Berry, D. L. (2015). Patient cues and symptoms of psychosocial distress: What predicts assessment and treatment of distress by oncology clinicians. *Psycho-Oncology, 24*, 1020–1027.

So, W. K., Chan, C. W., Choi, K. C., Wan, R. W., & Mak, S. S. (2013). Perceived unmet needs and health-related quality of life of Chinese cancer survivors at 1 year after treatment. *Cancer Nursing, 36*(3), E23–E32.

Song, Y., Lv, X., Liu, J., Huang, D., Hong, J., Wang, W., et al. (2016). Experience of nursing support from the perspective of patients with cancer in mainland China. *Nursing & Health Sciences, 18*(4), 510–518.

Soussain, C., Ricard, C., Fike, J. R., Mazeron, J. J., Psimaras, D., & Dlattre, J. Y. (2009). CNS complications of radiotherapy and chemogherapy. *Lancet, 7*(374), 1639–1651.

Stone, P. C., & Minton, O. (2008). Cancer-related fatigue. *European Journal of Cancer, 44*, 1097–1104.

Tang, S. T., Liu, T. W., Lai, M. S., Liu, L. N., Chen, C. H., & Koong, S. L. (2006). Congruence of knowledge, experiences, and preferences for disclosure of diagnosis and prognosis between terminally-ill cancer patients and their family caregivers in Taiwan. *Cancer Investigation, 24* (4), 360–366.

Uitterhoeve, R., Bensing, J., Dilven, E., Donders, R., de Mulder, P., & van Achterberg, T. (2009). Nurse-patient communication in cancer care: Does responding to patient's cues predict patient satisfaction with communication. *Psycho-Oncology, 18*(10), 1060–1068.

Uitterhoeve, R., Bensing, J. M., Grol, R. P., Demulder, P. H. M., & van Achterberg, T. (2010). The effect of communication skills training on patient outcomes in cancer care: A systematic review of the literature. *European Journal of Cancer Care, 19*(4), 442–457.

Weis, J. (2015). Psychosocial care for cancer patients. *Breast Care, 10,* 84–86.

Welton, J. M. (2016). Nurse staffing and patient outcomes: Are we asking the right research question? *International Journal of Nursing Studies, 63,* A1–A2.

Wong, W. S., Fielding, R., Wong, C., & Hedley, A. (2009). Confirmatory factor analysis and sample invariance of the Chinese Patient Satisfaction Questionnaire (ChPSQ-9) among patients with breast and lung cancer. *Value in Health, 12*(4), 597–605.

Wu, L. F., Koo, M., Tseng, H. C., Liao, Y. C., & Chen, Y. M. (2015). Concordance between nurses' perception of their ability to provide spiritual care and the identified spiritual needs of hospitalized patients: A cross-sectional observational study. *Nursing & Health Sciences, 17*(4), 426–433.

Zhang, J. E., Wong, F. K., You, L. M., & Zheng, M. C. (2012). A qualitative study exploring the nurse telephone follow-up of patients returning home with a colostomy. *Journal of Clinical Nursing, 21*(9–10), 1407–1415.

Zheng, M. C., Zhang, J. E., Qin, H. Y., Fang, Y. J., & Wu, X. J. (2013). Telephone follow-up for patients returning home with colostomies: Views and experiences of patients and enterostomal nurses. *European Journal of Oncology Nursing, 17*(2), 184–189.

Zheng, R., Johnson, J., Wang, Q., & Hu, J. (2014). A need for cancer patient education from the perspective of Chinese patients and nurses: A comparison study. *Supportive Care in Cancer, 22*(9), 2457–2464.

Part II
Health Communication
in Patient-provider Contexts in Asia

Examining Patient Preferences for Integrative Chinese-Western Colorectal Cancer Care in Hong Kong

Wendy Wong, Herbert H. F. Loong, Allyson K. Y. Lee,
Ambrose H. N. Wong, C. H. Sum, Jessica Y. L. Ching,
Justin C. Y. Wu, and Z. X. Lin

Abstract Cancer patients seek help from both Western medicine (WM) and Traditional Chinese Medicine (TCM). This study explored what patients with colorectal cancer (CRC) in Hong Kong (HK) expect from TCM to WM. Twenty purposively sampled CRC patients were interviewed and audio-taped. Interviews were transcribed verbatim in Cantonese. Data were analyzed using the Interpretative phenomenological analysis. Results showed that CRC patients' goal expectation on WM was not specific. In contrast, the 16 patients who had used TCM had specific goals that stemmed from their desire or requests for treatment continuation. These expectation differences affected their motivation of compliance to the treatment schedule. The motivation for WM patients came from their faith in biomedicine and family, and the desire to live. The motivation for TCM patients' compliance came from their belief in TCM and its effectiveness and provision of mental support. Although TCM was not the main treatment cancer patient received in HK, their expectations from it were high. Thus, TCM may be more than palliative in cancer treatment. Perceived WM status may hinder TCM development. More resources to ensure safe and effective interdisciplinary collaboration for the development of TCM cancer treatment can assist patients along the pathway of patients of CRC for effective communication.

W. Wong (✉) · J. Y. L. Ching · Z. X. Lin
School of Chinese Medicine, The Chinese University of Hong Kong, Shatin, New Territories, China
e-mail: wendy.wong@cuhk.edu.hk

H. H. F. Loong
Department of Clinical Oncology, The Chinese University of Hong Kong, Shatin, New Territories, China

W. Wong · A. K. Y. Lee · C. H. Sum · J. Y. L. Ching · Z. X. Lin
Hong Kong Institute of Integrative Medicine, The Chinese University of Hong Kong, Shatin, New Territories, China

A. H. N. Wong · J. C. Y. Wu
Department of Medicine & Therapeutics, The Chinese University of Hong Kong, Shatin, New Territories, China

© Springer Nature Singapore Pte Ltd. 2020
B. Watson and J. Krieger (eds.), *Expanding Horizons in Health Communication*,
The Humanities in Asia 6, https://doi.org/10.1007/978-981-15-4389-0_5

Keywords Colorectal cancer · Western medicine · Traditional chinese medicine

1 Introduction

Globally, colorectal cancer (CRC) is the second most common cancer in women and the third most common in men (Bray, Ren, Masuyer, & Ferlay, 2013; WHO, 2018). CRC is currently the fourth leading cause of mortality from all cancers in the world (Ferlay et al., 2013; Torre, Siegel, Ward, & Jemal, 2016). Among all cancers in Chinese populations, CRC ranks first in incidence and second for related deaths for both sexes in Hong Kong (Hong Kong Hospital Authority, 2016; Sung, Lau, Goh, & Leung, 2005; Torre et al., 2016). Current conventional treatments include surgical resection of primary tumors, often followed by adjuvant or palliative fluorouracil (Ku et al., 2012). In settings with enhanced health care resources, chemotherapy regimens utilizing multiple drugs such as FOLFOX and FOLFIRI, and monoclonal antibodies such as bevacizumab, cetuximab, and panitumumab, may also be offered depending on subsidies provided by the government (Ku et al., 2012).

Despite advances in conventional oncological care, mortality from CRC is high (Shin, Jung, & Won, 2013) and patients suffer from related and often unaddressed complaints of gastrointestinal, urinary, and sexual dysfunction, as well as pain and fatigue (Appleton, Goodlad, Irvine, Poole, & Wall, 2013; Cotrim & Pereira, 2008; El-Shami et al., 2015; Sahay, Gray, & Fitch, 2000). More advanced stages of the disease are associated with significant decreases in quality of life (Wong, Lam, Poon, & Kwong, 2013). Chinese Herbal Medicine (CHM) is commonly used among cancer patients who are also receiving conventional oncological care. CHM is reportedly used by 14.2% of CRC patients in the US, 55% in China, and 64% in Taiwan (McQuade, Meng, Chen, Wei, Zhang, & Bei, 2012; Su & Li, 2011).

A recent systematic review and meta-analysis of 83 randomized control trials (RCTs) of cancer patients taking CHM showed positive effects in terms of decreasing the incidence of leucopenia and potential prophylactic benefits in relation to white blood counts (Ma, Ai, Li, & Vardy, 2015). Some herbs were found to be effective in improving quality of life, relieving side effects of chemotherapy, and radiation therapy such as poor appetite, diarrhea or radiation-induced pneumonitis (Qi et al., 2010; Sałaga, Zatorski, Sobczak, Chen, & Fichna, 2014; Tao et al., 2010; Yang, Chen, & Xu, 2008; Zhong, Chen, Cho, Meng, & Tong, 2012). In vitro and in vivo studies have confirmed that CHM can inhibit CRC growth (Fan et al., 2012; Liang et al., 2012; Zhang et al., 2015); decrease CRC cell viability (Lin et al., 2013), suppress metastasis (Fan et al., 2015), reverse drug resistance (Sui et al., 2014), increase animal survival (Lin et al., 2014), and enhance chemotherapy potency (Deng et al., 2013).

The concurrent use of CHM for cancer treatment remains controversial since herbs (e.g. St. John's wort or *Gingko blioba* or *Panax ginseng*) have been found to potentially interfere with the efficacy of chemotherapy or lead to associated toxicities (Chiu, Yau, & Epstein, 2009; Meijerman, Beijnen, & Schellens, 2006;

Sparreboom, Cox, Acharya, & Figg, 2004). The quality of evidence for many studies involving CHM is poor due to a lack of blinding, randomizing, and publication bias (Sałaga et al., 2014; WHO, 2013). The theory of Traditional Chinese Medicine (TCM), however, emphasizes personalized interventions based on syndrome differentiation for Chinese medicine diagnoses. This makes conducting randomized controlled trials of TCM difficult (Bensoussan et al., 1998; WHO, 2002). With the standardization of the International Classification of Diseases-11 (ICD-11), the use, safety, and standard of care provided by TCM in cancer care are important (Lindmeier, 2018; Wong et al., 2017). There are significant differences in the way in which TCM and CHM are used in different countries (WHO, 2018). China is the only country that incorporates Chinese Medicine into the mainstream medical system with the corresponding support from the policy and public health care planning (WHO, 2013). This is different from other countries like the US, UK, and Hong Kong where WM and Traditional Medicine are two separate ethnomedicine systems (WHO, 2013). In addition, there is no official referral system among the Hong Kong health care system for cancer care such that concurrent use of WM and CHM would bring risk to patients' health with any potential unknown herbs' toxicity, herb–drug interaction or missing the prime time for treatments of cure of cancer.

The goal of the study reported in this chapter was to examine the communication about CRC, cancer with high incidence in the Chinese population, and to explore the communication gap from the patients' perspective to understand the underlying philosophies of care. With the complexity of cancer communication and comorbidities, the medical industry has always focused on the efficacy of drug treatments and qualitative studies of patients' needs are uncommon. This chapter reports on a qualitative study of the "pull and push factors" (Kelner & Wellman, 1997) which influence patients' expectations and decision making in relation to the use of WM and TCM in the treatment of their CRC. These "push and pull" factors influence patients to seek non-conventional healthcare treatments. These are usually because patients are dissatisfied with (pushed away) the conventional Western Medicine and/or because they are attracted to (pulled towards) inherent principles of non-conventional treatments (Kelner & Wellman, 1997). In this study, structured qualitative interviews were conducted to identify patients' perceptions of current treatments of CRC for the purpose of identifying possible strategies to improve patient-centered communication in the context of CRC treatment and survivorship among Chinese populations. Decision-making about cancer treatment is context-dependent and is influenced by various social and cultural factors. This chapter, therefore, begins by examining the relative role and position of TCM and WM within Hong Kong and mainland China. The chapter then moves to specific details and discussion of the methods and findings of this research. The chapter concludes by arguing for continued research in this area and, importantly, the inclusion of Chinese patients within such work. Despite recent initiatives from the medical industry to involve patients throughout the research (Richards & Godlee, 2014; Thorne et al., 2014) the Chinese population remains underrepresented (Ng et al., 2017).

2   TCM and WM in Hong Kong and Mainland China

Hong Kong's medical system maintains a good reputation for medical standards across different health care systems and the region is reported as having the highest life expectancy in the world (United Nations, 2019). However, this reputation does not extend so easily to TCM practitioners in Hong Kong. The Chinese Medicine Ordinance was passed in 1999 to regulate TCM practice in Hong Kong (CMCHK, 2008). Chinese Medicine Practitioners with the qualification of Bachelor of Chinese Medicine obtained in Hong Kong or mainland China were given the option to complete a licensing examination in order to practice locally. However, this license allowed them only to prescribe Chinese herbs. Despite the introduction of the ordinance, 2,600 out of the 10,047 CMPs neither provided the proof of 10 years of clinical practice nor passed the qualifying examination. Despite these attempts at regulation, there is no way for patients to identify CMPs who are qualified to provide cancer care (Social Survey Section, 2002). Consequently, the situation in relation to cancer care communication in colorectal cancer patients across diagnoses, disease progression, and palliative care support in the Chinese population remains complicated (Davis, Oh, Butow, Mullan, & Clarke, 2012). There is a need to facilitate mutual understanding and identify the communication barriers in cancer care (Cotrim & Pereira, 2008; Xu, Towers, Li, & Collet, 2006). Open communication and collaboration among CRC patients, oncologists, and CMP need to be more established than it currently is given: (1) increasing evidence on TCM treatment modalities addresses that there are gaps in current CRC treatment regimen; (2) CRC patients continue to use TCM, despite lack of support from oncologists; and (3) the possibility that TCM provides a more cost-effective strategy compared to WM alone in the treatment of CRC patients.

China is the only country that allows Chinese Medicine Practitioners to prescribe Western medication or conduct surgery in the hospital settings and allows Western medical doctors to prescribe Chinese herbs (Hesketh & Zhu, 1997; WHO, 2013). McQuade et al. conducted a survey on utilization of and attitudes towards TCM therapies from patients and physicians in the People's Republic of China (PRC) and found that physicians had very high rates of belief in the utility of TCM treatment (McQuade et al., 2012). It should be noted that the study was conducted at a center in PRC where the integration of TCM in cancer care was already established. TCM has been widely accepted by mainland Chinese physicians due to the history, culture, and politics of the People's Republic of China, with 98% receiving TCM training (Harmsworth & Leiwith, 2001). However, this raises questions about the quality of Western or Chinese medical training competency for cross-disciplinary prescriptions. The World Health Organization (WHO), for example, is reluctant to recommend TCM without evidence (Lindmeier, 2018; WHO, 2013). With these issues in mind, the following qualitative study was conducted.

3 Method

This exploratory qualitative study is reported in compliance with the Standards for Reporting Qualitative Research (Tong, Sainsbury, & Craig, 2007). Ethics approval was obtained from the Joint Chinese University of Hong Kong–New Territories East Cluster Clinical Research Ethics Committee (Ref no. 2016.307). Twenty purposively sampled colorectal cancer patients were recruited and interviewed. Research participants had CRC, at various stages, different age groups, different genders and received treatment from TCM and/or WM practitioners and doctors, were invited. The interviews were audio-taped and transcribed verbatim in Cantonese for analysis. All data were managed by NVivo 11 plus. Data were analyzed using an interpretative phenomenological analysis approach to identify and compare the expectations of CRC patients using WM and TCM. All participants (i.e., patients and family members) gave informed and written consent and understood the nature of the study.

3.1 Participants

A purposive and convenience sampling strategy was used to recruit patients with diagnosed CRC (Jane, Jane, Gilliam, Rosalind, & Nilufer, 2014). In three cases, their accompanying family member also attended the interviews. Chinese Medicine Practitioners and oncologists were also interviewed, but these results are not reported within this chapter. As the research was a pilot study, a sample size of 20 was set (Jane et al., 2014).

The inclusion criteria for participation in the study was as follows:

(i) Aged 18 years or over;
(ii) Diagnosed with CRC;
(iii) Experience with either WM or TCM for treatment of CRC;
(iv) Cognitively able to give written, informed consent for participation. Participants were identified by a unique code which is provided in the excerpts T.

Potential participants were excluded from the study if they were abusing alcohol or drugs at the time of the interview, cognitively impaired (i.e., unable to complete screener questions), or refused to provide written informed consent for participation.

Of the 20 participants, 60% ($n = 12$) were aged between 60 and 69 years, with a mean age of 62.1 years (S.D. = 8.98) and 50% were female. All patients had undergone surgery and 85% of them ($n = 17$) had also undergone chemotherapy treatment. Six patients (30%) had radiotherapy while two had undergone target therapy. Target therapy works by targeting the cancer's specific genes, proteins, or the tissue environment that contributes to cancer growth and survival (Cancer.Net

Editorial Board, 2019). Eighty percent of patients (n = 16) had consulted TCM practitioners and had taken CHM as part of their cancer treatment or recovery.

Twenty-five percent (n = 5) took CHM concurrently with their chemotherapy, 80% took CHM after their chemotherapy was completed, and 5% (n = 1) used CHM when the WM treatment was no longer able to stop cancer from growing or spreading to other body parts. Twenty percent (n = 4) had never used CHM during their treatment for CRC. The three family members who accompanied the CRC patients were also invited to participate in the interview (Bell, 2014).

3.2 Data Collection

Patient interviews were conducted at either the Cancer Center of the Prince of Wales Hospital, Shatin, Hong Kong or the Central Integrative Medical Centers, Faculty of Medicine, the Chinese University of Hong Kong, Hong Kong. The Principal Investigator (PI) was a CMP and the Co-Investigator (Co-I) was a medical oncologist who had regular contact with potential participants. As such, eligible patients were identified during initial or follow-up consultations at the respective clinical sites where they practiced. One patient could not be contacted to schedule an interview and was withdrawn from the study.

Data were collected through face-to-face audio-recorded, semi-structured interviews. Interviews were conducted in Cantonese by a trained research assistant. Interviews lasted between 14 and 66 min. An interview guide was used to facilitate the interviewing process while maintaining the flexibility for probing questions to elicit more details (Ritchie, Lewis, McNaughton Nicholls, & Ormston, 2014; Yeo et al., 2014). Both open and closed questions were used in this study. While open questions allowed participants to provide content, closed questions were used to clarify participants' meaning.

3.3 Data Analysis

Interpretative phenomenological analysis (IPA) was adopted in this analysis to explore how participants made decisions along their CRC journey from the perspective of either WM, TCM, or both (Smith, 1996; Smith, Flowers, & Larkin, 2009). After reading all transcripts, the authors identified emergent themes from the phrases of each individual patient and extracted significant phrases. The familiarization stage involved all authors. The authors discussed the themes and the connection between themes by different patients across CRC patients in different states. The data sources were cross-checked among the transcripts for mapping and interpretation with the same journey of participants to assess whether sufficient evidence in participants' actual disclosure. All authors then checked the original transcripts to assess whether comparable concepts were arranged into subcategories and then subcategories were collapsed into major categories when appropriate.

4 Results

Results indicate that Hong Kong Chinese colorectal cancer patients had different expectations of WM and TCM. Patients' expectations of WM were categorized into two key themes—faith in biomedicine and no expectation. The two diversified themes implied that patients needed to accept the reality of having cancer but at the same time, they had to understand that the treatment options offered by WM had minimal success rates and the potential for adverse effects. Therefore, when patients could not get a definite answer from the WM, they found hope in continuing treatment using TCM. Patients understood that they needed to accept that their chances of curing the cancer were unclear. Subthemes are summarized in Table 1.

Table 1 Themes related to patients' expectations of different treatment regimens

WM theme	Subtheme	Direct quotation from patients	Translated quotation
Faith in biomedicine	Cure from surgery and chemotherapy	期望緊係根治啦, 做手術啦希望 ... 做完手術可以切左出黎 (P23)	*"Expectation of course is complete cure, do surgery, get the tumor out after the surgery"* (P23)
	Authoritative status	有期望, 咪, 照西醫講, 點講就點做咯 (P29)	*"I have expectation, like, listen to the WMD, I will do what he says"* (P29)
No expectation		因為對呢方面本身係太認識, 亦都唔多了解, 所以其實, 唔會大, 即係有一個大期望會係點樣既, 即係總然之醫生講出黎果個療程, 或者佢講出黎覺得, 係合符果個本身所諗果個預期既話呢, 都係照根據佢咁講去做架 (P33)	*"because I am not too familiar with this area, and I have limited knowledge, so, actually, [my expectation] won't be high, won't have a high expectation on what happens, as long as what the WMD says about the treatment fits my anticipation, then I will follow his words"* (P33)
TCM			
Continuing treatment	Only remaining options when WM has failed or finished	外科話唔做, 咁我就睇中醫囉唯有 (P23)	*"Surgeon said there was nothing he could do, so I can only seek help from TCM"* (P23)

(continued)

Table 1 (continued)

WM theme	Subtheme	Direct quotation from patients	Translated quotation
	Holistic treatment	你知道西藥係發散嘅, 你只係醫你一時, 唔係睇到你嘅, 即係話長久, 對於你身體唔係幾, 幾, 幾平衡好呀 因為如果你食中藥嘅呢, 係醫咗你個質, 體質先, 然後你體質恢復啦, 你先係有個抵抗能力 (P36)	*"you know, western medicine is very strong, it can only treat you for a while, it's not for long-term use, and it's not, not, good for your body's balance. If you take CHM, however, it's treating your body constitution, and your body constitution will restore back to normal, then you will have the immunity back"* (P36)
	Prevention of recurrence and complete recovery	我希望可以幫到有改善啦, 希望姐係真係, 姐係會…點講呀, 可唔可以切底治療囉 (P39)	*"I hope it can help improving [my situation], I hope it really, how should I say it, see if it can completely cure it"* (P39)
	Relief of side effects	希望, 希望提升番下我個身體囉, 姐係就化療期間, 幫我就唔好甘辛苦囉. 姐係你化療好辛苦嫁嘛, 化療 (P37) 幫我快啲恢復我個, 唔好腳震啦, 最緊要 (P36)	*"I hope, hope it can boost my body a bit, I mean during chemotherapy, see if it can help me to relief some of the sufferings, you suffer a lot during chemotherapy"* (P37) *"help me with my, leg trembling, that's the most important"* (P36)

5 Participants' Expectation of WM

5.1 Patients' Faith in Biomedicine

Analysis indicated that the themes of "faith in biomedicine" and "no expectation" (i.e., I have to accept it) dominate patient's expectations of WM. The codes related to "faith in biomedicine" were informed by the Western medical doctors. The biomedicine approach associated with the WM doctors involved surgery, chemotherapy or radiotherapies to eliminate the tumor inside the body. Comments often related to the participants expressed *faith* in biomedicine. They believed that treatments provided by WM, namely surgery and chemotherapy, could eliminate (cure) all their cancer. The authoritative status of WM is shown in patients' perception that it is the rational choice for safe treatment with clinical evidence. The decreasing readings of biomedical markers focused on the histology reports (e.g., CEA, blood sample test or pathos-histological report) provided evidence to the patients that their cancer cells were clearing.

The other significant theme identified related to the notion of the patients having "no expectation" of WM in relation to their cancer prognosis. Although the patients had faith in biomedicine that surgery or chemotherapy or radiotherapies could help, the patients were well informed by the WM doctors that every intervention has potential limitations in terms of its ability to eliminate all cancer cells in the body. The patient needed to accept to a certain extent that the cancer cell would not respond perfectly to all the suggested treatments (Table 1). For example, one patient stated, "*[My] expectation of course is complete cure, do surgery, get the tumor out after the surgery*" (*P23*). More than 70% of patients expressed thoughts that were coded as "elimination" or "cure" and this indicates that patients believed surgery was most likely to lead to a complete cure. Once the tumor had been taken out, they would be clear of the disease. Chemotherapy was another common treatment patients anticipated, and this term mapped onto 50% of the conversations containing the word "surgery" if CRC were metastasized to the lymphatic system. This view implied when cancer cells spread to the lymph node, patients would receive chemotherapy that surgery cannot remove. Three patients said that they were informed by a WMD that chemotherapy after metastasis to the lymph nodes had a success rate of only 10–20% in terms of killing all cancer cells. To play safe from the chance of failure of chemotherapy, patients would like to or pushed for alternative treatment options to manage their uncertainty. In parallel, Chinese Medicine which is regulated by the Hong Kong government and rooted in Chinese culture, was their alternative choices.

6 Acceptance of Disease, Progression, Treatment Failures or Death

Many patients expressed that they had expectations of WM treatments, but given their lack of medical knowledge, they could not elaborate or discuss further with their corresponding WMD what their specific expectations were. They would then divert their answers to express their trust in the WMD. Nearly 75% of patients made comments such as, "*I have expectation, like, listen to the WMD, I will do what he says*" (*P29*). Ten cancer patients who had undergone WM treatments expressed that they had uncertainties. One explained that "*because I am not too familiar with this area, and I have limited knowledge, so, actually, [my expectation] won't be high, won't have a high expectation on what happens, as long as what the WMD says about the treatment fits my anticipation, then I will follow his words*" (*P33*).

The expectation to be cured and hope are often closely linked. Patients expressed that they had expectations of WM but these were negative because they knew about WM's available treatment options and the low success rate from the information that they found on the internet. In other words, the data and evidence were readily available for them to read and digest. Patients' understood and perceived the chance of success with WM was low or lost hope on WM because of the empirical data did not give them hope. One of the patients said, *"I have expectation [on WM] at the beginning, but now, I don't have any ... [the information on WM treatment] can all be found on the internet ... whenever I was waiting for the report of my check-up, you can get the report before you go inside to see the doctor, you can see what's written in the conclusion, there really is no point in going into see him ... I, WM is giving no hope. WM, I think it ... it does not have an effective treatment on cancer"* (P31). This quote suggests that the patient understood the risk of the interventions and the corresponding limitations. Therefore, they needed to face the reality of long-term disease or death. The patients were deferential to the authoritative status of WMDs at the beginning of the journey. In parallel, they were also looking for a relationship of healing where the doctor gave hope to them and could walk with them in their journey. However, it would appear it seems most patients lost hope in the WMD from data they found on the internet. This fragmented the doctor–patient relationship and patients often sought out TCM practitioners to increase their hope of survival.

7 Participants' Expectations of TCM

7.1 Patients Hope to Continue Treatment

Patients' responses showed that they hoped to continue consulting TCM as it offered options for on-going treatment. Within this theme, four subthemes were identified: (1) TCM was the only remaining options when WM had failed or WM treatments had been completed, (2) TCM could help prevent recurrence and aid complete recovery, (3) TCM could provide a holistic treatment, and (4) TCM could relieve side effects from WM treatments and specific cancer-related symptoms.

TCM often described as the last resort for patients with advanced cancers. There were four conditions in which patients said they would seek TCM to limit disease progression. One patient said that, *"Surgeon said there was nothing he could do, so I can only seek help from TCM"* (P23). On the other hand, four patients who had completed their WM treatment decided to use TCM because they wanted to take control over their disease and their body. Eighty-five percent expressed the view that once the WM treatment was completed, there would be no pills to take and TCM could provide them with specific herbs that may help the body self-regulate in ways that WM cannot. This was closely related to the next subtheme.

Patients knew TCM used a holistic approach in treatment. Eleven out of the sixteen (4 did not try TCM) patients mentioned they sought TCM for this purpose. The word "hope" was repeated, in that they hoped TCM could help them to regulate and supplement their body. As one patient put it, *"you know, western medicine is very strong, it can only treat you for a while, it's not for long-term use, and it's not,*

not, good for your body's balance. If you take CHM, however, it's treating your body constitution and your body constitution will restore back to normal, then you will have the immunity restored" (P36). Patients expected TCM could help with putting their impaired body back to normal after receiving WM treatments as they considered WM treatments to be effective in fighting the cancer cells but to impair other body functions at the same time.

Prevention of relapse and aiding complete recovery was also another aspect of patients' expectations from TCM (10 out of 16). Patients expressed that they hoped TCM could continue to aid the complete cure of their disease. Although patients could not give any evidence in terms of chances that TCM could decrease the likelihood of recurrence, they still believed there was a possibility. Although chemotherapy assists in treating cancer, its side effects also affect patients 'quality of life' such as gastrointestinal, urinary, and sexual dysfunction, pain or fatigue. Patients believed that TCM could help relieving irreversible neurotoxicity (i.e., limb tremors or numbness) bought by chemotherapy. Patients who received acupuncture or took prescribed herbs were found to have some relief from pain or improved sensation. However, some patients did not elaborate on how TCM could help them but only that it could help.

8 Discussion

8.1 Expectation Control Is Important for CRC Patients Who Will Seek TCM

Rao and colleagues have proposed two patterns of what they describe as a hierarchy of resort that is acculturative and counter-acculturative (Rao, 2006). Acculturative hierarchy of resort refers to when allopathic medicine, or biomedicine, is the first resort then followed by the so-called traditional medicine, while counter-acculturative hierarchy of resort begins with the traditional medical system. The patient moves on to the next resort if the first one is considered to have failed or has not satisfied their needs fully. Most patients follow the acculturative path and move down the hierarchy only when biomedicine fails to satisfy all of their needs. With regards to the unmet needs, some of the unmet needs of cancer survivors identified in previous research have been described in the following terms: (1) physical symptoms such as pain, (2) information (i.e., lack of knowledge regarding follow-up care, self-care, surveillance or prevention, etc.), (3) personal control (i.e., maintain autonomy), and (4) system of care (i.e., constraints and flaws that affect treatment, follow-up care, continuity of care, etc.) (Burg et al., 2015). Perceived beneficial response and wanting control are two of the main reasons why cancer patients consult complementary alternative medicine (Smithson, Britten, Paterson, Lewith, & Evans, 2012; Verhoef, Balneaves, Boon, & Vroegindewey, 2005). The results of the current study are consistent with this previous work in that when CRC patients believe TCM can provide something WM cannot, they then moved down the hierarchy. Patients expected TCM to relieve the side effects bought by WM treatment or other cancer-related symptoms to resolve their major unmet needs. Patients recognized that in the existing medical system, they cannot get information or treatment on any follow-up care, self-care, and prevention, thus they expected TCM to provide all of the above. Additionally, actively seeking care from TCM provided patients with a sense of empowerment or enablement for self-care and respect.

In this study, patients clearly understood that they have the choice of having surgery or chemotherapy as a cure for their disease, which was in contrast to the specific expectations they had from TCM. That is, TCM was expected to provide holistic treatment that helped restore the constitution of the body, regulate and supplement their damaged body, prevent recurrence of cancer, and relieve side effects from WM treatment and cancer-symptoms. Ten patients out of 20 who had received treatment from WM expressed that they did not have specific expectations. One patient explained that she did not have any expectations of WM because she has accepted her situation and believed that the WMD would try their best to help her. However, of the 16 patients who had sought help from TCM, none of them stated that they had specific expectations from CMP. What is the reason behind this discrepancy in expectations? The lack of clinical trial data (i.e., successful treatment rates or information on underlining toxicity are not clear) and evidence related to TCM hinders the communication between CMPs and WMDs and thus limits the integration of TCM into the conventional medical system. It may also be one of the reasons that TCM gives advanced cancer patients hope, albeit sometimes exaggerated hope. Compared to WM, TCM has less reliable data due to the poor quality of research studies. As noted above this is because of the lack of blinding, randomization, and potential publication bias (Kotsirilos, Vitetta, & Sali, 2011; Sałaga et al., 2014; WHO, 2013). However, patients regained their trust in TCM as an alternative when they heard successful stories from well reputed CMPs. Data from pragmatic clinical trials or observational studies provided them with additional evidence. Unfortunately, there is still a lack of reliable data and patients can easily fall prey to incompetent CMP who exploit cancer patients by promising unrealistic treatment outcomes with a cure.

Patients expected oncologists to remove the tumor and prescribe chemotherapy while they expected CMP to restore the body and prevent recurrence. The latter expectation is bigger and vaguer in scale. Without a solid and tangible goal like those that patients have for WM, they are more vulnerable to deception. As previously discussed in this chapter, there is no specialty training in TCM on cancer care and there is no accredited authority to evaluate the competence, performance or quality of CMPs in relation to best practice for the care of cancer patients. To complicate the matter even further, CHM prescriptions are based on syndrome differentiation and are personalized based on an individual patient's body constitution (林洪生, 2014). With little reliable information on how TCM can treat cancer and what exactly it is treating, patients' expectations, and hopes are open for individual interpretation and easily targeted by malicious exploitation.

8.2 An Integrative Cancer Model Is Needed to Preserve the Patients or Family's Dignity

Medical pluralism not only describes a situation in which multiple medical systems coexist, but it is also characterized by the dominance of biomedicine over alternative medicines, for instance, TCM (Ember, Thomson, Human Relations Area Files inc, Gale Group, & Gale and Ember Melvin, 2004) in Chinese culture. Since the British colonization in the nineteenth-century, biomedicine has dominated a local health system that can trace its roots back to Tung Wah hospital, a hospital that at its conception provided TCM service only (Leung & Wong, 2017). TCM regained some of its authority through the establishment of the Chinese Medicine ordinance in 1997 but it is still considered complementary and alternative in Hong Kong as it is still not incorporated fully in public hospital health care systems and over 80% of the CMP work in the private sector (Food and health Bureau Healthcare Planning and Development Office, 2017). TCM is still criticized for lacking clinical trial, data, evidence, and standardized guidelines.

Three types of medical systems can be found in Hong Kong: local, regional, and cosmopolitan (Ember et al., 2004). TCM belongs to the regional medical system because it is adopted by a relatively large population in a small area since it rooted in Hong Kong from Chinese culture. WM belongs to the cosmopolitan medicine as it is a world-wide system adopted by a majority of countries after it emerged in Hong Kong which was colonized. The effectiveness and efficiency of WM are reflected in some of the patients' comments in this paper and demonstrates that WM still holds a strong and credible position in Hong Kong (Our Hong Kong Foundation, 2018). Surgery and chemotherapy are the two powerful tools of WM and they were often mentioned by interviewees in this study. Cancer patients thought the removal of the tumor would guarantee cure, and chemotherapy was a powerful treatment even though it had a low success rate (20–30%) (Davis et al., 2017). Patients' expectations of WM were built on their confidence in biomedicine and statistics (Appleton et al., 2013; Sahay et al., 2000; Smithson et al., 2012). One similarity across interviewees in relation to those who had expectations of WM and those who did not have any expectations was that they all trusted WM and their course of action was based on this trust. Patients who had expectations of WM reflected that they would follow the WMD's instructions because they trust their authoritative status and credibility even though they did not provide any specific reason why they trusted WM in that way. Similarly, for those who did not express any expectations of WM, they explained that it was because they had little knowledge of WM, but they would still follow WMD's instruction on their treatment regimen (Smithson et al., 2012; Verhoef et al., 2005). It seems that patients' trust in WM is not the result of understanding how WM treatment works or clinical data but because they are affected by the dominant status of WM in Hong Kong society.

The authoritative status of WM has been established by the HK government through a top-down approach which has created a monopoly over other medical systems (Ember et al., 2004), including TCM. As TCM is still not incorporated into the major healthcare system and is not subsided by the government, means Hong Kong Chinese population have to pay themselves to see CMP as 90% practice in the private market (Hong Kong Legislative Council, 2018; Shae, Fung, & Lam, 2017). Different medical systems within a society could either have a cooperative or competitive relationship, but people are often capable of "dual use" of distinct systems (Ember et al., 2004). In spite of the current medical system's structure, whenever there are unmet needs that the dominant medical system fails to fulfill, patients will proactively move on to the alternative system that has roots in their culture according to their hierarchy of resort.

With a high demand for TCM among cancer patients, there is an urgent need for a monitored, well-managed, and safely integrative medical system. Patient safety and treatment effectiveness are the two main issues that any medical system should focus on improving. Instead of forcing patients to choose CMP from an unregulated market due to the absence of a referral system which could highly increase the chances of herb–drug interaction and negatively affect patients' survival, it is wise to develop an integrative medical model that brings the best from WM to TCM together to benefit cancer patients. The purpose of any medical system should not hinder any patients from assessing optimal treatment and care that are appropriate and safe. In order to do this, both WMDs and CMPs have to start communicating with each other. Both parties have to be willing to learn the knowledge that is outside their realm of expertise. WMD should be willing and eager to learn the principles of TCM on how they treat cancer while CMP has to take specialty training to improve their knowledge on western medical drugs and potential herb–drug interactions and complications. By recognizing the complementary and supplementary nature of the different medical systems a better integrative system can be developed for the benefit of the patient.

In this study, of the 20 patients who had received WM treatments, 16 of them adopted TCM treatments during their cancer journey. Owing to the history of Hong Kong for pursuing globalization of evidence-based medicine, it is a city of medical pluralism in which multiple ethnomedical systems coexist and patients can adopt more than one medical system for any illnesses (Wade, Chao, Kronenberg, Cushman, & Kalmuss, 2008). Despite biomedicine being the mainstream in the Hong Kong medical system, findings of this study, as well as many other international studies, reflected that many cancer patients seek consultation from TCM in parallel (WHO, 2015). Cancer patients proactively sought help from outside the realm of WM when WM failed them or when it had no more to offer (Leng, Lei, Lei, & Gany, 2014). From the establishment of the development strategies by WHO in 1994, TCM has had a clear role in countries in terms of regulation, research, and development (WHO, 2013). However, TCM is not yet fully incorporated into the Hong Kong public healthcare system but is rather subcontracted by the Hospital Authority (HA) to non-governmental organizations (NGO). Under the scheme of HA Tripartite Chinese Medicine Centre for Training and Research (CMCTR), 18 CMCTRs have been established, with each operated by an NGO, supported academically by a university, subsidized, and monitored by HA. The CMCTRs accounted for 12% of the TCM consultations in the primary care settings. Other than the CMCTRs, patients can find 90% of private CMP in the clinics affiliated with Hong Kong universities or in the private markets (Wong et al., 2017).

There is neither a referral system under the HA nor any special training for CMP. Additionally, patients are unable to differentiate whether or not a particular CMP is focused on cancer care. Since there is no referral system, patients are left on their own to search for and choose their own CMP. While some CMP insists that it is safe to use CHM and WM concurrently and that using CHM can enhance chemotherapy potency (Deng et al., 2013), oncologists argue that because there is a lack of evidence and clinical trials on potential herb–drug interaction, to ensure cancer patients' safety they should not be used at the same time. Although TCM is proven to be beneficial in treating cancer, cancer-related symptoms, relieving side effects of chemotherapy, and general recovery (Liang et al., 2012; Ma et al., 2015; Qi et al., 2010; Sałaga et al., 2014; Tao et al., 2010; Ting et al., 2012; Yang et al., 2008; Zhong et al., 2012, 2015), it is not without risk. It is not the aim of this paper to argue which system has greater merits, but to point out the fact that in reality, a considerable number of patients are actively seeking help from TCM in a WM dominated society.

Concurrent use of CHM and WM has long been debated among physicians. This debate reflects concerns for the quality of herbs, the lack of best clinical research, or best practice of CMP, a lack of support of CMP to access the medical record of the laboratory and the blood results of specific patients to promote continuity of care. The practical clinical guidelines that show a good communication platform adopted by China in the incorporation of American Society of Clinical Oncology (ASCO) and National Comprehensive Cancer Network Care (NCCN) (So et al., 2019) have demonstrated the best practice and the alignment of protecting the patients' safety which at the same time reserves the tradition of Chinese Medicine in the cancer care context. The lack of communication between WMD and CMP, compounded by differences in treatment philosophies, has caused patients to be sandwiched between the two systems. It could be alleviated by a communication platform which incorporates best practice and clinical guidelines.

Some progress that has improved communication has been made. A multi-disciplinary cancer care platform supported by the Hong Kong SAR government and HA promoting integrative cancer care approaches has enhanced the communication skill set of CMP from diverse educational backgrounds (Hong Kong Insitute of Integrative Medicine, 2019). This platform encourages direct communication across the medical industry by connecting the surgeon, basic biomedical scientist, oncologist, and CMP. Furthermore, the establishment of the electronic health record sharing system by the Hong Kong SAR government in 2022 will also facilitate communication between patients and their choices of WMD or CMP (Hong Kong Food and Health Bureau, 2019). This e-Health platform, with patients' consent, will potentially inform WMD about patient's CHM usage, and therefore, allow the two approaches to become complementary. This could avoid the sub-optimal clinical scenario in which patients do not disclose their drug use information during active WM treatment or Chinese herbs use. This poses significant patient safety risks from current use of both Western and Chinese medicine without communicating with each other along different phrases of cancer care in a health care system (Farooqui et al., 2012; Grace, Bradbury, Avila, & Du Chesne, 2018; Leng et al., 2014). Further research is needed to determine if this enhanced communication will improve the quality of care.

9   Conclusion

This study found that patients' expectations of WM primarily related to the provision of surgery and chemotherapy which they believed were key to curing cancer. Their trust and confidence stemmed from their faith in biomedicine which is, in fact, a product of the domination of biomedicine in the modern, pluralist medical system in Hong Kong. The patient's health-seeking behavior or even adherence to the treatment regimen was highly influenced by the authoritative status of the WMD. On the other hand, patients expected TCM to fulfill their unmet needs which WM often failed to satisfy. They expected TCM to provide continuing treatment, or to be the only treatment when WM ran out of options, a holistic treatment that contributes to the prevention of recurrence and complete recovery and to relieve side effects of WM treatments and cancer-related symptoms.

In this study 16 out of 20 patients interviewed had received TCM treatments. Despite WM being the first resort for many patients, in Hong Kong, TCM also occupies an important role in cancer patient's journey of recovery and the demand is high. It is crucial to ensure patient safety by developing oncology specialty training for CMPs, as well as to construct a referral system within the local public hospitals. Accountability and regulation have to be introduced into the system for it to minimize potential risks to cancer patients. Similarly, WMDs have to take up initiatives to learn more about TCM treatment principles. Harmony is built on the principle of mutual understanding. For the common good, namely cancer patients' benefit, both CMPS and WMDs have to change the way they are operating now. Recognizing cancer patients' needs and understanding their current health-seeking behavior is important in building a better medical system. As this study shows, an integrative medical system is a solution that will bring two seemingly opposed medical systems together. A patient-centered approach with cross-disciplinary communication is essential to the provision of the best colorectal cancer care. With transparent communication of different disciplines of medicine facilitated by good clinical practice and clinical guidelines, patients can ultimately get benefitted from a better quality of care in the near future.

Funding Funding for this study was provided to the lead author from the Chinese University of Hong Kong (Ref: 2015.2.012).

References

Appleton, L., Goodlad, S., Irvine, F., Poole, H., & Wall, C. (2013). Patients' experiences of living beyond colorectal cancer: A qualitative study. *European Journal of Oncology Nursing, 17*(5), 610–617. https://doi.org/10.1016/j.ejon.2013.01.002.

Bell, L. (2014). Patient-centered care. *American Journal of Critical Care, 23*(4), 325. https://doi.org/10.4037/ajcc2014383.

Bensoussan, A., Talley, N. J., Hing, M., Menzies, R., Guo, A., & Ngu, M. (1998). Treatment of irritable bowel syndrome with Chinese herbal medicine. *JAMA, 280,* 1585–1589.

Bray, F., Ren, J., Masuyer, E., & Ferlay, J. (2013). Estimates of global cancer prevalence for 27 sites in the adult population in 2008. *International Journal of Cancer, 132*(5), 1133–1145. https://doi.org/10.1002/ijc.27711.

Burg, M. A., Adorno, G., Lopez, E. D. S., Loerzel, V., Stein, K., Wallace, C., et al. (2015). Current unmet needs of cancer survivors: Analysis of open-ended responses to the American Cancer Society Study of Cancer Survivors II. *Cancer, 121*(4), 623–630. https://doi.org/10.1002/cncr.28951.

Cancer.Net Editorial Board. (2019). Understanding targeted therapy. Retrieved from https://www.cancer.net/navigating-cancer-care/how-cancer-treated/personalized-and-targeted-therapies/understanding-targeted-therapy.

Chiu, J., Yau, T., & Epstein, R. (2009). Complications of traditional chinese/herbal medicines (TCM)—A guide for perplexed oncologists and other cancer caregivers. *Supportive care in cancer: Official journal of the Multinational Association of Supportive Care in Cancer, 17*(3), 231–240.

CMCHK. (2008). Chinese medicine ordinance—Chinese Medicine Council of Hong Kong. Retrieved from http://www.cmchk.org.hk/cmp/eng/#../../eng/main_ord.htm.

Cotrim, H., & Pereira, G. (2008). Impact of colorectal cancer on patient and family: Implications for care. *European Journal of Oncology Nursing, 12*(3), 217–226. https://doi.org/10.1016/j.ejon.2007.11.005.

Davis, C., Naci, H., Gurpinar, E., Poplavska, E., Pinto, A., & Aggarwal, A. (2017). Availability of evidence of benefits on overall survival and quality of life of cancer drugs approved by European Medicines Agency: Retrospective cohort study of drug approvals 2009–13. *BMJ, 359,* j4530. https://doi.org/10.1136/bmj.j4530.

Davis, E., Oh, B., Butow, P., Mullan, B. A., & Clarke, S. (2012). Cancer patient disclosure and patient-doctor communication of complementary and alternative medicine use: A systematic review. *Oncologist, 17,* 1475–1481.

Deng, S., Hu, B., An, H., Du, Q., Xu, L., Shen, K., ... Wu, Y. (2013). Teng-Long-Bu-Zhong-Tang, a Chinese herbal formula, enhances anticancer effects of 5–Fluorouracil in CT26 colon carcinoma. *BMC Complementary and Alternative Medicine, 13* (128).

El-Shami, K., Oeffinger, K. C., Erb, N. L., Willis, A., Jennifer, K. B., Pratt-Chapman, M. L., et al. (2015). American cancer society colorectal cancer survivorshop care guidelines. *American Cancer Society, 65*(6), 427–455.

Ember, C., Thomson, G., Human Relations Area Files inc, Gale Group, & Gale and Ember Melvin. (2004). *Encyclopedia of medical anthropology [electronic resource]: health and illness in the world's cultures.*

Fan, Y., Jin, S., He, J., Shao, Z., Yan, J., & Feng, T. (2012). Effect of β, β-dimethylacrylshikonin on inhibition of human colorectal cancer cell growth in vitro and in vivo. *International Journal of Molecular Sciences, 2012*(13), 9184–9193.

Fan, L., Li, Y., Sun, Y., Yue, Z., Meng, J., Zhang, X., et al. (2015). Paris saponin VII inhibits metastasis by modulating matrix metalloproteinases in colorectal cancer cells. *Molecular Medicine Reports, 11*(1), 705–711.

Farooqui, M., Hassali, M. A., Abdul Shatar, A. K., Shafie, A. A., Farooqui, M. A., Saleem, F., et al. (2012). Complementary and alternative medicines (CAM) disclosure to the health care providers: A qualitative insight from Malaysian cancer patients. *Complementary Therapies in Clinical Practice, 18*(4), 252–256. https://doi.org/10.1016/j.ctcp.2012.06.005.

Ferlay, J., Soerjomataram, I., Ervik, M., Dikshit, R., Eser, S., Mathers, C., & Bray, F. (2013). Cancer Incidence and Mortality Worldwide: IARC CancerBase No. 11. *GLOBOCAN 2012 v1.0.*

Food and health Bureau Healthcare Planning and Development Office. (2017). Strategic Review on Healthcare Manpower Planning and Professional Development. Retrieved from http://www.hpdo.gov.hk/doc/srreport/c_chapter1.pdf.

Grace, S., Bradbury, J., Avila, C., & Du Chesne, A. (2018). 'The healthcare system is not designed around my needs': How healthcare consumers self-integrate conventional and complementary healthcare services. *Complementary Therapies in Clinical Practice, 32*, 151–156. https://doi.org/10.1016/j.ctcp.2018.06.009.

Harmsworth, K., & Leiwith, G. (2001). Attitudes to Traditional Chinese Medicine amongst Western trained doctors in the People's Republic of China. *Social Science and Medicine, 52*(1), 149–153.

Hesketh, T., & Zhu, W. X. (1997). Health in China: Traditional Chinese medicine: One country, two systems. *BMJ, 315*(7100), 115–117. https://doi.org/10.1136/bmj.315.7100.115.

Hong Kong Food and Health Bureau. (2019). *eHRSS records millionth registrant: new milestones, new horizon*. Hong Kong Retrieved from https://www.ehealth.gov.hk/en/publicity_promotion/ehealth_news_18/millionth_registrant.html.

Hong Kong Hospital Authority. (2016). *Hong Kong cancer registry*. Hong Kong Retrieved from http://www3.ha.org.hk/cancereg/statistics.html.

Hong Kong Insitute of Integrative Medicine. (2019). Latest development on gastrointestinal cancer: integrative approaches in diagnosis and treatment [Press release]. Retrieved from http://cmk.ha.org.hk/zh-cht/information-index/index/pa/2019hkiimhighlights.

Hong Kong Legislative Council. (2018). *Panel on Health Services LC Paper No. CB(2) 349/18–19: Role and operation of Chinese Medicine Centres for training and Research*. Hong Kong: Hong Kong SAR Government Retrieved from https://www.legco.gov.hk/yr17-18/english/panels/hs/minutes/hs20180430.pdf.

Jane, R., Jane, L., Gilliam, E., Rosalind, T., & Nilufer, R. (2014). *Designing and selecting samples* (2nd ed). Los Angeles, California: SAGE.

Kelner, M., & Wellman, B. (1997). Health care and consumer choice: Medical and alternative therapies. *Social Science and Medicine, 45*(2), 203–212.

Kotsirilos, V., Vitetta, L., & Sali, A. (2011). *A guide to evidence-based integrative and complementary medicine*. Sydney, N.S.W.: Elsevier Churchill Livingstone.

Ku, G., Tan, I., Yau, T., Boku, N., Laohavinij, S., Cheng, A., et al. (2012). Management of colon cancer: Resource-stratified guidelines from the Asian Oncology Summit 2012. *The lancet Oncology, 13*(11), 470–481. https://doi.org/10.1016/S1470-2045(12)70424-2.

Leng, J., Lei, L., Lei, S., & Gany, F. (2014). Chinese American Cancer Patients: Use of Traditional Herbal Chinese Medicine and communication with providers about such use. *Psycho-Oncology, 23*, 386–387.

Leung, T. H., & Wong, W. (2017). Development of integrative medicine in Hong Kong. *Chinese Journal of Integrative Medicine, 23*(7), 486–489. https://doi.org/10.1007/s11655-017-2815-z.

Liang, L., Wang, X.-Y., Zhang, X.-H., Ji, B., Yan, H.-C., Deng, H.-Z., et al. (2012). Sophoridine exerts an anti-colorectal carcinoma effect through apoptosis induction in vitro and in vivo. *Life Sciences, 91*(25–26), 1295–1303. https://doi.org/10.1016/j.lfs.2012.09.021.

Lin, X., Yi, Z., Diao, J., Shao, M., Zhao, L., Cai, H., & Sun, X. (2014). ShaoYao decoction ameliorates colitis-associated colorectal cancer by downregulating proinflammatory cytokines and promoting epithelial-mesenchymal transition. *Journal of Translational Medicine, 12*(105).

Lin, W., Zheng, L., Zhuang, Q., Zhao, J., Cao, Z., & Zeng, J. (2013). Spica prunellae promotes cancer cell apoptosis, inhibits cell proliferation and tumor angiogenesis in a mouse model of colorectal cancer via suppression of stat3 pathway. *BMC Complementary and Alternative Medicine, 13*(144). https://doi.org/10.1186/1472-6882-13-144.

Lindmeier, C. (2018 June 18). WHO releases new international classification of diseases (ICD-11). *World Health Organization.*

Ma, L., Ai, P., Li, H., & Vardy, J. (2015). The prophylactice use of Chinese herbal medicine for chemotherapy-induced leucopenia in oncology patients: A systematic review and meta-analysis of randomized clinical trials. *Supportive Care in Cancer: Official Journal of the Multinational Association of Supportive Care in Cancer, 23*(2), 561–579.

McQuade, J., Meng, Z., Chen, Z., Wei, Q., Zhang, Y., & Bei, W. (2012). Utilization of and attitudes towards Traditional Chinese Medicine therapies in a Chinese cancer hospital: A survey of patients and physicians. *Evidence-Based Complementary and Alternative Medicine, 2012,* 504507.

Meijerman, I., Beijnen, J., & Schellens, J. (2006). Herb-drug interactions in oncology: Focus on mechanisms of induction. *The Oncologist, 11*(7), 742–752.

Ng, G. W. Y., Pun, J. K. H., So, E. H. K., Chiu, W. W. H., Leung, A. S. H., Stone, Y. H., et al. (2017). Speak-up culture in an intensive care unit in Hong Kong: A cross-sectional survey exploring the communication openness perceptions of Chinese doctors and nurses. *British Medical Journal Open, 7*(8), e015721. https://doi.org/10.1136/bmjopen-2016-015721.

Our Hong Kong Foundation. (2018). A health system for the 21st Century—Research Report [Press release]. Retrieved from https://www.ourhkfoundation.org.hk/sites/default/files/media/pdf/ohkf_research_report_digital_1201.pdf.

Qi, F., Li, A., Inagaki, Y., Gao, J., Li, J., Kokudo, N., et al. (2010). Chinese herbal medicines as adjuvant treatment during chemo- or radio-therapy for cancer. *Bioscience Trends, 4*(6), 297.

Rao, D. (2006). Choice of medicine and hierarchy of resort to different health alternatives among Asian Indian migrants in a metropolitan city in the USA. *Ethnicity & Health, 11*(2), 153–167. https://doi.org/10.1080/13557850500460306.

Richards, T., & Godlee, F. (2014). The BMJ's own patient journey. *BMJ, 348,* g3726. Retrieved from https://www.bmj.com/content/348/bmj.g3726.

Ritchie, J., Lewis, J., McNaughton Nicholls, C., & Ormston, R. (2014). *Qualitative research practice: A guide for social science students and researchers* (2nd ed). Los Angeles, California: SAGE.

Sahay, T. B., Gray, R. E., & Fitch, M. (2000). A qualitative study of patient perspectives on colorectal cancer. *Cancer Practice, 8*(1), 38–44.

Sałaga, M., Zatorski, H., Sobczak, M., Chen, C., & Fichna, J. (2014). Chinese herbal medicines in the treatment of IBD and colorectal cancer: A review. *Current Treatment Options in Oncology, 15*(3), 405–420.

Shae, W.C., Fung, H. L., & Lam, C.W. (2017). *Medical Hegemony and Hong Kong medical system* (醫學霸權與香港醫療制度), Chung Wah Book Co. Ltd.

Shin, A., Jung, K., & Won, Y. (2013). Colorectal cancer mortality in Hong Kong of China, Japan, South Korea, and Singapore. *World Journal of Gastroenterology, 19*(7), 979–983. https://doi.org/10.3748/wjg.v19.i7.979.

Smith, J. (1996). Beyond the divide between cognition and discourse: Using interpretative phenomenological analysis in health psychology. *Psychology and Health, 11,* 261–271.

Smith, J., Flowers, P., & Larkin, M. (2009). *Interpretative phenomenological analysis: Theory, Method and Research.* Los Angeles: SAGE.

Smithson, J., Britten, N., Paterson, C., Lewith, G., & Evans, M. (2012). The experience of using complementary therapies after a diagnosis of cancer: A qualitative synthesis. *Health, 16*(1), 19–39. https://doi.org/10.1177/1363459310371081.

So, T. H., Chan, S. K., Lee, V. H., Chen, B. Z., Kong, F. M., & Lao, L. X. (2019). Chinese medicine in cancer treatment—How is it practised in the East and the West? *Clinical Oncology, 31*(8), 578–588. https://doi.org/10.1016/j.clon.2019.05.016.

Social Survey Section. (2002). *Thematic household survey report no. 8.* HKSAR.

Sparreboom, A., Cox, M., Acharya, M., & Figg, W. (2004). Herbal remedies in the United States: Potential adverse interactions with anticancer agents. *Journal of Clinical Oncology: Offical Jounal of the American Society of Clinical Oncology, 22*(12), 2489–2503.

Su, D., & Li, L. (2011). Trends in the use of complementary and alternative medicine in the United States: 2002–2007. *Journal Health Care Poor Underserved, 22*(1), 296–310.

Sui, H., Pan, S., Feng, Y., Jin, B., Liu, X., Zhou, L., — Li, Q. (2014). Zuo Jin Wan reverses P-gp-mediated drug-resistance by inhibiting activation of the PI3K/Akt/NF-kappaB pathway. *BMC Complementary and Alternative Medicine, 14*(279).

Sung, J. J., Lau, J. Y., Goh, K. L., & Leung, W. K. (2005). Increasing incidence of colorectal cancer in Asia: Implications for screening. *The Lancet Oncology, 6*(11), 871–876. https://doi.org/10.1016/s1470-2045(05)70422-8.

Tao, L., Zhu, Y., Lu, X., Gu, Y., Zhao, A., Zheng, J., et al. (2010). Clinical study on survival benefit for elderly patients with resected stage II or III colorectal cancer based on traditional Chinese medicine syndrome differentiation and treatment. *Journal of Chinese Integrative Medicine, 8*(12), 1159–1164.

Thorne, S., Hislop, T. G., Kim-Sing, C., Oglov, V., Oliffe, J. L., & Stajduhar, K. I. (2014). Changing communication needs and preferences across the cancer care trajectory: Insights from the patient perspective. *Supportive Care in Cancer, 22*(4), 1009–1015. https://doi.org/10.1007/s00520-013-2056-4.

Ting, F., Hong, L., Jiao, Y., Zhenjun, S., Jun, H., Yingying, F., et al. (2012). Effect of β, β-dimethylacrylshikonin on Inhibition of Human Colorectal Cancer Cell Growth in Vitro and in Vivo. *International Journal of Molecular Sciences, 13*(7), 9184–9193. https://doi.org/10.3390/ijms13079184.

Tong, A., Sainsbury, P., & Craig, J. (2007). Consolidated criteria for reporting qualitative research (COREQ): A 32-item checklist for interviews and focus groups. *International Journal for Quality in Health Care, 19*(6), 349–357. https://doi.org/10.1093/intqhc/mzm042.

Torre, L. A., Siegel, R. L., Ward, E. M., & Jemal, A. (2016). Global cancer incidence and mortality rates and trends—An Update. *Cancer Epidemiology, Biomarkers and Prevention, 25* (1), 16–27. https://doi.org/10.1158/1055-9965.Epi-15-0578.

United Nations. (2019). *United Nations—World population Prospects 2019.*

Verhoef, M. J., Balneaves, L. G., Boon, H. S., & Vroegindewey, A. (2005). Reasons for and characteristics associated with complementary and alternative medicine use among adult cancer patients: A systematic review. *Integrative Cancer Therapies, 4*(4), 274–286. https://doi.org/10.1177/1534735405282361.

Wade, C., Chao, M., Kronenberg, F., Cushman, L., & Kalmuss, D. (2008). Medical pluralism among American women: Results of a national survey. *Journal of Women's Health (2002), 17* (5), 829–840. https://doi.org/10.1089/jwh.2007.0579.

WHO. (2002). *WHO traditional medicine strategy*, 2002–2005.

WHO. (2013). *WHO traditional medicine strategy: 2014–2023.*

WHO. (2015). *Cancer—Fact sheet.* Retrieved from http://www.who.int/mediacentre/factsheets/fs310/en/.

WHO. (2018). Cancer. Retrieved from http://www.who.int/mediacentre/factsheets/fs297/en/.

Wong, W., Lam, C. L. K., Bian, X. Z., Zhang, Z. J., Ng, S. T., & Tung, S. (2017). Morbidity pattern of traditional chinese medicine primary care in the Hong Kong Population. *Scientific Reports, 7*, 7513. Retrieved from https://www.nature.com/articles/s41598-017-07538-5.epdf?author_access_token=O0vhymqX6SQVJY6gHakhudRgN0jAjWel9jnR3ZoTv0MZEcLlQ2QBiEu7epqMcdQt58sqTPNlYD6AA5GdxUWVtfSx9nXz8WEYCUniVI2AXchzEZB6QpWSt3S8rXtOW1W-0k9dMLJgtttQSYDybOyk6A%3D%3D.

Wong, C., Lam, C., Poon, J., & Kwong, D. (2013). Clinical correlates of health preference and generic health-related quality of life in patients with colorectal neoplasms. *PLoS ONE, 8*(3), e58341.

Xu, W., Towers, A. D., Li, P., & Collet, J. P. (2006). Traditional Chinese medicine in cancer care: Perspectives and experiences of patients and professionals in China. *European Journal of Cancer Care, 15*, 397–403.

Yang, Y., Chen, Z., & Xu, Y. (2008a). Randomized controlled study on effect of Quxie capsule on the median survival time and quality of life in patients with advanced colorectal carcinoma. *Zhongguo Zhong Xi Yi Jie He Za Zhi, 28*, 111–114.

Yang, Y., Ge, J., Wu, Y., Xu, Y., Liang, B., & Luo, L. (2008b). Cohort study on the effect of a combined treatment of traditional Chinese medicine and Western medicine on the relapse and metastasis of 222 patients with stage II and III colorectal cancer after radical operation. *Chinese Journal of Integrative Medicine, 14,* 251–256.

Yeo, A., Legard, R., Keegan, J., Ward, K., McNaughton Nicholls, C., & Lewis, J. (2014). In-depth interviews. In J. Ritchie, J. Lewis, C. McNaughton Nicholls, & R. Ormston (Eds.), *Qualitative research practice : A Guide for social science students and researchers* (2nd ed). Los Angeles, California: SAGE.

Zhang, M., Sun, G., Shen, A., Liu, L., Ding, J., & Peng, J. (2015). Patrinia scabiosaefolia inhibits the proliferation of colorectal cancer in vitro and in vivo via G1/S cell cycle arrest. *Oncology Reports, 33*(2), 856. https://doi.org/10.3892/or.2014.3663.

Zhong, L. L. D., Chen, H.-Y., Cho, W. C. S., Meng, X.-M., & Tong, Y. (2012). The efficacy of Chinese herbal medicine as an adjunctive therapy for colorectal cancer: A systematic review and meta-analysis. *Complementary Therapies in Medicine, 20*(4), 240–252. https://doi.org/10.1016/j.ctim.2012.02.004.

林洪生. (2014). 惡性腫瘤中醫臨床指南, *Clinical practice guidelines of Chinese Medicine in Oncology*: 人民衛生出版社.

Framing Boundaries of Medical Interactions: Data from China

Ying Jin

Abstract There has been extensive research on doctors' preference to foreground the medical frame over the medical interactions, however, little attention has been paid to how different frames are entered and closed at the boundaries of medical talk. Much less is known about the situation in traditional Chinese medicine, causing a great amount of speculation and unwarranted claims. This article uses frame analysis to investigate the opening and closing stages of 45 visits of doctor–older patient consultations in Mainland China, focusing on how participants in both traditional Chinese medicine and western medicine practices collaborate in and navigate between the construction of medical and relational frames of talk. All interactions were audio-recorded and transcribed verbatim. Findings reported in this chapter show variations between different clinical practices in relation to sequential attributes and framing priorities. It is suggested that these variations could possibly be explained by broader clinical differences in pathology and philosophy.

Keywords Medical interactions · China · Frame · Communication

1 Introduction

Extract 1

Context: The patient entered the consultation room and put the physical examination report onto the desk.

D: 胃镜在哪儿做的 where did you have the gastroscopy

P: 今天做的 i had it today

D: 今天做的啊 today

Y. Jin (✉)
International Research Center for the Advancement of Health Communication,
Department of English, The Hong Kong Polytechnic University, Hong Kong, China
e-mail: 15902575r@connect.polyu.hk

© Springer Nature Singapore Pte Ltd. 2020
B. Watson and J. Krieger (eds.), *Expanding Horizons in Health Communication*,
The Humanities in Asia 6, https://doi.org/10.1007/978-981-15-4389-0_6

P: 哎（.）刚做的刚做的他拿来的 yes（.）just now just now he just got this （（for me））

This short exchange raises a number of issues that will be explored in this chapter. At first glance, it is an example of a medical talk between a doctor and a patient. However, a closer inspection of the exchanges suggests a sense of "oddness"—the topic under discussion is not prototypical talk of medical openings (see Coupland, Robinson, & Coupland, 1992, 1994). With no ritual greeting, no relational work, and not even a "perfunctory exchange of 'hi-how-are-you-I'm-fine'" (Roter & Hall, 2006: p. 3), the doctor opened the conversation with serious medical talk by asking the patient about her recent physical examination.

As an example of institutional talk, medical interviews are goal-oriented with embedded routinized activities. These activities feature distributional asymmetries between participants in various matters such as roles and identities, access to knowledge and resources, and participation in interaction (See Drew & Heritage, 1992). While extensive work has been reported in the literature in relation to doctor-patient communication, much of this body of work uses the openings and closings as data sources for the investigation of medical interviews. Research on medical openings has been sparse (Coupand et al., 1992, 1994; Gafaranga & Britten, 2003; Rindstedt, 2014; Robinson, 1998). Even less attention has been paid to medical closings (Defibaugh, 2018; Robinson, 2001). Nevertheless, investigations in how participants open and close medical visits are important for a better understanding of, for example, (i) the structure of social practices (ii) participants' roles and identities, and (iii) relationships between participants. As Schegloff (1986) rightly notes, the openings supply "a metric of sorts for the introduction of various tellable" (p. 117). In addition, prior studies on medical openings and closings are mostly situated in western medicine (WM) practices, leaving us ignorant of other medical practices in the broad field of healthcare (refer to Yip & Zhang in this edition for their unique contribution to the study of communication in Traditional Chinese Medicine). To remedy this lack of knowledge and to join the burgeoning research on communication in other medical practices (i.e., traditional Chinese medicine) (Chang & Lim, 2019; Ting et al., 2016; Tu, Kang, Zhong, & Cheng, 2019), this study examines the first and the final phases of doctor–older patient encounter in both traditional Chinese medicine (TCM) and WM practiced in Mainland China.

The primary goal is to analyze how the boundaries of medical interactions—openings and closings—between doctors and older adults are achieved. The study focuses on (1) how participants orient to and collaborate in the work of entering and closing medical talk, and (2) how the framing of medical discourse in different clinical practices could reflect broader clinical differences in both philosophy and pathology. This chapter begins by reviewing the literature on medical openings in WM, identifying the niche, and making a case for the value of the present investigation. Next, analytical frameworks and methodological approaches will be elaborated.

2 Medical Openings and Closings

As Drew and Heritage (1992) note in their discussion of institutional talk, conversational openings and closings are often "shaped through a standard series of sequences" (p. 43). Scholarship on medical openings in WM has consistently observed that the opening phase of a medical interview usually consists of some "phatically designed talk" (Coupland et al., 1994: p. 92), including phatic communion (in the sense of Malinowski, 1923) and various forms of small talk (in the sense of Coupland, 2000).

A point of departure is Coupland et al.'s (1994) work on geriatric outpatients. These scholars discussed several components of medical openings: summons (usually offered by nurses), greeting-greeting exchanges (mostly initiated by the doctor), dispositional communication (e.g., getting the patient to sit down), the indication of familiarity (mostly initiated by the doctor), and a "how-are-you" exchange. According to Coupland and her colleagues, these activities are conventionalized and together constitute a relational-oriented frame of medical openings. As they stated, "even our most instrumental, transactional encounters [...] involve far more than the transmission and reception of factual (e.g., diagnostic or prescriptive) information" (p. 93). Robinson (1998) extends Coupland et al.'s (1994) work by investigating participants' nonverbal behaviors, gaze, and body orientation to be more specific, during the openings of general practice medical consultations. Similar to Coupland et al.'s findings, regular components of medical openings include greetings, dispositional talk, patient identity confirmation, and determination of patients' chief concerns. In a study of outpatient consultations in a Chinese cancer hospital, Tu et al. (2019) observed that medical openings are primarily comprised of activities of a minimal greeting (i.e., "hello") and identity confirmation.

Moreover, different kinds of talk in medical openings have been examined, such as the "how-are-you" (hereafter, HAY) sequences (Coupland et al., 1992) and small talk (Jin, 2018). Sacks (1975) described the HAY sequences as a substitute for greeting. In other words, the HAY sequences foreground the relational or phatic function of communication rather than aiming for a literal, factual response. In medical openings, however, different interpretations were observed. For example, Coupland et al. (1992) observed the HAY openings in medical encounters, focusing on how participants negotiate the work of phatic communion. Central to their discussion is the degree to which patients' responses to the HAY elicitation designates phaticity. Of particular value in their findings is the observation of a systematic ambiguity (i.e., being phatic and factual) in patient response, and this ambiguity seems to be a mutually intelligible activity that is co-constructed by both conversational parties.

In agreement with, but more importantly, as an extension of Coupland and colleagues' (1992) work, Díaz (2000) observed the structures of medical openings and the solutions to the HAY ambiguity (see also Silverman, 1987; Frankel, 1990) in adult oncological patient encounters. Congruent with Coupland et al.'s (1992) observation, medical openings in Díaz's (2000) observation were mostly initiated with greetings which consist of personal introduction and a familiarity sequence. Common to both Díaz's (2000) and Coupland et al.'s (1992) studies is the consideration of the ambiguity in the HAY type of elicitation, as well as the observation of factuality in patient response. Findings from these scholars thus provide evidence of the "clinical use" (Díaz, 2000: p. 373) of HAY elicitation and add weight to Schegloff's (1986: p. 118) notion of "overt topic-priority relevance" embedded in the HAY sequences. Of particular value in Díaz's (2000) study is the discussion of doctors' disambiguation of what is the expected response in patient disclosure (see also Rindstedt, 2014 on multiparty disambiguation of the HAY sequence in doctor-child-parent encounters). Other variations of the HAY sequences include, for example, "what can I do for you?" and "how are you getting on?" (see Gafarange & Britten, 2003).

While the HAY sequences in medical openings may implicate both phaticity and factuality in the sense of first concern elicitation, small talk in medical openings usually fulfills the functions of relationship building and transition to serious medical talk (Benwell & Creaddie, 2016; Hudak & Maynard, 2011). Walsh (2007), for example, observed a mutual engagement of participants in small talk before the initiation of therapy tasks in speech-language pathology encounters. In nurse-patient encounters, Defibaugh (2018) examined small talk in the opening and closing sequences. According to Defibaugh (2018), the engagement of participants in the HAY sequences and non-work talk at the beginning of the visit mainly serves the function of indicating familiarity and building rapport. Of particular value is her investigation of small talk at the closings of medical visits. While humor and jokes were observed, Defibaugh (2018) argued that by creating a positive relationship, small talk at medical closings lays the groundwork for future visits and creates a continuity of care.

Drawing on these findings, this study investigates the opening and the closing stages of medical consultations in both TCM and WM practiced in Mainland China. The findings reported here contribute novel insights to (1) knowledge of how WM is practiced in Mainland China, and (2) the understanding of the differences between TCM and WM practices in relation to communication.

3   Frame Analysis

A discursive framework informed by frame analysis (Goffman, 1986) is used for the present analysis. The concept of frame or framing is used to describe instances of talk, how medical openings and closings are initiated and closed, how participants shift between medical and relational talk and the implications of participants' orientation towards the forthcoming discourse. Goffman (1986) described the frame as the basic elements of experience for organizing and interpreting social activities. The analysis of the frame allows people to answer questions such as "what is it that's going on here" (Goffman, 1986: p. 8). The frame can be identified by footing

—the "alignment, or set, or stance, or posture, or projected self" that participants "take up" to themselves and others in the giving and receiving of messages (Goffman, 1981: p. 128). For example, a person sitting on a deckchair with sunglasses and a straw hat might evoke the frame of beach experience. In this sense, the frame is metacommunicative as it provides the listener with instructions in his/her interpretation of the messages generated within the frame (Bateson, 1972). Frame not only shapes meaning but also organizes the involvement of individuals in the interaction (Goffman, 1986). For example, frames like hospitals prescribe different involvement of health professionals and clients in terms of the extent to which they are to be engaged in medical activities.

During the course of interaction, participants may change their footing, and hence, they change the frame for the ongoing activity. Goffman (1981) demonstrated how participants constantly change their footing (e.g., tones, postures, or giving up the floor in a conversation) and that such changes shape/influence the nature of the natural talk. Likewise, in medical conversations, participants may change footing, through different "cues and markers" (Goffman, 1981: p. 157), and align themselves to different roles (Sarangi, 2010) in talk. The present study attempts to locate cues and markers that reflect participants' orientation to the frame that characterize their interaction. Two broad frames are under discussion: medical and relational frames (see also Coupland et al., 1994; Mishler, 1984). While understanding the difficulty in setting up a clear-cut dichotomy between medical and relational frames (Ragan, 2000), the qualitative analysis here mainly addresses participants' foregrounding of goals. Decisions in relation to participants' communicative goals (i.e., medical- or relational-oriented) are made based upon how the recipient of the utterance(s) responds.

4 Data and Methodology

This chapter draws on data from a larger study of doctor–older patient communication at one state-owned 3A hospital (see Eggleston et al., 2008 for hospital classification in China) in Mainland China. Data discussed in this chapter were collected between December 2016 and January 2016. Data were collected through the observation of 45 consultations between doctors of both TCM and CM and their patients. Six doctors (3 WM and 3 TCM) participated in the study. Patients were recruited from the outpatient department of the Divisions of Gastroenterology and Traditional Chinese Medicine, which were both located on the same floor of the hospital.

To be eligible, patients had to be (1) at least 50 years old, (2) formally diagnosed chronic gastritis, and (3) capable of independent communication, with no cognitive disorders. Chronic gastritis was chosen as the specific disease condition because it is a common disease of older adults. It is also a key specialism of the hospital.

Ethical approval was granted by both the Ethical Committee of the hospital and the researcher's home university.[1] The patients were approached in the waiting areas outside the two divisions. Informed consent was obtained from all the participants prior to the consultation. The participant response rate was 37.5%. A total of 45 patients (15 males, 30 females) agreed to participate, with an age range from 50 to 84 years (average was 64 years). All the participants were Mandarin Chinese speakers and had visited the hospital before. None of the patients were initial visitors, i.e., they had seen the individual doctors before.

For the purpose of this study, medical consultations were divided into three phases of opening, medial, and closing. This paper only concentrates on the opening and closing stages. Medical openings primarily consist of the tasks of greeting, checking identity, acknowledging presence, and eliciting the patient's initial concern (Robinson, 1998). Medical closings include tasks of prescribing, making next appointments, and leave-taking. Though it is not always easy to draw a clear-cut line between different phases of talk, as in some situations, new activities occur in the closing stage, medical conversations in this study are orderly. The 45 consultations were thus divided into 135 fragments, 90 out of which constitute the data reported here. All the conversations were transcribed verbatim following the conventions of conversation analysis (Jefferson, 1984, 2004). The data reported here were translated into English for illustrative purposes, but the content was analyzed in the original language (i.e., Mandarin Chinese).

5 Results

5.1 Types of Consultation and Clinical Environment

All the consultations were repeated visits. Most of the patients stated that they had seen the same doctor more than five times. Given the nature of chronic illness which, to some extent, requires continuity of care, each consultation serves as a follow-up of the preceding consultations and probably a precedent for potential subsequent consultations. In some consultations, patients came with their families. In the observation of the WM encounter, two types of consultations were identified: medication refills and regular visits.

Observation of the medical interviews suggests a clinical difference in relation to the environment within which consultation takes place. In TCM, a patient saw a doctor in the presence of other patients who were waiting for their own appointments inside the consultation room. Those waiting patients talked with each other and thereby shared their own medical information and experiences. In contrast, patients waiting for WM appointments sat and waited on the chairs in the waiting area until they were called. Usually, the nurse called two to three patients at the

[1]Reference No. HSEARS20161101001.

same time. While one was seeing the doctor, the other two waited outside the door of the consultation room. Thus, the environment in WM was less noisy and more spacious than that in TCM. In each of the following extracts, D stands for the doctor, P stands for the patient, and F stands for the family.

5.2 Activities in WM Openings

The way the doctors and patients open their conversations reveals their attitudes towards the social activities being undertaken, their roles within the activities, and their social relations (Rindstedt, 2014). In contrast to what has been reported in the literature, observation of the data revealed that medical openings in the present study were quite goal-oriented with less relational work. This is particularly the case in WM openings, which mostly opened with an on-topic talk with no phatic communion, no familiarity sequences, and not even a scripted HAY exchange. Activities in WM openings primarily included reading patients' physical test reports, eliciting patients' initial concerns, and patient problem presentation. Stated differently, what was observed here in medical openings feature what elsewhere will be considered characteristic of the history-taking stage of the medical consultation.

Extract 1: WM-regular

Context: the patient entered into the room and passed her physical test report to the doctor.

1 D 你的内镜比较() Your gastroscopic report is relatively ().

2 P 哎对对对 Yes, right, right, right.

3 D 现在什么地方痛 Where do you feel painful?

Extract 2: WM-regular

Context: The patient passed the physical test report to the doctor.

1 P 医生(.)喏(.) Doctor, here.

2 P 这个地方(.)左边盖个章 Stamp here, on the left. ((the doctor stamped as requested))

3 D 怎么以前做过的喽 So you did this before?

Extract 3: WM-regular

1 P 开一个胃镜 I want a gastroscopic test.

2 D 好的 Ok.

3 F 你胃怎么不舒服 What's wrong with your stomach?

4 P 呃： Um.

5 D： 胃痛啊 Stomachache?

One of the unmarked activities observed in WM openings is the negotiation of
the patient's physical test, as exemplified in Extracts 1–3. All extracts occurred just
as the patient entered the consultation room. Here in Extracts 1 and 2, the patients'
passing of the physical test report to the doctor reflects their prioritization of the
medical frame for consultation openings. This orientation seems to be well accepted
and co-constructed by both participants. In Extract 1, the doctor's awareness of the
patient's preference to talk about the gastroscopic test is apparent at the beginning
of the extract. The doctor responded to the patient's passing behaviour by reading
and evaluating the test report. The co-construction of the medical frame is also
evidenced by the doctor's next turn when she asked, "where do you feel painful,"
marking a transition to the history-taking stage. The forthcoming discourse
involved exchanges of information collection. In Extract 2, the patient initiated the
conversation by addressing the doctor. Instead of engaging in greetings, the patient
immediately indicated her orientation to the medical frame by "directing" the doctor
to stamp her physical test. The doctor's responsive behavior (i.e., stamping the test
report) and inquiry (asking the patient if he had had this test before) demonstrated
her co-construction of the medical frame at the opening stage of the interview. In
addition, the doctor's inquiry also marked a transition to the history-taking stage, as
evidenced by the use of the word 以前 (before) and the tense marker 过 (indicating
past tense). This inquiry later invoked extensive discussions regarding the patient's
preceding physical examinations. In Extract 3, the patient entered the room and
directly announced his chief concern, namely that he wanted to have a gastroscopic
test. Interestingly here is the doctor's immediate agreement with no probing of the
reasons why the patient would like the test. It was rather the patient's family who
invoked discussions of the patient's health problems (line 3) (see Laidsaar-Powell
et al., 2013 for a review of the companion's role in medical interviews), marking a
shift to the history-taking stage.

Alternatively, WM interviews also frequently opened with patient problem
presentation sequences (e.g., doctors' elicitation of patients' initial concerns and
patient information giving). The patient problem presentation sequences could
either be initiated by the doctor or the patient. Consider Extracts 4 and 5.

Extract 4: WM-regular

1 P 那个贫血已经好几年了 I've had anemia for years.

2 P 我知道的 I know that.

3 P 我们在那[个 we were at the

4 D [你查过没有 Have you checked?

Extract 5: WM-regular

1 D 是怎么 What's wrong?

2 P 肚子胀 I feel bloated.

3 D 嗯 Um.

4 P 小腹胀(.)就下面 Abdominal bloating, just here. ((The patient pointed the doctor her abdomen))

In Extract 4, the patient's problem presented at the beginning of the interview reflected her stance to prioritize the medical frame. This prioritization was accepted and, in fact, further developed by the doctor, as evidenced by the doctor's inquiry asking if the patient had checked before. Note that the doctor's inquiry actually "impeded" on the patient's turn by interrupting the patient's extension (line 3), which could be either medical-related (e.g., describing where and how did she noticed her anemia) or relational (the recalling might invoke some non-medical talk). Therefore, the doctor's interruptive turn here reflected her co-construction of talk on physical tests. Similarly, in Extract 5, a strictly medical frame was co-constructed by both the doctor and the patient. In line 1, by saying that "what's wrong," the doctor displayed her preference for the medical frame for the ongoing discourse at the initial stage of the consultation. The patient's complaint of her abdominal bloating and the subsequent extension on the details of her health problem were indicators of her agreement and alliance to the medical frame.

One interesting phenomenon observed throughout Extracts 1–5 is the absence of the patient identity confirmation sequence (Heath, 1981; Robinson, 1998). Robinson (1998) described two reasons for the importance of securing the patient's identity at medical openings: to make sure that the doctor is treating the right patient and to confirm that the doctor has the appropriate records. Coupland et al. (1994) also pointed out that identity confirmation serves the function of rapport building, although the doctor has access to the patient's identity either/both through the medical records or/and the attendance list shown on the screen.

The absence of patient identity confirmation was particularly noted in medication refill visits. Consider Extracts 6 and 7.

Extract 6: WM-medication refill

1 P 给我开个药就行了 Just give me some medicine

2 P 这个老胃病又犯了(.)又犯起来 My old gastric problem is flaring up again. It is flaring up again.

3 P 给我开个金奥康吧 Give me some *jin'ao'kang* ((name of the pill)).

4 D 平时吃的就是金奥康哦 Do you take *jin'ao'kang* normally? ((The doctor was reading the patient's medical record on the screen))

Extract 7: WM-medication refill

1 P 医生(.)我就是配那个(.)呃(.)那个(.)耐信 Doctor, I am just, I want some *Nai'xin* ((name of the medicine))

2 D 你耐信刚配过的哎？You just had some not long ago. ((The doctor was reading the patient's medical record on the screen))

WM consultations for medication refills in this study were all initiated by the patient. The opening request, as exemplified in both extracts, was formulated in a directive. In so formulating, the patients displayed their orientation towards the medical frame at the beginning of the consultation. The doctors were probably aware of their patients' needs, which in this situation was more task- than relational-oriented and responded by co-constructing the task of prescription.

5.3 Activities in TCM Openings

Similar to WM consultations, some of the TCM consultations also opened with patient problem presentation. Consider Extracts 8 and 9.

Extract 8: TCM

1 P 情况不是很好 I am not good. ((The patient was speaking in a low tone))

2 D 怎么了 What's wrong?

3 P 头晕(.)晕乎乎的 I feel dizzy. My head is swimming.

Extract 9: TCM

1 D 咳嗽怎么样了 How's your cough?

2 P 没好(.)一点也没好 Not good. Not even any better.

3 D ↑一点也没好? Not even any better?

4 P 嗯(.)晚上起来哦咳的我肋骨都疼了 Yes(.) I coughed so hard at night that my ribs hurt.

In both extracts, medical interviews opened with patient problem presentation sequences. In Extract 8, the patient entered the room with a negative evaluation of her situation, indicating a preference of the medical frame for the forthcoming interview. She was probably so concerned about her health that her tone sounded low and sad. The doctor's awareness of the woman's sadness and her preference to take the medical frame was apparent in line 2, where the doctor invited patient extension on the details of the problem. Similarly, in Extract 9, a medical-oriented consultation opening was operationalized as both participants' communication demonstrating a preference for the serious discussion of the patient's cough.

Contextualization cues reflecting this mutual preference include (1) the doctor's use of a symptom-specific question requesting symptomological details (Heritage & Robinson, 2006), (2) the patient's use of diminutive ("not any"), and (3) the patient's subsequent elaboration on his symptom. Here, both participants indicated an attempt to shift out of the opening phase into a different activity (i.e., history taking).

One notable difference between TCM and WM openings, at first glance, is the observation of greeting exchanges and the HAY sequences in TCM consultations. Nevertheless, these activities were not present in all TCM openings and were only minimally engaged in by doctors and patients. Consider Extracts 10–12.

Extract 10: TCM

1 D 嘿?你好 Hey, hello.

2 P (姓)医生 Doctor (surname).

3 D 最近还好吧 How are you these days?

4 P () ((The patient's response is barely audible))

5 D 胸痛啊这方面怎么样啊 How's your chest pain?

Extract 11: TCM

1 P (Surname)医生 Doctor (Surname) ((The patient's voice is hoarse and he kept coughing))

2 D 你好(.)感冒了啊 Hello(.) You got a cold?

3 P 哎(.)感冒了 Yes, I got a cold.

4 D 今天很厉害嘛 It looks very serious today.

5 P 哎(.)昨天晚上特别厉害 Yes. It was very serious last night.

Extract 12: TCM

1 D (name the patient) ((twice))

2 P 哎 Yes.

3 D 坐到这里来 Sit down here.

4 P (0.3) ((the patient sat down))

5 D 你最近怎么样啊 How are you these days? ((The doctor reads the patient's record.))

6 P 肿瘤医院叫我做化疗 The Cancer Hospital asked me to take the chemotherapy.

Medical openings exemplified by Extracts 10–12 feature a different communication style as those in Extracts 1–9, a style that is consistent with what has been documented in the literature (Coupland et al., 1992, 1994; Díaz, 2000; Rindstedt,

2014; Robinson, 1998). In Extract 10, the doctor took a polite stance: she greeted the patient while the patient was entering the room. Note here the tonal increase (marked by '?'), which showed the doctor's surprise at seeing the patient and also indicated, to some extent, the previous acquaintance between the doctor and the patient. The marked "hey" at line one thus could be understood as a tool reflecting the doctor's attempt to build relational work. In addition, given the acquaintance, the "hey" also served the function of identity confirmation. The announcement of familiarity was immediately followed by a greeting ("hello") indicating politeness. The patient's addressing of the doctor with her surname was not only an acknowledgment of the doctor's greeting but also an indicator of intimacy and functioned as relationship building. In summary, the "hey"-initiated sequence accomplished multiple relational tasks: confirming the patient's identity, indicating familiarity, and greeting. Here, both participants oriented to the relational frame of the medical interview. This orientation was extended by the doctor's HAY inquiry, which could be understood as designating phaticity and aiming for "clinical" response (see Díaz, 2000 for the notion of the clinical use of HAY sequences). While determination on the function of the doctor-initiated HAY type of inquiry here was not made, as the patient response was not audible (line 4), it is very likely that the phaticity of the HAY inquiry was prefaced and understood, evidenced by the doctor's subsequent symptom-specific question. As Díaz (2000) pointed out, one strategy to solve the ambiguity of HAY is by "respecifying" (p. 373) the HAY. Here, in Extract 10, the doctor's specification on the patient's chest pain could be understood as her attempt to solve the ambiguity of HAY. It also indicates a shift out of the HAY phaticity into its factuality. In other words, the doctor's symptom-specific inquiry marked a transition from the relational frame to the medical frame.

In Extract 11, the patient entered the room with a serious cough and a hoarse voice. After an initial exchange of phaticity by greeting each other, the doctor shifted to the medical frame of the interview. She was probably aware that the patient was weak and fragile, and therefore, foregrounded the medical frame by discussing the patient's health problem. In addition, the fact that the doctor's question is built on an observation of the patient (his symptom, his countenance, and probably the way he sat down, e.g., bending over the back when coughing) displayed the doctor's technical expertise and personal care (as what would be expected in casual conversations) to the patient. In other words, the placement of the symptom-specific inquiry accomplished both relational and medical tasks and achieved a seamless transition between phaticity and factuality. This understanding is also evidenced by the patient's response which, rather than giving a detailed extension of his medical experience, showed only a minimal agreement to the doctor's observation. That is, the way the patient responded to the doctor's inquiry probably reflected his understanding of the doctor's question as a more relational attempt. The medical attempt of the doctor's inquiry was resumed and enhanced in her subsequent turn, after which elaboration on the seriousness of the patient's cough was made possible.

The doctor's naming of the patient was observed in Extract 12. The naming occurred immediately after the patient entered the room. The doctor named the patient twice as there were too many people waiting inside the room, talking with their families or other patients. Disposition communication (Coupland et al., 1994) was observed when the doctor directed the patient to sit down. The doctor's HAY elicitation occurred in line 5. While the doctor left the patient to decide on the clinical or phatic use of the HAY elicitation, the patient seemed to foreground the clinical reading by telling the doctor that she was advised by another hospital (a cancer specialty hospital) to take the chemotherapy. This patient-initiated frame shift displayed the patient's preference to foreground the medical tasks at the beginning of the interview, possibly due to the fact that the patient's health problem was so serious. From line 6 onwards, the discourse was all about the patient's medical history and treatment negotiation.

Another observation in TCM openings is the presence of small talk (for more discussions, see Jin, 2018), mainly serving the functions of relationship building and easing the transition to the medical frame. Consider Extracts 13 and 14.

Extract 13: TCM

1 D 你几点到的医院啊(.)什么时候到的啊(surname)阿姨 When did you arrive? Aunt (Surname), when did you arrive?

2 P ()到的 At().

3 D 7.30到的啊 7.30?

4 P 嗯 Yes.

5 ((The doctor asks the assistant to write the medical record))

6 D 现在感觉怎么不好 How do you feel? What's the problem?

7 P 现在感觉就是肚子有点胀 I feel I had some abdominal bloating.

Extract 14: TCM

1 D 你这回来啦 You came back.

2 P 哎回来了 Yes, I came back.

3 D 好玩不啦 Is it interesting?

4 P 都是个人 Too many people.

5 D 最近口干不干 Do you feel thirsty these days?

In both extracts, the medical opening was operationalized, and the relational frame foregrounded the medical frame. In Extract 13, the doctor opened the consultation by asking the older woman when she arrived. The doctor's question was apparently relational rather than medical. It is a conventional practice that patients need to make appointments before they see a doctor. Patients could either make an appointment online or at the end of each visit. Alternatively, which is, in fact, very common in many of the state-owned hospitals, patients can also come in person in the early morning to see if there are still vacancies. The doctor's question on the time of arrival thus served multiple relational tasks: as phatic as a greeting and/or as relational as showing care and concern. The doctor's orientation to foreground the relational frame is also evidenced by her addressing of the older adult as Aunt (Surname), which demonstrated respect and politeness. It not until lines 5 and 6 that the doctor announced a shift from relational building to serious medical talk. Thus, the small talk here served the functions of easing the patient and "oil[ing] the interpersonal wheels" (Holmes, 2000: p. 49) in serious medical talk.

Extract 14 demonstrates a similar pattern. The participants' preference to take the relational frame was apparent at the beginning of the extract. The doctor was obviously familiar with the patient when she stated, "You came back," from which two levels of meanings can be interpreted. First, the doctor knows the patient well. Second, the patient's leaving was made known to the doctor. Therefore, the doctor's statement of "you came back" at the beginning of the interview can be treated as a substitute for the familiarity sequence and patient identity confirmation. The doctor's attempt to foreground the relational frame is more evident at her next turn, where she extended the current phatic communion to a form of social talk (Holmes, 2000; Ragan, 2000) by asking, "Is that interesting?". This suggests that both participants had a shared knowledge of what "that" refers to. In other words, the doctor not only knew the patient had left but where and/or why she had left. In so asking, the doctor claimed her intimacy with the patient. And while the doctor was foregrounding the relational task at the opening stage, the patient also actively engaged in the co-construction of medical openings as more relational by acknowledging the presence of herself and complaining that there were too many people (it is very likely that the patient was talking about a trip). It was not until line 5 that the doctor perceived a need to shift out of the current relational frame into the serious medical talk, and thus announcing a shift to the history-taking stage.

5.4   Activities in WM Closings

Robinson (2001: p. 641) stated that the objective of ending medical interviews is "verbally and nonverbally ending a spate of interaction" between the participants. Similar to the observation in medical openings, one in medical closings demonstrates an equally systematic way of how doctors and older patients co-construct the work of closing a medical frame of talk. One almost ubiquitous activity in medical closings in both TCM and WM interviews is the sound of the printing machine, indicating that the doctor is printing the prescription and creating some kind of "closing-relevant environments" (Robinson, 2001: p. 4). Consistent with Robinson's (2001) observation, activities commonly observed in the closing stage of WM interviews comprised arrangement sequences and patient treatment education. The arrangement sequences in the present data included two main practices:

arrangement for future appointment and arrangement for payment. Consider Extracts 15 and 16.

Extract 15: WM-regular

Context: The doctor was typing.

1 P 那我就15号再来好了哦 Then I could come on 15th right?

2 (0.3) ((The doctor was printing the prescription))

2 D 半个月以后 In half a month.

3 P 半个月以后啊(.)哦 Half a month? Oh.

4 (0.7) ((The doctor signed on the prescription and passed it to the patient))

5 P 好谢谢哦 Okay, thank you.

6 D 没事 No problem.

((The patient exited the room.))

Medical closing in Extract 15 was operationalized as an activity in which a future appointment was made possible. Here, the doctor's typing was an indicator of entering into the closing stage. This contextualization cue was well accepted and understood by the patient, as evidenced by her inquiry about the arrangement of the next appointment. This negotiation of appointment making was co-constructed by the doctor who provided the patient with proposals regarding when the patient was to visit the doctor next. Once accepted by the patient (marked by the patient's 'oh' acknowledgment), the doctor indicated her orientation towards the end of the interaction by signing the prescription and passing it to the patient, which functioned as a pre-closing (Schegloff & Sacks, 1973). These pre-closing cues were positively responded to by the patient with acceptance (marked by "okay") and gratitude showing ("thank you"). Extract 15 thus illustrates how the doctor and the patient collaborate in the closure of the medical interview and, in doing so, create an environment in which future appointment making is a relevant activity in the closing stage.

Extract 16: WM-regular

Context: The printing machine is now working. The patient was recommended to take a gastroscopic test next week.

1 D 那给你这个(.)先去 <付完钱以后先去预约 Take this((the prescription)). Make an appointment after you paid.

2 P 先去预约是吧=今天付款以后就去预约 Make an appointment first right? I will make an appointment today after I paid.

3 D 付款以后旁边有个预约台(.)每周二周四做的哦 There is an appointment desk next to the cashier. ((The physical examination)) is on every Tuesday and Thursday.

4 P 哦(.)不用再回过来了哦 Oh. I don't need to come back later, do I?

5 D 不用回来了 No, you don't.

((The patient stood up and left the room.))

Extract 16 illustrates how participants collaborate both in closing the work of payment and in the projected orientation to the closure of the medical interview. The patient was advised to take a gastroscopic test next week. In line 1, the doctor's passing of the prescription to the patient can be interpreted as a pre-closing and an indicator of her orientation towards the end of the interaction. Immediately following that, the doctor initiated an arrangement sequence by directing the patient where to pay, how to make the next appointment, and the schedule of the hospital's gastroscopy center. This arrangement can be viewed as a mutually-accepted and co-oriented activity in a closing-relevant environment. Evidence of the patient's understanding of the doctor's arrangement and orientation towards medical closure includes his confirmation of the doctor's information (line 2), acceptance of the arrangement (lines 2 and 4), and his question asking if he needs to come back later (line 4). The patient's question can be understood as a substitute for "Can I leave directly," and therefore, strongly projected a shift into the closure of the interaction. This was supported by the doctor's confirmation that the patient did not need to come back.

Extract 17 illustrates how participants co-construct the work of patient education regarding treatment as a relevant activity in medical closings.

Extract 17: WM-regular

Contexts: The printing machine is now working.

1 D 两种是饭前两种是饭后哦(.)别看错了 Two are pre-meal and two are after-meal. Don't mess them up.

2 P 哦(.)一个小时哦 = 两种都是一个小时是吧 Oh. One hour right? One hour for both right?

3 D 对 Yes.

((The patient stood up and exited the room.))

The sound of the printing machine marked a transition to the closing stage of the medical interview. In line 1, the doctor initiated a sequence regarding patient treatment education. While both participants demonstrated a preference for the medical frame by discussing medical drug-taking, the fact that the doctor informed the patient about the different categories of medical drugs can also be an indicator of care and concern. This care demonstration is even more pronounced when the doctor reminded the patient not to mess them up (line 1). Evidence of the patient's acceptance of the doctor's advice includes her immediate acknowledgment ('oh') and repetition for confirmation (line 2). Interesting here to note that after the doctor's confirmation ("yes") of the patient's question, the patient exited the room. The closure of medical interaction with the doctor's acknowledgment in this extract is, in fact, a powerful indicator of the participants' collaboration in making patient treatment education the last relevant activity in medical closings.

Extract 18: WM-regular

Context: The printing machine is now working. The doctor passes the prescription to the patient.

1 P 可以了啊 Is that okay?

2 D 嗯 Um.

((The patient left the room))

One notable feature of WM closings detected in this study and illustrated in Extracts 16 to 18, is the absence of a leave-taking sequence (also called a terminal exchange by Schegloff & Sacks, 1973) in most (nearly 60%) of the WM consultations. In the classical piece of conversational closings, Schegloff and Sacks (1973) noted that one of the two crucial components for the achievement of a proper closing is the terminal exchange. They pointed out that this terminal exchange accomplishes the collaboration of termination. The observation of the absence of such terminal exchanges in most of the WM interviews possibly reflects a communication style that is accepted by both the doctor and the patient (See Extract 18). Other forms of a leave-taking sequence observed in the rest of the WM data include a thank-you-my-pleasure exchange (Extract 15) and a goodbye exchange.

5.5 Activities in TCM Closings

While participants in WM closings demonstrated a preference for a more medical frame by engaging in tasks such as patient education and arrangement of the next appointment, participants in TCM closings co-constructed actively in both the medical and relational frames by engaging in both medical-related tasks and non-medical small talk. Activities included in TCM closings are primarily negotiation on how to concoct the herbs (Extract 19), small talk, and relational work (Extract 20), and patient education on lifestyles (Extract 21).

Extract 19: TCM

Context: The doctor writes the prescription.

1 D 自己煎还是代煎 Do you prefer to concoct the herbs by yourself or by the hospital?

2 P ↑自己煎自己煎 By myself, by myself.

3 D 我还希望你自己煎呢 I would also prefer you to do that by yourself.

4 P 嗯(.)有那个买的 Um, I can buy that.

5 D 电的啊 Electronic?

6 P 嗯 Um.

7 D 你哪里买啊 Where do you buy it?

8 P 网上有卖的 I can buy it online.

9 D 我和你讲啊这个电的啊不要给它煎到停 Listen, when you use the electronic cooker, not to wait until it stops.

10 P 半个小时啊 Half an hour?

11 D 半个小时可以了(.)你就闹钟闹一下哦 Half an hour is enough. You can set an alarm.

12 P 我好像有个定时器的 I think I have a timer.

13 D 对啊定时一下 Yes, you can set a timer.

14 D 煎到停时间太长了 It would be too long if you wait until it stops.

15 P 它可以拨时间的 I can set a timer.

16 D 嗯 Um.

17 ((Some patients walking in))

18 P 那(姓)医生我走了啊 So now I am leaving doctor (Surname).

19 D 嗯(.)走好啊 Um. Bye and safe.

((The patient exits the room.))

In Extract 19, talk regarding how to concoct the herbal medicine accomplished both medical and relational tasks. The closing was initiated by the doctor's writing of the prescription. While writing the prescription, the doctor asked the patient whether he preferred to concoct the herbs on his own or by the hospital. Negotiation on this matter is a typical practice in TCM closings, the initiation of which can be treated as the announcement of the transition to medical closings. Interestingly here is the patient's response with a marked increasing tone (↑) and a repetitive claim of his preference. The way the patient responded to the doctor displayed his strong dispreference of concocting the herbs by the hospital. Here, the patient's indication of his preference constituted a sufficient response to accomplish the co-construction of the current medical talk. The patient's dispreference was noted by the doctor, who immediately responded by saying, "I would also prefer you to do that by yourself." Here, rather than contributing to the collaboration of the previous medical talk, the doctor's turn can be treated as rapport building, showing understanding and agreement to the patient's decision. The doctor's attempt at relation-building was immediately accepted by the patient who collaborated in the construction of relational work by initiating talks on the electronic cooker. Although, at first glance, talk on the electronic cooker is relevant to previous medical talk to the extent that the cooker is used to concoct the herbs, the place it was invoked suggests that it was not pronounced for the sake of medical task completion, but rather for relationship building. The invocation of the topic next to the doctor's agreement served as an explanation of the patient's previous decision (i.e., to concoct the herbs on his own). The patient might be aware that his response in line 2 could be "offensive" to the doctor as hospital staff. Thus, the invocation of the electronic cooker could be an indicator of the patient's foregrounding of the relational frame. Similarly, the subsequent discussion on where to buy the cooker seems to be less related to medical task completion, but rather an indicator of participants' collaboration in relationship building.

Patient education on treatment was also observed in this extract. From line 9 onwards, the doctor and the patient actively co-constructed the work in patient education, mainly concerning the time appropriate to concoct the herbs. Medical interviews were closed by a leave-taking sequence initiated by the patient. Note here that rather than using the conventional "goodbye" or "bye-bye," the patient said, "so doctor (surname) I am now leaving," providing the doctor an opportunity of repair (e.g., the provision of new information). Therefore, the patient's addressing of the doctor with her surname and the formulation of leave-taking in a manner of informing provide evidence to the patient's preference to relationship building at the end of the interview. Being aware of the patient's orientation, the doctor collaborated in the work of relationship-building by acknowledging his leave-taking and saying "bye and safe." Extract 19 thus illustrates participants' collaboration in the negotiation of both medical and relational frames at the closing stage of TCM interviews.

Extract 20: TCM

Context: The doctor writes the prescription.

1 P 这个药7天还是几天啊 How long is the treatment? 7 days or?

2 D 7天 Seven days.

3 P 看好以后下个星期再来 I come again next week after this treatment?

4 D 哎(.)可以 Yes. You can.

5 P 那么我走了啊(.)谢谢啊 So I am now leaving. Thank you.

6　　P=你给我预约下个礼拜(.)二(.)下个礼拜我再来看你(.)好预约吗
Could you arrange me with next appointment on next Tuesday? I

would like to come again next week. Can I make an appointment on that day?

7 D 可以的 Okay.

8 P 老婆都好预约了不要说看病了 Nowadays, even your wife can be booked, let alone a medical appointment.

9 D 啧(.)乱讲 Tut, you are talking all sorts of nonsense.

10 P 不是吗(.)你一生出来你老婆就阎王那边预约好这辈子娶哪个老婆了(.)这就是姻缘哈哈 Isn't that true? Since your birth, the Yama has already decided whom you're going to marry with. So marriage is predestined. Huh Huh.

11 D 哈哈 huh huh(.)

12 P 好了哦 Is that okay?

13 D 好了你去好了 Okay, you can leave.

14 P 那我去了 Then I am leaving.

((The patient stands up and exits the room.))

Extract 20 more vividly illustrates how participants collaborate in the work of closing the current medical interview and how they are oriented to multiple medical and relational tasks (arrangement of next appointment, patient education on treatment, and relationship building) as relevant activities during the final stage of the interview. In Extract 20, the doctor's writing of the prescription was an indicator of the transition to the closing phase, which was immediately understood and accepted by the patient. The patient aligned with the doctor by asking the doctor how long the treatment lasts (line 1) and the appropriate time for the next appointment (line 3). After the doctor accepted the patient's proposal (that he will come next week), the patient indicated his leave-taking by informing the doctor that he is now leaving and showing gratitude. However, it seems that the patient immediately (marked by "=" line 6) realized that he forgot to negotiate with the doctor the specific date of the next appointment. Thus, he resumed his prior discussion about the next appointment with the doctor. Here, both participants oriented to the medical frame and demonstrated a preference for the negotiation of future appointments as a relevant activity during medical closings. Note that the task of arranging the next appointment was accomplished in line 7 with the doctor's agreement on the patient's proposed date. From line 8 onwards, the relational frame of the medical interview was foregrounded as participants collaborated in the work of some form of non-medical small talk. In line 8, by saying that "even your wife can be booked, let alone a medical appointment," the patient was using humor and displaying friendship. This understanding is more evident in the patient's next turn, where he extensively expressed his ideas on marriage and explained why he thought that a wife could be booked. Evidence of the doctor's collaboration in the relational work includes her negative evaluation of the patient's comparison between booking a wife and booking a medical interview (line 9). By saying, "Tut, you're talking all sorts of nonsense," the doctor engaged in the current non-medical small talk by expressing disagreement and negatively evaluating the patient's statement. In addition, the doctor's negative evaluation also functioned as an invitation for patient elaboration, as evidenced by immediate patient extension on why marriage is predestined. The joint laughter (lines 10 and 11) functioned as a marker of the success of the humor, additional evidence of participant's collaboration in relational work, and also an indicator of topic closing (Kangasharju & Nikko, 2009). This last function of joint laughter is also evidenced by the patient's turn asking for leave ("is that okay?"), and after the doctor's acknowledgment, the patient's departure.

Extract 21: TCM

Context: The doctor writes the prescription.

1 D 自己煎还是代煎 Do you prefer to concoct the herbs by yourself or by the hospital?

2 P 自己煎(.)上了年纪都在家里的 By myself. I am now old and spend most of the time at home.

3 D 所以就是说你要记牢一年四季冷冻的东西要少吃 So you need to remember that you should eat less cold food all year round.

4 P 就喝点羊肉汤啊 I drink some mutton soup.

5 D 嗯(.) Um.

6 P 阿娇啊 E'jiao ((a kind of supplement made by donkey-hide gelatin))

7 D 哎(.)这种好的 Yes. This kind of food is good for your health.

8 P 哦 Oh.

9 D 这里要不要预约(.)你都是自己约的哦 Do you want to make an appointment now? You make appointment on your own, right?

10 P 不要预约 No, not now.

11 D 好 Okay.

12 P 谢谢哦医生 Thank you doctor.

((The patient gets off the table and exits the room.))

Re-invocation of earlier-discussed lifestyles was frequently observed in TCM closings. In Extract 21, the doctor's writing of the prescription and her question about the patient's preference on how to concoct the herbs marked a transition to the closing phase of the interaction. In line 3, by saying "so you need to remember that you should eat less cold food all year round," the doctor invited the patient to join in the construction of lifestyle education. Evidence of the patient's collaboration includes her information giving on her recent diet (mutton and *e'jiao*) and acknowledgment of the doctor's evaluation. After completion of the current discussion about patient lifestyle education, the doctor and the patient participated in the construction of appointment arrangements. While the patient indicated her preference not to make an appointment at this stage, the doctor initiated a pre-closing ("okay"), providing the patient the last opportunity to raise concerns and also indicating her orientation towards the end of the interview. The patient accepted the doctor's proposal, as she acknowledged the doctor by showing gratitude, getting off the table, and leaving the room.

6 Discussion and Conclusion

The analysis presented in this chapter has provided some insights into how participants collaborate in the work of entering and closing medical talk in different clinical practices in Mainland China. One surprising finding is the scarcity of a greeting sequence in WM openings. Most of the interviews in the current WM corpus opened with an on-topic talk. Participants in WM encounters were goal-oriented by engaging in activities strictly related to the medical agenda of the interview. This finding is at odds with what has been reported in prior studies with similar clinical settings (e.g., Coupland et al., 1994; Díaz, 2000). One possible explanation is the medical environment in which patients see doctors. During the time when the data were collected, it was observed that doctors in the WM practice were very busy. The waiting area was full of people who arrived an hour before the official visit time started. In addition, as the patients in this research were older adults with chronic illness, they usually came with more than one health problem or a combination of different age-related symptoms. Doctors were often presented with a dilemma between spending more time on each patient and seeing more patients. Therefore, they lacked time to engage in relational work with their patients. As Tu and colleagues (2019) noted, outpatient interaction in Chinese hospitals is a short and problem-focused encounter with an emphasis on efficiency. This is also the case in TCM encounters, as some of the TCM interviews also opened with an on-topical talk. But, compared with WM, TCM openings in this study included more relational work. This is partly because when compared with WM, TCM consultations were more relaxing. As Lam (2001) stated, while WM is mainly used for the identification of illness, physical examination, and operation and treatment, TCM is used more frequently for recuperation, for "cut[ting] the tail of the illness" (p. 763). Participants in TCM encounters may be less stressed and thus more likely to engage in relational work such as greetings and small talk.

Observation of the medical closings reveals similar patterns. Compared with TCM, WM closings were more task-oriented, with participants collaborating in the construction of medical-related tasks such as appointment arrangement and patient education on treatment. One noted feature in WM closings is the absence of a leave-taking sequence, which could be equally explained, at least to some extent, by a large number of visits in WM practice. It was observed that usually before the first patient left the room, the next entered. On the other hand, while the relatively more active engagement of participants in small talk in TCM closings could be an indicator of a closer doctor-patient relationship, it could also be the result of a more casual clinical environment (e.g., the fact that many patients waiting inside the consultation room, talking with each other) in TCM than in WM encounters.

Another possible explanation for the clinical differences in relation to how participants enter and close medical consultations is grounded in the differences between TCM and WM in relation to clinical pathology and philosophy. TCM is conventionally understood as holistic medicine, emphasizing the integrity of physical organs to the outside environment (Luo et al., 2013). It holds the belief that the physical problems of the human body can be explained by a combination of internal and external factors. As Lu and colleagues (2004: p. 1855) argued, TCM highlights the "pathogenicity of social and natural factors". This understanding partially explains the reason that participants collaborate in patient lifestyle education and non-medical small talk at the closing stage of the TCM interviews. On the other hand, WM understands human diseases at more scientific levels, for example, by identifying molecular changes. This is not to claim that WM underestimates the value of non-biomedical causes of human diseases, but rather the two approaches to medicine place different weights on the importance of the external factors on health.

This chapter contributes to the empirical investigation of doctor–older adult conversations and has both theoretical and practical implications. One theoretical contribution concerns the understanding of the boundaries of medical conversation as highly institutionalized social activities that are goal-oriented. As Drew and Heritage (1992: p. 22) put it, "institutional talk is normally informed by goal orientations of a relatively restricted conventional form" and that such talk often involves "special and particular constraints on what one or both of the participants will treat as allowable contributions to the business at hand". In this sense, the findings reported here also contribute to understanding the clinical differences between TCM and WM practices in terms of their clinical "conventional forms" which shape participants' behaviors in communication. Understanding these differences is important as patients may have different expectations of doctors' communication behaviors, and this may, in turn, impact patient satisfaction. In addition, given the trend to provide integrated medicine (i.e., to combine both TCM and WM), knowledge of the clinical conventional forms may facilitate both intra-professional communication and professional-client communication.

It is important to note that this study had some limitations. First and foremost, given that only one hospital is included, it is likely that what is reported here is only a matter of institutional practice rather than a communication practice that is clinically-specific. In addition, given the difficulty of hospital access, the data were collected only from two divisions. Generalization of the findings should thus be cautious. In addition, the findings of communication in WM practice are only applicable to WM practiced in Mainland China. Future research focused on cross-cultural differences could combine current observation with what is observed in WM practice in other cultures.

Acknowledgments The author would like to thank the directors of the Division of Gastroenterology and the Division of Internal Traditional Chinese Medicine, and the participating doctors and patients for their support. The author would also like to thank Dr. Margo L. Turnbull for her advice on the draft of the paper.

References

Bateson, G. (1972). *Steps to an ecology of the mind.* New York: Ballantine.

Benwell, B., & McCreaddie, M. (2016). Keeping "small talk" small in healthcare encounters: Negotiating the boundaries between on- and off-task talk. *Research on Language and Social Interaction, 49,* 258–271.

Chang, L., & Lim, J. C. J. (2019). Traditional Chinese medicine physicians' insights into interprofessional tensions between traditional Chinese medicine and biomedicine: A critical perspective. *Health Communication, 34,* 238–247.

Coupland, J. (2000). Introduction: Sociolinguistic perspectives on small talk. In J. Coupland (Ed.), *small talk* (pp. 1–25). England: Pearson Education Ltd.

Coupland, J., Coupland, N., & Robinson, D. (1992). "How are you?": Negotiating phatic communion. *Language in Society, 21,* 207–230.

Coupland, J., Robinson, D., & Coupland, N. (1994). Frame negotiation in doctor-elderly patient consultations. *Discourse & Society, 5,* 89–124.

Defibaugh, S. (2018). *Nurse practitioners and the performance of professional competency: Accomplishing patient-centered care.* Cham: Palgrave Macmillan.

Díaz, F. (2000). The social organization of chemotherapy treatment consultations. *Sociology of Health & Illness, 22,* 364–389.

Drew, P., & Heritage, J. (1992). Analyzing talk at work: An introduction. In P. Drew & J. Heritage (Eds.), *Talk at work: Interaction in institutional settings* (pp. 3–65). Cambridge: Cambridge University Press.

Eggleston, K., Li, L., Meng, Q.-Y., Lindelow, M., & Wagstaff, A. (2008). Health service delivery in China: A literature review. *Health Economics, 17,* 149–165.

Frankel, R. (1990). Talking in interviews: A dispreference for patient-initiated questions. In G. Psathas (Ed.), *Interactional Competence* (pp. 231–262). New York: Irvington.

Gafaranga, J., & Britten, N. (2003). "Fire away": The opening sequence in general practice consultations. *Family Practice, 20,* 242–247.

Goffman, E. (1981). *Forms of talk.* Philadelphia: University of Pennsylvania Press.

Goffman, E. (1986). *Frame analysis: An essay on the organization of experience.* Boston: Northeastern University Press.

Heath, C. (1981). The opening sequence in doctor-patient interaction. In P. Atkinson & C. Heath (Eds.), *Medical work: Realities and routines* (pp. 71–90). Aldershot, UK: Gower.

Heritage, J., & Robinson, J. D. (2006). The structure of patients' presenting concerns: Physicians opening questions. *Health Communication, 19,* 89–102.

Holmes, J. (2000). Doing collegiality and keeping control at work: Small talk in government departments. In J. Coupland (Ed.), *Small talk* (pp. 32–61). England.

Hudak, P. L. & Maynard, D. W. (2011). An interactional approach to conceptualizing small talk in medical interactions. *Sociology of Health & Illness, 33,* 634-653.

Jefferson, G. (1984). Transcription notation. In J. M. Atkinson & J. Heritage (Eds.), *Structures of social action* (pp. ix–xvi). Cambridge and New York: Cambridge University Press.

Jefferson, G. (2004). Glossary of transcript symbols with an introduction. In G. H. Lerner (Ed.), *Conversation analysis: Studies from the first generation* (pp. 13–31). Philadelphia, PA: John Benjamins Publishing Company.

Jin, Y. (2018). Small talk in medical conversations: Data from China. *Journal of Pragmatics, 134*, 31–44.

Kangasharju, H. & Nikko, T. (2009). Emotions in organizations: Joint laughter in workplace meetings. *Journal of Business Communication, 46*, 100–119.

Laidsaar-Powell, R. C., Butow, P. N., Bu, S., Charles, C., Gafni, A., Lam, W. W. T., ... Juraskova, I. (2013). Physician-patient-companion communication and decision-making: A systematic review of triadic medical consultations. *Patient Education and Counseling, 91*, 3–13.

Lam, T. P. (2001). Strengths and weaknesses of traditional Chinese medicine and western medicine in the eyes of some Hong Kong Chinese. *Journal of Epidemiology and Community Health, 55*, 762–765.

Lu, A. P., Jia, H. W., Xiao, C., & Lu, Q. P. (2004). Theory of traditional Chinese medicine and therapeutic method of diseases. *World Journal of Gastroenterology, 10*, 1854–1856.

Luo, J., Xu, H., & Chen, K. J. (2013). Potential benefits of Chinese herbal medicine for elderly patients with cardiovascular diseases. *Journal of Geriatric Cardiology, 10*, 305–309.

Malinowski, B. (1923). The problem of meaning in primitive languages. In C. K. Ogden & I. A. Richards (Eds.), *The Meaning of meaning* (pp. 296–336). London: Routledge & Kegan Paul.

Mishler, E. G. (1984). *The discourse of medicine: Dialectics of medical interviews*. New Jersey: Ablex Publishing Corporation.

Ragan, S. L. (2000). Sociable talk in women's health care contexts:Ttwo forms of non-medical talk. In J. Coupland (Ed.), *Small talk* (pp. 269–287). England: Pearson Education Ltd.

Rindstedt, C. (2014). Conversational openings and multiparty disambiguations in doctors' encounters with young patients (and their parents). *Text & Talk, 34*, 421–442.

Robinson, J. D. (1998). Getting down to business: Talk, gaze, and body orientation during openings of doctor-patient consultations. *Human Communication Research, 25*, 97–123.

Robinson, J. D. (2001). Closing medical encounters: Two physician practices and their implications for the expression of patients' unstated concerns. *Social Science & Medicine, 53*, 639–656.

Roter, D. L. & Hall, J. A. (2006). *Doctors talking with patients/patients talking with doctors: Improving communication in medical skills* (2nd ed.). Westport: Praeger.

Sacks, H. (1975). Everyone has to lie. In M. Sanches & B. G. Blount (Eds.), *Sociocultural dimensions of language use* (pp. 57–79). New York: Academic Press.

Sarangi, S (2010). Recofiguring self/identity/status/role: The case of professional role performance in healthcare encounters. In G. Garzone & J. Archibald (Eds.), *Discourse, identities and roles in specialized communication* (pp. 33–54). Bern: Peter Lang.

Schegloff, E. A. (1986). The routine as achievement. *Human Studies, 9*, 111–151.

Schegloff, E. A. & Sacks, H. (1973). Opening up closings. *Semiotica, 8*, 289–327.

Silverman, D. (1987). *Communication and medical practice: Social relations in the clinic*. London: Sage.

Ting, X., Yong, B., Yin, L., & Mi, T. (2016). Patient perception and the barriers to participating patient-centered communication: A survey and in-depth interview of Chinese patients and physicians. *Patient Education and Counseling, 99*, 364–369.

Tu, J., Kang, G., Zhong, J. d., & Cheng, Y. (2019). Outpatient communication patterns in a cancer hospital in China: A qualitative study of doctor-patient encounters. *Health Expectations, 22*, 594–603.

Walsh, I. P. (2007). Small talk is "big talk" in clinical discourse: Appreciating the value of conversation in SLP clinical interactions. *Topics in Language Disorders, 27*, 24–36.

Understanding the Co-construction of Medical Consultations in Traditional Chinese Medicine: A Discourse Structural Analysis

Jesse W. C. Yip and Chenjie Zhang

Abstract Findings from previous research on Western medical consultations indicate that the doctor–patient relationship involved in these consultations is mostly asymmetrical. This asymmetry of relationship is clearly revealed in the analysis of participants' conversational dominance in doctor–patient interactions. This chapter argues that the doctor–patient relationship in Traditional Chinese Medicine (TCM) consultations may be different with that in Western medical consultations. With audio recordings and transcriptions of 28 conversations between TCM practitioners and patients, this chapter examines the sequential structure of TCM consultations and speech functions of doctors and patients in the TCM context. The findings show that small talk contributes to a more symmetrical doctor–patient relationship because both the TCM practitioners and patient are engaged in it. The prevalence of explanations indicates the feature of patient-centered approach in TCM consultations. Moreover, the statistical test in speech function frequencies of doctors and patients further supports the claim that the doctor–patient relationship in TCM consultations may be more symmetrical as insignificant differences of the frequencies are observed. Based on the analyses, this chapter further suggests that TCM consultations are co-constructed by both TCM practitioners and patients.

Keywords Discourse analysis · Doctor–patient relationship · Medical consultations · Traditional Chinese medicine

1 Introduction

Traditional Chinese Medicine (TCM) has evolved for more than 2000 years into the most advanced and comprehensive therapeutic approach to medicine in China. Medical providers have increasingly recommended TCM-based approaches as

J. W. C. Yip (✉) · C. Zhang
Department of English, Hong Kong Baptist University, Hong Kong, China
e-mail: jesseyipwaichi@life.hkbu.edu.hk

© Springer Nature Singapore Pte Ltd. 2020
B. Watson and J. Krieger (eds.), *Expanding Horizons in Health Communication*,
The Humanities in Asia 6, https://doi.org/10.1007/978-981-15-4389-0_7

alternative therapies. A growing number of medical schools have acknowledged the importance of concepts originating from TCM for use in disease prevention and holistic treatments. Approximately 75% of U.S. adults have tried holistic medicine. Due to its popularity, researchers from various disciplines, including communication, linguistics, and medicine, have focused on TCM discourse as a means of improving the quality and effectiveness of doctor–patient communication. However, few studies have explored communication in TCM consultations (e.g., Gu, 1996, 1999; Zhao, 1999), and even less research has considered contemporary practices in doctor–patient communication in these consultations. Following nearly two decades of rapid evolution, TCM practitioners' approaches to medical consultations likely differ from past forms of practice. This chapter critically examines communicative practice in TCM consultations, investigating the generic structure of TCM consultations and corresponding speech functions of practitioners and patients. Findings oppose the claims of an asymmetrical doctor–patient relationship in TCM consultations (Gu, 1996; Zhao, 1999), suggesting that the consultations are co-constructed by medical providers and patients.

2 Asymmetry in the Doctor–Patient Relationship

In the communication field, the doctor–patient relationship has been described as inequitable (Cordella, 2004; Harvey & Koteyko, 2013; Pilnick & Dingwell, 2011). This asymmetry is reflected in institutional contexts where the institutional organization endows the authority with power to pursue defined goals (Fisher & Todd, 1986). Doctors who are familiar with hospital or clinic operations can make informed decisions regarding their patients' health; conversely, patients are outsiders who may be unaware of the medical procedures involved in their treatment (Cordella, 2004). Moreover, doctors have received professional training, whereas patients seldom possess expertise around treating illness. Therefore, doctors assume a dominant role in patient interactions. The inherent asymmetry of the doctor–patient relationship has also been recognized in Chinese medical contexts. Pun, Chan, Wang, and Slade (2018) conducted an integrative review of doctor–patient communication in Asian contexts and suggested that a doctor-centered communication style was more common for Chinese patients. For example, Yin, Hsu, Kuo and Huang (2012) found that doctors in Taiwan displayed a lower level of politeness through using "bald-on-record, direct, and non-redressed" communication styles.

Despite a limited number of relevant studies, some research has indicated that the doctor–patient relationship in TCM is similar to that in Western medicine. Gu (1996) framed doctor–patient communication in TCM as a goal-centered interaction, wherein interlocutors shared a goal of treating a patient's illness but pursued the objective differently. Doctors approached this goal in a rather routinized manner, whereas patients tended to be guided by anxiety and folk beliefs (e.g., the importance of following doctors' advice and worries about death). Gu (1996) argued that realizing this common goal resulted in expectation disparities, over-informativeness about the consultation, and relational asymmetry. Zhao (1999) revealed such asymmetry by investigating sequencing, topic development, and diagnostic information in Chinese medical interviews, pointing out several patterns. First, medical practitioners mostly initiated questions but patients rarely asked them: out of 383 questions identified in diagnostic interviews, 87.4% were raised by doctors with only the remainder posed by patients. Second, doctors determined the topics appropriate for discussion and limited patients' contributions, jumping from topic to topic without negotiating with patients. This proposition was supported by a study by Ohtaki, Ohtaki and Fetters (2003), who argued that doctors in the U.S. and Japan controlled communication with patients by asking more questions than patients did. Lastly, Zhao (1999) found that doctors delivered diagnostic information, prescribed medicine, or suggested a follow-up consultation without any explanation.

However, this asymmetrical relationship in doctor–patient communication in Asian contexts appears to have undergone a gradual change in which patient autonomy, including the rights to be active participants in shared decision making, is becoming more prominent (Pun et al., 2018). Essentially, patient-centered care has begun replacing doctor-centered communication in medical consultations. Patient-centered care suggests that patients' preferences, needs, and beliefs should be elicited and that patients should be engaged and respected as informed participants (Slade et al., 2015). Despite relevant emerging trends in doctor–patient communication, no studies have provided empirical evidence to support these observations.

3 Sequential Structures, Speech Functions, and the Doctor–Patient Relationship

Investigating the sequential structure of medical consultations and participants' speech functions during consultations can enhance understanding of how consultations are constructed and offer insights into the doctor–patient relationship within such consultations. The structure of interactions includes various moves, and recognizing specific moves in consultations can reveal the general operation and sociocultural features of doctor–patient communication in a TCM context. Byrne and Long (1976) called interactional moves "phases", denoting a logical sequence of routine events. Relevant moves in medical consultations are driven by and composed of interlocutors' various speech functions. For example, the move of diagnostic examination in medical consultations can be initiated by doctors' speech functions of questioning or commanding and ended by patients' speech functions of compliance. Revealing moves and their related speech functions among participants provide two valuable insights. The first concerns a doctor's and patient's participation in each move; by identifying the frequencies of participants' speech functions in moves, researchers can observe which participant (doctor or patient) dominates which move. The second revelation involves uncovering the doctor–patient relationship in medical consultations based on speech functions (i.e., symmetrical or asymmetrical). In this context, the doctor–patient relationship refers to the extent to which each participant dominates the conversation rather than the social distance or intimacy between participants. For instance, small talk is a move indicating an equal relationship between a doctor and patient because the doctor no longer dominates the conversation based on his or her expertise and institutional authority in Western medicine or TCM consultations (see Jin, 2018). The supplementary speech functions of tracking and challenging reveal a relatively more equitable exchange between doctors and patients, such as in a study, wherein patients tracked and challenged doctors' statements during medical consultations in the Accident and Emergency Department of a Hong Kong hospital (Slade et al., 2016).

Studies investigating the sequential structure of medical consultations have suggested that most moves are doctor-dominant, which leads to an asymmetrical doctor–patient relationship. Byrne and Long (1976) examined 2500 medical interviews in England and New Zealand and generalized a phase model of six moves common in Western medical consultations: (a) establishing a doctor–patient relationship; (b) exploring the reason(s) for the visit; (c) conducting examinations; (d) evaluating the patient's condition; (e) outlining a treatment plan; and (f) terminating the consultation. Although Byrne and Long's study is over 40 years old, its findings remain influential and provide a paradigmatic routine for doctor–patient consultations. More recent studies on doctor–patient interactions have referenced that study (e.g., Mishler, 1984; Neighbour, 1987; Ohtaki et al., 2003). In particular, Ohtaki et al. (2003) compared moves in doctor–patient communication in the U.S. and Japan, noting that the move of social talk (occurring within non-problem-focused casual conversations) could be an addition to Byrne and Long's model. This new move implies that the sequential structure of medical consultations can evolve, and the doctor–patient relationship in medical consultations may change accordingly.

Despite several studies exploring the sequential structure and doctor–patient relationship in Western medical consultations, few have shed light on similar elements of TCM consultations. Gu (1996) illustrated the general structure of communication in TCM consultations in five phases, namely *jiezhen* (接診), *zhenduan* (診斷), *lifa* (立法), *chufang* (處方), and *tiaoli* (調理). *Jiezhen* entails eliciting and evaluating patients' reports of illness; *zhenduan* refers to diagnosing; *lifa* accounts for identifying principles to treat illness; *chufang* is prescription; and *tiaoli* captures recuperative measures. To the authors' knowledge, Gu's (1996) work remains the only research to highlight the communicative structure of TCM consultations. However, the study did not account for evolution in the doctor–patient relationship or the sequential structure of consultations over time as the Chinese health and medical system develops; thus, it is necessary to re-examine the structure of TCM consultations in contemporary practices. This study explores the sequential structure of TCM consultations by highlighting pertinent moves and their related speech functions among practitioners and patients to illustrate how TCM consultations are structured and how the doctor–patient relationship manifests in these sessions.

4 Methodology

4.1 Data Collection

Data collected for this study were taken from TCM consultations between Chinese healthcare practitioners and patients in a public hospital in Zhengzhou, Henan province, China. To consult a practitioner, people were required to register and queue up in a room that was divided into a waiting zone and consultation area. While one person was consulting with a practitioner, others were waiting in the waiting zone. People in the queue could chime in or otherwise interrupt conversations between the practitioner and the consulting patient. TCM practitioners tended not to immediately prohibit participation from patients who were waiting. A waiting patient who suffered from an illness similar to that of the consulting patient might express support for him or her, such as by encouraging the consulting patient to trust the practitioner, to comply with treatment recommendations, or to maintain a healthy lifestyle. Normally, waiting patients who joined the conversation would withdraw from the conversation quickly. Most consulting persons suffered from general or chronic illnesses, such as insomnia, stomachache, cold, or fever.

Consultations were recorded by the second author after obtaining ethnical consent from the hospital, 4 participating doctors, and 28 patients. Each practitioner met with seven patients. The entire recording procedure spanned 3 weeks in 2017. Consultations were held in Mandarin. The recordings totaled 6 hours and 4 minutes and were transcribed in simplified Chinese to compile a corpus of TCM consultations. The corpus consisted of 28 transcribed cases; dialogues with waiting patients were not included in the corpus.

4.2 Data Analysis

The authors initially read the data carefully and iteratively to obtain a general understanding of the conversations. The ensuing analysis was divided into two phases: move analysis and speech functions analysis. Move analysis was conducted to identify possible moves in medical consultations, whereas speech functions analysis aimed to disclose speech functions between a TCM practitioner and patient. Moves and speech functions are interrelated; a move can be initiated, maintained, and terminated by various speech functions.

4.3 Move Analysis

Move analysis enables researchers to define textual boundaries between moves in discourse on the basis of moves' content and linguistic criteria (Swales, 1990). In this study, a *move* is defined as a logical sequence of TCM consultations. All transcripts in the corpus were analyzed to reveal moves in the consultations. Transcripts were divided into moves and steps (i.e., sub-categories of moves). Analyses considered the rhythm and intonation of interlocutors' utterances. The authors began by analyzing complete conversations to generalize the basic sequence in medical consultations; such generalization helped to confirm that subsequent identification of moves and steps was valid and authentic. Before formal analysis, eight transcripts of cases were randomly selected from the corpus and analyzed independently by the authors. The authors compared the identified moves and steps in the chosen transcripts and generalized a schema for subsequent analyses. Contradictory codes were discussed and re-analyzed as necessary. Changes in the course of analysis (i.e., the addition, deletion, or sequence of moves) were marked to obtain a final move structure across all transcripts. The authors concurred on the final coding of all transcripts.

4.4 Analysis of Speech Functions

The second phase of data analysis involved identifying the speech functions in conversations according to the Initiation-Response-Follow-up (IRF) model. Drawing upon knowledge of Systemic Functional Linguistics (Halliday & Matthiessen, 2014), the model was proposed by Pun, Matthiessen, Williams, and Slade (2017), who suggested coding exchanges for three main types of speech functions: initiating, responding, and following up. The current authors selected eight random samples from the corpus of TCM consultation cases to conduct a pilot study using IRF analysis. The IRF model appeared to oversimplify exchange structures in TCM consultations, which contained speech functions other than initiation, response, and follow-up. Modifications were made to increase the applicability of the model. As interlocutors used several speech functions to extend the continuity of a given topic, extension was incorporated into the model as a speech function category. The "follow-up" category in the original scheme was eliminated due to overlap with the "extension" sub-category. Accordingly, this study focuses on three speech functions in analysis: Initiation (I), Extension (E), and Response (R).

The extension category consisted of three sub-categories: development, register, and rejoinder. *Development* refers to an expansion of what another interlocutor uttered; *register* refers to repetition of the words of the interlocutor or a news marker (e.g., "Really?") to encourage the interlocutor to continue speaking; and *rejoinder* refers to checking or challenging what the interlocutor said (Eggins &

Slade, 1997). The "follow-up" category was omitted to avoid categorical overlap with the sub-category "register". Given the above alterations, the authors proposed the IER model as better suited to analyzing conversations in TCM consultations. This model allows exchanges among doctors and patients in TCM consultations to be coded for initiation, extension, and response as three main speech function categories. The added category of *extension* and its sub-categories accounted for the speech functions speakers are used to extend the continuity of speech. All transcripts in the corpus were coded according to the modified IER model; Table 1 provides a model summary and examples.

Table 1 IER model in the context of TCM consultations

Initiation (I)	Extension (E)	Response (R)
Statement 中医讲此皆聚于肺 (胃) 观于胃 (肺). 你的病好像是咳嗽在肺, 但是是胃上的事 In TCM theory, external evil invades the stomach, and it leads to illness in the lungs. Your illness looks like a cough from the lungs, but its root is your stomach	*Development* 那我得饮食上注意了看来 Then I need to pay attention to my diet *Register* 真的啊? Really? *Rejoinder* 胃的问题? Problems with my stomach?	*Acknowledgement* 好的 Okay *Contradiction* 这听着还挺奇怪了 That sounds strange
Offer 开7天的药啊 I will provide herbal medicine for 7 days		*Acceptance* 行 OK *Rejection* 太多了呀 That's too much.
Question 夜里咳不咳? Do you cough at night?		*Answer* 有时候夜里也咳 Sometimes I also cough at night *Disclaimer* 我也记不清了 I can't remember
Command 晚上最多熬到十点, 就不要再晚了 You may stay up until 10 pm at most, but no later than that		*Compliance* 行,我明白了 OK, I see *Refusal* 那都不现实. 我太忙了 That is impossible. I am too busy
Greeting/Degreeting 你好/再见 Hello/Bye		*Response to greeting* 你好/再见 Hello/Bye

Inter-coder reliability was assessed to ensure coding accuracy and consistency. The first and second authors coded 14 transcripts independently according to the IER model. Coded transcripts were later compared. The authors discussed differences between codes and agreed on approximately 97% of classifications. The authors consulted two professors whose specializations were Discourse Analysis and Systematic Functional Linguistics about every case where the authors had not agreed on the codes, discussed and eventually reached consensus on all the coding. Frequencies for each identified speech function of the IER model in transcripts were counted and used in a *t*-test to compare the frequencies of speech functions in the moves between practitioners and patients in the 28 consultations. A *t*-test is a measure to determine the likelihood of difference between two sets of data. The test was employed in this study to determine whether the speech functions of TCM practitioners and patients during moves in TCM consultations were significantly different.

5 Findings

The findings of this study are divided into two main parts: move analysis and analysis of speech functions in moves. The first part investigates the sequential structure of TCM consultations and reveals the moves and steps in consultations. The second part compares speech function frequencies between TCM practitioners and patients according to the IER model and relates the frequencies to the identified moves.

5.1 Move Analysis

This section opens with a move analysis to reveal the moves involved in TCM consultations to manifest the basic move structure of consultations. The following sub-sections focus on specific moves and their steps with corresponding examples.

Excerpt 1

Context: The patient, a middle-aged woman, had a fever with symptoms including cough, dizziness, and insomnia. This was a follow-up TCM consultation:

1. Patient: 上礼拜发烧了，39 度。烧了，就光干咳样了。头晕，睡不着。

   I had a high fever last week, 39 degrees centigrade. The fever, just like the dry cough. I feel dizzy and can't fall asleep.

2. Doctor: 你也是光想给孩子吃好的，你也跟住吃好了。

   You always want to prepare fatty foods for the children. Then you eat with them.

3. Patient: 还是吃太好了。

   Because I eat too much fatty food.

4. TCM Practitioner: 烧了几天？

   How long did you have the fever?

5. Patient: 烧了三天。

   For three days.

6. TCM Practitioner: 你吃了什么药？

   What medicine did you take?

7. Patient: 我？我都不吃药。正好今天过来了。要不然我都不来了。

   Me? I usually take nothing. I was just nearby today. Otherwise, I would not have visited you.

8. TCM Practitioner: 你不吃药你咋好啊? 哈哈。

How did you recover if you did not take any medicine?

Ha-ha.

9. Patient: 烧，就让它烧。烧到最后喝喝水，喝喝汤。

Let the fever run its course. I drank water and soup afterwards.

10. TCM Practitioner: 咦，这也是个法子哈哈。

Oh, what a solution, ha-ha.

11. Patient: 38 度，然后就 39 度。烧的浑身冷，胳膊和指头缝里都觉得冷。

12. 最后鼻子里的气儿我觉得都难受都是热的，身上冒的气儿感觉都 13. 是热的。

38 degrees Celsius, and then 39 degrees Celsius. The fever made my whole body cold, even my arms and fingers. Eventually, it felt like the air from my nose was hot and the air around my whole body was hot, too.

14. TCM Practitioner: 那还不给妞妞送到奶奶那?

Then, why not take [your granddaughter] to her grandmother's place?

15. Patient: 那不是想着她周六才回来再给她送过去。她家人少，在屋里不是

16. 急。

What I was thinking was that I would take her there after her mother came back Saturday. There were only a few family members home, and she might be bored.

17.　　　(8s)

18. TCM Practitioner: 我看你舌头。

　　　　　　　Let me look at your tongue.

19. Patient:　　那还是吃菜少。

20.　　　　　(5s)

　　　　　I still eat too few vegetables.

21.　　　　　还得吃菜，抓紧吃菜。

22.　　　　　(3s)

　　　　　I need to eat more vegetables immediately.

23. TCM Practitioner: 吃青菜是好事啊。高维生素啊。

　　　　　　　Eating vegetables is good. They are rich in vitamins.

24. Patient: 那天李伟说："人家中医大夫也喝酒啊，我以为中医都不喝酒

25. 了。早知道我给人家弄点送点好酒了。"

　　　　　　One day, Li Wei said, "The TCM doctors also drink wine. I

　　　　　　assumed that TCM doctors did not drink. If I had known that, I

　　　　　　would have given them bottles of good wine."

26. TCM Practitioner: 他那喝酒的人，那么小的量，他坚持不了。

　　　　　　　A man who likes drinking wine as much as him cannot

　　　　　　　control himself with a small regular amount.

27. Patient:　　　嗯，他说蚊子都不咬他，因为血里都是酒。

　　　　　　　　Yes, he said the mosquitos did not bite him because his blood contained lots of wine.

28. TCM Practitioner: 哈哈哈。

　　　　　　　　Hahaha.

29.　　　　　　　（29s）

30. Patient:　　　就那干咳样了，一阵一阵的，也不勤反正。

　　　　　　　　Just the dry cough, intermittent, not frequent anyway.

31.　　　　　　　（3s）

32.　　　　　　　烧那两天，天天咳反正。

　　　　　　　　I cough every day when I suffer from a fever.

33.　　　　　　　（43s）

34. TCM Practitioner: 开一周？

　　　　　　　　I'll give you a one-week prescription?

35. Patient:　　　嗯，下礼拜我再来。

　　　　　　　　Yes, I will see you next week.

The consultation was initiated by the patient who described her symptoms of illness (Line 1), after which the TCM practitioner explained the illness in a humorous way (Line 2). The following move (Lines 4–10) was a diagnostic examination, wherein the practitioner probed the patient's situation. The practitioner asked questions about how long the patient had had a fever, whether she had taken medicine, and how she had dealt with her sickness. The patient described her symptoms in greater detail in Lines 11–13. Interestingly, the practitioner engaged in seemingly off-topic small talk in Line 14; the practitioner asked why the patient did not bring her granddaughter to the other grandmother's place. The patient did not appear surprised with the immediate switch of topic and responded to the practitioner in Lines 15–16. Then the practitioner conducted a physical examination by checking the patient's tongue in Line 18. The diagnostic examination ended at this time. Notably, the patient proposed her own advice in Lines 19 and 21. The practitioner then affirmed the advice in Line 23, signaling co-construction of advice in Lines 19 and 21. Additional small talk occurred in Lines 23–28, during which the interlocutors discussed drinking alcohol and family anecdotes. Afterwards, the patient emphasized her symptom of a cough in Lines 30 and 32. At the end of the consultation, the practitioner prescribed herbal medicine for the patient (Line 34) in an interrogative. The consultation closed when the patient answered the practitioner's question about the treatment period and scheduled a subsequent appointment in Line 35.

Several moves were identified in the above analysis, including information elicitation (Line 1; Lines 11–13; Lines 30–32), diagnostic examination (Lines 4–10; Line 18), treatment planning (Lines 19–23; Line 34), small talk (Lines 14–16; Lines 23–28), and explanation (Lines 2–3). Steps appeared in some of the moves; specific steps are discussed in the analysis of each move below. This move structure was a common and logical sequence; slight variances were observed on a case-by-case basis. The identified moves and steps could be postponed, advanced, or repeated throughout a consultation for various reasons. No absolute sequence of moves and steps was identified in the corpus. The basic move structure of TCM consultations is generalized in Table 2.

Table 2 shows the predominant move structure of doctor-patient conversations in TCM consultations. Information elicitation, diagnostic examination, and treatment planning were predominant, appearing in 75% or more of analyzed TCM consultations. Most prevalent moves occurred when investigating patients' illnesses

Table 2 Moves and steps in TCM consultations

Moves	Descriptions	Number of cases ($N = 28$)	Percentage (%)
1. Information elicitation	Probing for information about consulting persons' illness symptoms and lifestyle	21	75
2. Diagnostic examination	Conducting an examination, which may consist of inspection, auscultation and olfaction, inquiry, and pulse-feeling and palpation (*wang wen wen qie*, 望闻问切)	28	100
3. Treatment planning	Proposing treatments (e.g., herb composition/dosage; various Chinese medical therapies)	26	92.8
4. Closing	Ending conversations and reminding the consulting persons of advice from the consultation	12	42.9
Small talk[a]	Off-topic interactions	24	85.7
Explanation[a]	Explaining causes of sickness, proposed treatments, and prescriptions	28	100

[a]Side moves occurring within the other four moves

and health status. The diagnostic examination move occurred in all consultations. Small talk and explanation constituted side moves within the four main moves. Small talk played a unique role in TCM consultations, as the frequency of this move was much higher in TCM consultations than in Western medical consultations (Ohtaki et al., 2003). Frequent occurrences of explanation indicated that TCM practitioners were willing to help patients understand the causes of illness as well as the rationale behind recommended treatment and prescriptions.

5.1.1 Information Elicitation Move

Information elicitation is vital in medical consultations because medical providers must collect sufficient information to diagnose illnesses and prescribe medicine accordingly.

Excerpt 2

1. Patient: 好多了，痰也能吐出来了。然后，咳嗽胸也没那么疼了。但是还

2.   是这个星期比较明显，就是到...下午四五点那会儿，有时候感觉头

3.   有点晕，身上没劲。上午没事，上午有时候出去然后都没事，但

4.   是下午有时候可能会觉得身上没劲。然后我下午都睡觉。

I feel much better. The phlegm can be spit out. My chest is not as painful as [it was] before when coughing. But it was more distinct this week at 4 or 5 pm. I'll sometimes feel dizzy and exhausted [around that time]. I feel fine in the morning, even if I go out. But I feel exhausted in the afternoon. And I often sleep in the afternoon.

5. TCM Practitioner: 那你等过两天上班了下午也睡觉啊？

So, did you take a nap several days later when you went back to work?

6. Patient: 那肯定不行了，所以我说这不知道怎么回事。

That's certainly impossible, so I said I didn't know what happened.

The above example demonstrates that the patient provided information by actively describing her symptoms, such as a severe cough and dizziness (Lines 1–4). The practitioner requested more details about the patient's life related to her symptoms in Line 5, which she provided in Line 6.

5.1.2 Diagnostic Examination Move

TCM practitioners emphasize diagnostic methods of Chinese medicine, particularly four steps (*sizhen*, 四診): inspection (*wang*, 望), auscultation and olfaction (*wen*, 聞), inquiry (*wen*, 問), and pulse-feeling and palpation (*qie*, 切) (Wu & Lu, 2007). Whereas biomedical physicians approach diagnosis by referring to a patient's personal history, physical symptoms, and blood or urine samples (as part of laboratory tests), TCM practictioners tend to diagnose through observations of the tongue and pulse (Zwickey & Schiffke, 2007). The diagnostic examination in TCM consultations includes two steps, verbal examination and discussing lifestyle and other conditions.

Table 3 shows that the selected TCM practitioners tended to conduct verbal examinations. Chinese medicine is akin to experiential medicine in that it does not depend on scientific medical examinations, such as electrocardiograms, blood tests, and X-rays. Li (2011) termed the practice of TCM a "thought experiment", whereas Western medicine is a "scientific experiment". TCM practitioners in this study asked questions about patients' conditions when conducting examinations; nearly 80% of consultations involved discussing lifestyle and other conditions. This step indicated that practitioners cared about the lifeworld of patients, which is thought to affect overall health from a TCM perspective.

Verbal examination is important for TCM practitioners to diagnose patients' illness or disease, as this step enables them to learn more about patients' medical conditions.

Table 3 Steps of diagnostic examination

Steps	Number of cases ($N = 28$)	Percentage (%)
Verbal examination	16	57.1
Discussing lifestyle and other conditions	22	78.5

Excerpt 3

1. Patient: （咳嗽）咳嗽。

   (Cough) Cough.

2. TCM Practitioner: 夜里咳不咳啊？

   Do you cough at night?

3. Patient: 夜里有时候也咳，好像嗯...

   Yes, I cough at night. It's like...Umm.

4. TCM Practitioner: 后半夜还是白天咳？不是，后半夜前半夜咳？

   Cough at midnight or in the daytime? No, cough early in the
   night or near dawn?

5. Patient: 不一定哪一会儿都是。

   Just coughing irregularly.

6. TCM Practitioner: 以前咳...以前经常咳嗽么？

   You coughed before... Have you coughed for a while?

7. Patient: 没有。

   No.

8. TCM Practitioner: 没有，就是说喘的...胸口的气出不来的。

   No, it's labored breathing... difficult to release air in the chest.

9. Patient: 就是好像...嗯...有气往上顶了。

   It's like... Umm.... There is air stuck inside.

Verbal Examination Step

The above example illustrates a typical verbal examination in medical consultations, wherein doctors often want to know the duration of patients' illness and which medicines they have taken, if any. In Excerpt 3, the TCM practitioner dug deeply into the patient's symptom, a cough. Once the patient told the practitioner she had coughed in Line 1, the practitioner asked consecutive questions related to specific features of the cough in Lines 2, 4, and 6. A preliminary diagnostic judgment based on the preceding verbal examination came in Line 8, at which point the practitioner speculated that the patient was in fact experiencing labored breathing.

Discussing Lifestyle and Other Conditions Step

The emphasis of TCM on patients' lifestyle largely differentiates this practice from Western medicine. TCM practitioners believe they can diagnose illness more accurately through knowledge of the patient's lifeworld, which is presumably related to human health.

Excerpt 4

1. TCM Practitioner: 最近有点累着了是不是？

   You have been a little tired recently, right?

2. Patient: 嗯，累。

   Umm, tired.

3. TCM Practitioner: 有点累着了。

   A little tired.

The TCM practitioner in Excerpt 4 inferred that the patient had been tired recently to discover the patient's current condition (Line 1), confirmed by the patient's agreement (Lines 2–3). In another example, the practitioner also paid attention to the patient's mental health. The following instance shows the practitioner asking if the patient was in a good mood (Line 1) and then verifying the patient's mood stability (Line 3).

Excerpt 5

1. TCM Practitioner: 你情绪心情有没有好一点？

   Are you in a good mood?

2. Patient: 心情我觉得一直都觉得还可以。

   I think my mood is usually fine.

3. TCM Practitioner: 还行 哈？

   It is fine, right?

4. Patient: 嗯。心情一直都挺好的。

   Umm. Mood is fine.

   上班回去啊，觉得，下班再回去歇歇啊，吃点……有时候饭都不吃，

   我就吃水果。就吃吃，吃不少晚上的。

   When going home after work, I think I can rest and eat

   something...sometimes I do not have dinner, just fruit. I keep eating and eat

   a lot in the evening.

Causes of a disease in Chinese medicine are related to external and internal pathogenic factors (Ody, 2014). External factors refer to living conditions, such as climate and weather, which can invade the body from the outside to result in disease; internal factors include emotions, such as joy, anger, and sadness, which may attack relevant organs (Ody, 2014). Thus, TCM practitioners must possess knowledge of patients' daily lives for the diagnostic examination move. In Excerpt 5, the TCM practitioner was concerned with the patient's mood in Line 1 and then confirmed its stability in Line 3.

5.1.3 Treatment Planning Move

Treatment planning was the most prevalent move in TCM consultations, appearing in more than 90% of analyzed conversations. The move includes two steps, namely giving a prescription and giving advice.

Table 4 Treatment planning steps

Steps	Number of cases ($N = 28$)	Percentage (%)
Offering advice	25	89.3
Giving prescription	21	75

As revealed in Table 4, the "offering advice" step occurred relatively more frequently than the "giving prescription" step; this may be due to TCM practitioners' emphasis on advising patients to apply dietary and lifestyle changes to promote recovery and overall health.

Offering Advice Step

Advice giving was a common step in the treatment planning move, in which practitioners offered lifestyle-related suggestions (e.g., recommended modifications to patients' eating habits).

Excerpt 6

TCM Practitioner: 坚持运动。

                  Keep exercising.

Patient: 我运动着了啊。一三五我都坚持都没停。

           I often exercise. I exercise regularly with no breaks every Monday,

           Wednesday, and Friday.

Excerpt 7

TCM Practitioner: 血糖这个不要轻易吃西药。

                  For the blood sugar, please don't take Western medicine without

                    careful consideration.

Patient: 嗯，我不想看西医。

           Yes, I don't want to visit a Western Medicine doctor.

As shown in the above excerpts, practitioners recommended that patients exercise regularly (Excerpt 6) and be cautious about taking Western medicine to treat blood sugar problems (Excerpt 7). This move highlights differences between TCM and Western medicine; whereas Western medicine doctors tend to prescribe drugs and supplements, TCM practitioners prescribe herbal compositions and provide advice regarding patients' diet and lifestyle. Such advice often assumed an imperative form.

Giving Prescription Step

Selected practitioners applied TCM theories and experiential knowledge to formulate appropriate, effective herbal compositions and dosages for their patients.

Excerpt 8

1. TCM Practitioner: 我这个月给你化化湿啊。

   I will prescribe an herbal composition to eliminate your dampness

   this month.

2. TCM Practitioner: 你家里有薏米么？

   Do you have Job's-tears seeds at home?

3. Patient: 有。

   Yes.

4. TCM Practitioner: 你加点薏米进去。我就不给你开了。

   Add some Job's-tears seeds to the medicine. Then, I

   will not need to write them on the prescription.

5. Patient: 好啊。

   OK.

5.1.4 Small Talk Move

Studies have outlined several major functions of small talk. Malinowski (1972) suggested that small talk is a form of phatic communication with an aim of achieving companionship. Laver (1975, p. 217) later proposed three social functions of small talk: a "propitiatory function" to avoid silence-led hostility, an "exploratory function" for interlocutors to reach a consensus, and an "initiatory function" to complete business. Regardless of the specific function of small talk in medical consultations, a general purpose of small talk is phatic communication. A recent comparison of small talk between Western and Chinese medical visits (Jin, 2018) found that more frequent small talk at different conversational stages in TCM consultations indicated greater acquaintance between doctors and patients. The following excerpt demonstrates functions of small talk in TCM consultations.

Excerpt 9

1. TCM Practitioner: 你这回是自个煮 (药) 了不是？自己煮的吧？

    Did you boil the herbal medicine by yourself last time? You

    boiled it yourself?

2. Patient: 自己煮。

    By myself.

3. Patient: 我买了一个自动锅，可好用了。

    I bought an automatic pot, really convenient.

4. TCM Practitioner: 行。

    OK.

5. Patient: 就那个自动壶，紫砂壶，特别好用。

    The electronic pot is a teapot. It's really user-friendly.

6. TCM Practitioner: 放那就行了也煮不干？

    You can just leave it and it won't run out of water?

7. Patient: 放那就好，煮不干。它煮到一定时候它叫唤，一叫唤，你正好篦出

8.   半碗水来。特别好。

    Right, it won't. It will alert you at a certain time. When it

    beeps, you just pour out a half-bowl of liquid. Extremely good.

9. TCM Practitioner: 嗯。

    Hmm.

10. Patient: 我都用第二个了。特别好用。

   It's my second one. Very convenient.

11. TCM Practitioner: 有点咳嗽。干咳么？

   You have a little cough. Dry cough?

12. Patient: 干咳嗽。

   Dry cough.

Excerpt 10

TCM Practitioner: 十天半月熬的夜都过不来劲。晚上最多熬到十点，就不要再晚

了。第二天早上六点五点起床都没事。这就是夜里，就是叫你休息了。你任何

与自然不配合，气候啊等等，不听话熬夜，那身体它不会太好。

You may not recover in even 10 days or half a month after staying up too late. You

should only stay up until 10 pm at most. Don't stay up later than that. It is okay if you

get up at 5 or 6 am the next morning. You should sleep at night. Any behaviors that

go against nature, such as the climate and so on – if you stay up late without obeying

nature, it may make the human body unhealthy.

   The small talk in Excerpt 9 was initiated by the patient (Line 3) after telling the practitioner that she could boil the herbal medicine by herself (Line 2). Lines 1 and 2 comprise a complete adjacent pair: the topic of small talk was derived from the previous topic (Lines 1–2), which was related to how the patient could take medicine (boiling it in the hospital or at home). In small talk (Lines 3–10), the interactants discussed the usefulness of the patient's newly purchased electronic pot. Topics in small talk are often "non-controversial" (Holmes, 2005). In Line 10, the practitioner terminated small talk and shifted the topic to the patient's symptoms, after which the conversation entered the diagnostic examination move. This pattern aligns with Holmes' (2000, p. 53) claim that the superior party in an interaction usually has the power to "minimize, or cut off small talk and get on to business". Although doctors may temporarily inactivate their professional role and treat a patient as a friend through more casual conversation (Ribeiro, 2003), the TCM practitioner in Excerpt 9 stopped small talk to continue the medical consultation.

5.1.5 Explanation Move

Explaining is a necessary side move in TCM consultations. As shown in Table 2, all consultations in this study involved this move. Its prevalence is contrary to Zhao's study (1999) in which doctors often delivered diagnostic information, prescribed medicine, or suggested a follow-up consultation without any explanation. In TCM practice, the need to explain patient-centered recommendations or treatments tends to be related to the concept of *holism*, wherein a patient's lifestyle, social life, and environment are mutually influential to health.

In Excerpt 10, the practitioner advised the patient not to stay up late and explained that anything contradictive to nature or climate could harm the human body. This explanation was based on a holistic view in Chinese medicine, "nature and humans in one" (*tian ren he yi*, 天人合); this perspective posits that humans and the natural environment are integrated in the world, which is derived from five elements—metal (*jin*, 金), wood (*mu*, 木), fire (*huo*, 火), earth (*tu*, 土), and water (*shui*, 水)—and that humans' organs are connected to these elements. For example, the liver is connected with wood and the kidney is connected with water. Within this link, humans who behave unnaturally, such as by staying up excessively late, are likely damaging their bodies. In short, the explaining move often involves principles and philosophy of Chinese medicine and tends to be dominant among TCM practitioners. The following section explicates speech functions of selected TCM practitioners and patients.

6 Speech Functions in Moves

A *t*-test was used to compare the frequencies of speech functions between TCM practitioners and patients to gauge the doctor–patient relationship in consultations (i.e., as either symmetrical or asymmetrical).

As revealed in Table 5, the frequencies of major speech functions, including initiation, extension, and response, were not significantly different among practitioners and patients. First, regarding conversational dominance, Eggins and Slade (1997) stated in their speech function theory that initiation is an important element reflecting interlocutor dominance in a conversation. As shown in Table 5, initiation frequencies between TCM practitioners and patients were not significantly different. Thus, practitioners and patients both had opportunities to dominate conversations, despite discrepant mechanisms of domination; for example, patients produced more statements to initiate moves and doctors tended to use commands. In terms of extension, the speech functions of development and register denote the extent to which speakers accept previous speakers' propositions (i.e., speakers express themselves by building on and expanding previous speakers' propositions) (Eggins & Slade, 1997). Table 5 indicates that the frequencies of extension speech functions among participants were not significantly different, implying that participants demonstrated a similar degree of acceptance toward each other's propositions. Lastly, the speech function of response indicates speakers' attitudes toward previous speakers' propositions. Supporting responses include speech functions of acknowledgement, acceptance, response, and compliance; confrontational responses include contradiction, rejection, disclaimer, and refusal. The t-test results in Table 5 reveal that TCM practitioners and patients were not distinct in their frequencies of supporting or confronting one another's propositions. Overall, the findings in Table 5 suggest that the relationships between TCM practitioners and patients were largely symmetrical, since both parties' participation was analogous in terms of speech function frequencies. This finding challenged the claim that TCM practitioners played a dominant role in medical consultations, leading to asymmetrical relationships with patients (Gu, 1996; Zhao, 1999). Analyses of

Table 5 Comparison of speech functions of TCM practitioners and patients

Speech functions	TCM Practitioners		Patients			Significant
	Mean	SD	Mean	SD	t-test value	Difference
Initiation	25.90	28.34	18.90	17.17	0.35[*]	No
Statement	9.15	10.47	18.90	17.17	0.04[#]	Yes
Offer	0.00	0.00	0.05	0.22	0.33[*]	No
Question	11.65	15.52	5.90	6.64	0.14[*]	No
Command	4.80	4.79	0.70	1.45	0.00[#]	Yes
Greeting/Degreeting	0.35	0.49	0.15	0.37	0.15[*]	No
Extension	9.75	3.13	10.45	7.07	0.68[*]	No
Development	7.95	3.05	9.25	6.61	0.43[*]	No
Rejoinder	0.85	1.35	0.75	1.12	0.8[*]	No
Register	0.95	1.05	0.45	0.69	0.084[*]	No
Response	12.30	11.66	20.80	26.71	0.20[*]	No
Acknowledgement	2.95	3.46	4.45	6.61	0.38[*]	No
Contradiction	3.15	3.79	1.45	1.88	0.08[*]	No
Acceptance	0.00	0.00	0.00	0.00	0.00	N/A
Rejection	0.05	0.22	0.00	0.00	0.33[*]	No
Answer	5.55	6.13	12.70	17.64	0.10[*]	No
Disclaimer	0.05	0.22	0.00	0.00	0.33[*]	No
Compliance	0.40	1.14	1.85	2.58	0.03[#]	Yes
Refusal	0.00	0.00	0.10	0.31	0.16[*]	No
Response to greeting	0.05	0.22	0.20	0.41	0.16[*]	No

Note SD = standard deviation; [*]$p > 0.05$ (two-tailed); [#]$p < 0.05$ (two-tailed)

speech functions in this study revealed that practitioners' activeness in consultations was not highly discrepant from that of patients.

Even so, significant differences were identified in three speech functions: statement, command, and compliance. Patients produced more statements during conversations than practitioners; practitioners issued more commands to patients; and patients complied with practitioners more frequently. Lastly, practitioners offered feedback to patients and terminated moves or steps more often. Table 6 presents practitioners' and patients' speech functions in the identified moves.

Table 6 provides a comparison of the frequencies of different speech functions, revealing the dominance of TCM practitioners and patients in the identified moves and steps. As shown, practitioners mainly initiated the treatment planning move through the statement speech function and initiated the explanation move through the command speech function. TCM practitioners who acquired medical knowledge through training are expected to be competent in offering advice to patients during the treatment planning move. Their professional knowledge also enables them to explain TCM and general medicine concepts to patients. Accordingly, the diagnostic examination and treatment planning moves were inevitably initiated or dominated by TCM practitioners due to their professional competence and the purpose of medical consultations (i.e., to treat patients' illnesses).

Conversely, patients often complied with practitioners in the offering advice step. Patients tend to assume a relatively passive position when processing practitioners' advice in medical consultations due to limited professional medical knowledge (Cordella, 2004). Most commonly, patients accepted and followed practitioners' advice. There are many reasons for this acceptance, and they include trust in the practitioner's competence, anxiety about their health condition, and their desire to be cured.

Notably, patients primarily initiated the information elicitation move through the statement speech function. In Western medical consultations, this move is traditionally dominated by doctors who lead the consultations (Harvey & Koteyko, 2013). However, patients in TCM consultations seemed motivated to initiate this move; the pattern could be attributed to the symmetrical doctor–patient relationship, which enabled patients to take an active role in their consultations. Patients

Table 6 Speech functions in moves

Move/step	Statement		Command		Compliance	
	TCMP	P	TCMP	P	TCMP	P
Information elicitation		81				
Diagnostic examination	8	7				
Treatment planning	9	3	34	10	9	28
Step: offering advice	9	3	28			25
Step: giving prescription			6	10	9	3
Small talk	9	24				
Explanation	31	15	1			1

TCMP = TCM Practitioners; P = Patients

frequently used the statement speech function when describing symptoms, and the TCM practitioners seldom interrupted them. Such behavior may be rooted in TCM's tenet of holism, such that practitioners must gather comprehensive patient information (e.g., about their lifeworld). Patients also initiated small talk move actively through statements; they were willing to share personal life events with practitioners to establish a closer doctor–patient relationship. Using the statement speech function, patients could switch from an ongoing move to provide room for TCM practitioners to participate in small talk.

7 Conclusion

Health communication in Asian contexts is an emerging research field, and the number of studies on medical communication in a Chinese medicine context remains small. This study challenges arguments from previous research on doctor–patient communication in TCM consultations (e.g., Gu, 1996; Zhao, 1999), which suggested that doctors played a dominant role in conversations with patients amidst an asymmetrical doctor–patient relationship. This study contends that TCM consultations may be co-constructed by practitioners and patients via a primarily symmetrical relationship.

The move analysis revealed that two side moves, namely explanation and small talk, reflected nuances in TCM consultations. These moves are neither emphasized nor prevalent in Western medical consultations (see Byrne & Long, 1976; ten Have, 1989; Cheng, 2011) but play significant roles in TCM consultations. TCM practitioners tended to explain the philosophy behind suggested prescriptions and advice. This move exemplified patient-centered care, specifically that patients should be informed and their wish to understand medical advice should be addressed (Slade et al., 2015). Moreover, the small talk move indicated that the doctor–patient relationship was not entirely asymmetrical; TCM practitioners and patients both engaged in this move. The power hierarchy between interlocutors could be further minimized when doctors temporarily inactivated their professional role and treated patients as friends (Ribeiro, 2003). These moves shifted the doctor–patient relationship from asymmetrical to more symmetrical.

Statistical tests in this study indicated that the speech function frequencies of participating TCM practitioners and patients did not differ significantly. Consultations were co-constructed by patients and practitioners rather than dominated by practitioners. Patients were active in information elicitation and small talk; they often took initiative in describing symptoms, thereby introducing the information elicitation move. Thus, patients generally played active roles in TCM consultations, as they did not wait for practitioners to lead conversations. The patients also frequently initiated the small talk move through the statement speech function, sharing personal life events with practitioners. This finding further substantiated the importance of small talk in balancing the relationship between TCM practitioners and patients. Several moves, including diagnostic examination and offering advice, were inevitably initiated and led by TCM practitioners given their expansive professional knowledge about Chinese medicine. This chapter is the pioneering and preliminary research that sheds light on doctor–patient relationship in TCM consultations from a discourse structure perspective. Further studies digging deeper into the relevant issues in TCM contexts are much encouraged.

References

Byrne, P. S., & Long, B. E. L. (1976). *Doctor talking to patients: A study of the verbal behaviour of general practitioners consulting in their surgeries*. London, UK: H.M.S.O.

Cheng, K. (2011). Asymmetrical doctor-patient relationship in Hong Kong: A discourse analytical study, Doctoral dissertation, Hong Kong Baptist University, Hong Kong. Retrieved from https://repository.hkbu.edu.hk/etd_ra/1255/.

Cordella, M. (2004). *The dynamic consultation: A discourse analytical study of doctor-patient communication*. Amsterdam, The Netherland: John Benjamins.

Eggins, S., & Slade, D. (1997). *Analysing casual conversation*. London, UK: Cassell.

Fisher, S., & Todd, A. (Eds.). (1986). *Discourse and institutional authority: Medicine, education and law*. Norwood, USA: Ablex.

Gu, Y. (1996). Doctor-patient interaction as goal-directed discourse in Chinese sociocultural context. *Journal of Asian Pacific Communication, 7*(3–4), 156–176.

Gu, Y. (1999). A brief introduction to the Chinese health care system. *Health Communication, 11* (3), 203–208.

Halliday, M. A. K., & Matthiessen, C. M. I. M. (2014). *An introduction to functional grammar* (4th ed.). London, UK: Routledge.

Harvey, K., & Koteyko, N. (2013). *Exploring health communication: Language in action*. New York, USA: Routledge.

Holmes, J. (2000). Doing collegiality and keeping control at work: Small talk in government departments. In J. Coupland (Ed.), *Small talk* (pp. 32–61). New York, USA: Pearson Education Ltd.

Holmes, J. (2005). When small talk is a big deal: Sociolinguistic challenges in the workplace. In M. H. Long (Ed.), *Second language needs analysis* (pp. 344–371). Cambridge, UK: Cambridge University Press.

Jin, Y. (2018). Small talk in medical conversations: Data from China. *Journal of Pragmatics, 134*, 33–34.

Laver, J. (1975). Communicative functions of phatic communion. In A. Kendon, R. M. Harris, & M. R. Key (Eds.), *Organization of behavior in face-to-face interaction* (pp. 215–238). Paris, France: Mouton.

Li, T. (2011). Philosophic perspective: A comparative study of traditional Chinese medicine and western medicine. *Asian Social Science, 7*(2), 198–201.

Malinowski, B. (1972). Phatic communion. In J. Laver & S. Hutcheson (Eds.), *Communication in face-to-face interaction* (pp. 146–152). Harmondsworth, UK: Penguin Books.

Mishler, E. (1984). *The discourse of medicine: Dialectics of medical interviews*. Norwood, USA: Ablex.

Neighbour, R. (1987). *The inner consultation*. Oxford, UK: Radcliffe Medical Press.

Ody, P. (2014). *Chinese medicine for everyday living*. London, UK: Bounty Books.

Ohtaki, S., Ohtaki, T., & Fetters, M. D. (2003). Doctor–patient communication: A comparison of the USA and Japan. *Family Practice, 20*(3), 276–282.

Pilnick, A., & Dingwell, R. (2011). On the remarkable persistence of asymmetry in doctor/patient interaction: A critical review. *Social Science and Medicine, 72*, 1374–1382.

Pun, J., Matthiessen, C., Williams, G., & Slade, D. (2017). Using ethnographic discourse analysis to understand doctor-patient interactions in clinical settings. SAGE Research Methods Cases.

Pun, J., Chan, E. A., Wang, S., & Slade, D. (2018). Health professional-patient communication practices in East Asia: An integrative review of an emerging field of research and practice in Hong Kong, South Korea, Japan, Taiwan, and Mainland China. *Patient Education and Counseling, 101*(7), 1193–1206.

Ribeiro, B. T. (2003). Conflict talk in a psychiatric discharge interview: Struggling between personal and official footings. In C. R. Caldas-Coulthard & M. Coulthard (Eds.), *Readings in critical discourse analysis* (pp. 179–193). New York, USA: Routledge.

Slade, D., Manidis, M., McGregor, J., Scheeres, H., Olandler, E., Stein-Parbury, J., et al. (2015). *Communicating in hospital emergency departments*. Heidelberg, Germany: Springer.

Slade, D., Matthiessen, C. M. I. M., Lock, G., Pun, J., & Lam, M. (2016). Patterns of interaction in doctor-patient communication and their impact on health outcomes. In L. Ortega, A. E. Tyler, H. I. Park, & M. Uno (Eds.), *The usage-based study of language learning and multilingualism* (pp. 235–254). Washington, District of Columbia: Georgetown University Press.

Swales, J. M. (1990). *Genre analysis: English in academic and research settings*. Cambridge, England: Cambridge University Press.

Ten Have, P. (1989). Talk and institution: A reconsideration of the 'asymmetry' of doctor-patient interaction. In D. Boden, & D. Zimmerman (Eds.), *Talk and social structure: Studies, in ethnomethodology and conversation analysis* (pp. 138–163). Cambridge, UK: Polity.

Wu, Z., & Lu, Q. (2007). The discourse of Chinese medicine and westernization. In X. Shi (Ed.), *Discourse as cultural struggle* (pp. 155–176). Hong Kong: Hong Kong University Press.

Yin, C. P., Hsu, C. W., Kuo, F. Y., & Huang, Y. T. (2012). A study of politeness strategies adopted in pediatric clinics in Taiwan. *Health Communication, 27*(6), 533–545.

Zhao, B. (1999). Asymmetry and mitigation in Chinese medical interviews. *Health Communication, 11*(3), 209–214.

Zwickey, H., & Schiffke, H. C. (2007). Genetic correlates of Chinese medicine: In search of a common language. *The Journal of Alternative and Complementary Medicine, 13*(2), 183–184.

Instructions as Actions for Initiating Exercise Therapy in Physiotherapy in Hong Kong

Veronika Schoeb and Adrian Yip

Abstract Background: Instruction in exercise therapy aims at patients being able to correctly perform exercises. The analysis of instructional sequences (i.e., questions) examines the achievement of social actions during exercise therapy. This study investigated physiotherapists' questions for patients' initiations of exercises and analyzed patients' verbal and embodied responses, focusing on actions performed by physiotherapists' question designs and patients' responses. Study findings add to the evidence of underrepresented Chinese population. Methods: Data were collected from two Hong Kong rehabilitation centers. Forty-seven consultations (6 physiotherapists; 16 patients) were video-recorded and analyzed using Conversation Analysis. Interactional features including verbal (e.g., vocabulary, grammar, turn-taking) and nonverbal aspects (e.g., gaze and gesture) were examined. Results: Ninety-eight questions were posed by physiotherapist during the initial phase of exercise. Five categories were identified: invitations, memory check, information seeking, understanding check, or adherence check. Physiotherapists' questions led to a variety of embodied and verbal outcomes. Implications: The multimodal analysis of exercise instruction demonstrates that initiations of exercises are situated in task-relevant actions. Physiotherapists set the agenda regarding the exercise choice. Overall, physiotherapists and patients orient to verbal and nonverbal resources without precedence from either. The importance of non-verbal communication during exercises is highlighted.

Keywords Instruction · Exercise therapy · Conversation analysis · Chinese

V. Schoeb (✉) · A. Yip
Department of Rehabilitation Sciences, The Hong Kong Polytechnic University, Hong Kong, China
e-mail: veronika.schoeb@hesav.ch

V. Schoeb
HESAV School of Health Sciences, HES-SO University of Applied Sciences and Arts, Western Switzerland, Lausanne, Switzerland

A. Yip
Department of Linguistics, Queen Mary University of London, London, UK

© Springer Nature Singapore Pte Ltd. 2020
B. Watson and J. Krieger (eds.), *Expanding Horizons in Health Communication*,
The Humanities in Asia 6, https://doi.org/10.1007/978-981-15-4389-0_8

161

1   Background

Physiotherapy is one of the health professions using exercises as therapeutic interventions. Instructing an exercise, however, is not just simply giving information to a patient. When physiotherapists work with patients on their exercise training program, it is their main task to correct faulty movement patterns and instruct exercises to address muscle weakness, pain, or limitation in a range of motions (Physioswiss, 2019). In a qualitative study on patients' perception with regard to exercises, patients reported that appropriate exercise and activity modification were important aspects for their management of their symptoms in the long run (Liddle, Baxter & Gracey, 2007). In addition, another study emphasized the importance of communication skills for exercise adherence: "the practitioner's core listening and interpretation skills may have as much of an influence on treatment outcomes as the technical aspects of treatment" (Slade, Patel, Underwood, & Keating, 2014, p. 1002). Exercise instruction can, therefore, be considered as a collaborative activity during which physiotherapists use various resources to make sure that patients can understand the exercises, follow instructions, and ultimately be competent in doing the exercises properly and independently. Throughout this process, patients need to be active participants during exercise instruction (Martin, 2004).

Instruction is at the heart of exercise therapy, during which adjacency pairs are generally employed. As described by Schegloff and Sacks (1973), this class of sequences consists of the following features: (i) two utterance length; (ii) adjacent positioning of component utterances; (iii) different speakers produce each utterance; (iv) a first pair part precedes a second pair part; and (v) the two parts belong to the same pair type. As far as the present study is concerned, instructional sequences are anchored in a "request"/"compliance with request" adjacency pair (Lindwall & Ekström, 2012) which means that physiotherapists instruct an exercise (request) that patients then perform (compliance with request). While the process of acquiring the instructed actions and various instructional/corrective sequences have been discussed in a physiotherapy context (Parry, 2004, 2005), communication of initial requests is apparently assumed to be straightforward and has not been explored. Nonetheless, exercises can be initiated through various formulations, and each can perform a different social action (Stivers et al., 2017). As Heritage (2010) indicated, questions are hardly neutral but loaded with the reasoning, beliefs, and expectations of questioners. Each question can be formulated to simultaneously set agendas, embody presuppositions, convey epistemic stance, and incorporate preferences (Heritage, 2010). Also, the sequential positioning of questions can affect its neutrality and the effectiveness of achieving the communicative goal (Robinson & Heritage, 2016).

In addition to specific linguistic devices (such as questions) to achieve social actions (complying with a request), the therapist's intervention during exercise therapy should ultimately aim at improving the patient's exercise performance. We know from neurophysiological research that learning a movement requires various high-level skills, and that feedback is important for skill acquisition (Lewthwaite &

Wulf, 2010). Learning or improving a skill/exercise/movement—the domain of physiotherapy—requires instruction and feedback, but also interpersonal and communication skills, such as encouragement, empathy, or non-verbal communication (O'Keeffe et al., 2016). In a study from a physiotherapy outpatient setting, Martin (2004) found that therapists use verbal instruction in conjunction with touch to improve the patient's performance of a new exercise. Martin's study highlighted the importance of co-construction during exercise therapy and the necessity of patient's increasing participation while learning.

While obtaining a correct movement during exercise therapy is key for optimal performance, another issue is at stake: exercise adherence. Exercise as a therapeutic modality can only be effective if it is performed on a regular basis. However, this is far from easy. Various factors have been identified to hinder or foster exercise adherence, and multiple interventions have been proposed to enhance participation in exercises (Essery, Geraghty, Kirby & Yardley, 2017). Most of these approaches focus on behavioral change. Yet, it has been pointed out by Rhodes and Fiala (2009) that cognitive behavioral approaches have had limited effect on patient's adherence to exercise prescription. Given the limited success of the currently dominant approach in rehabilitation, we argue that there seems to be a need for a shift to a more social interactive approach, based on a detailed analysis of the interactional aspects during exercise instructions.

The aim of this study is to identify physiotherapists' questions for patients' initiations of exercises and to analyze patients' verbal and embodied responses. In particular, it is important to consider the actions performed by physiotherapists' question designs and their implications on patients' responses. Additionally, this study adds to the literature by analyzing the underrepresented Chinese population. Despite the increasing popularity of patient-centered communication in Western countries, patients in this culture have been under-investigated. In the context of exercise participation, however, there might be a lot to learn. The Chinese population has the reputation of being more passive and more reluctant to ask questions out of respect for medical authority (refer to chapters by Jin and Chan in this edition for further discussion of the nature of communication between Chinese doctors and patients), and it is argued that they have the strong desire for a harmonious relationship with health care professionals (Kwok & Koo, 2017). This chapter, therefore, sheds light on the ways physiotherapists initiate exercises and their respective outcomes in the Chinese context.

2 Methods

Data were collected from one public and one private rehabilitation clinic in Hong Kong between November 2015 and May 2016. Ethical approval was obtained by the Hong Kong Polytechnic University Review (No HSEARS20150902001) and the Hospital Authority Hong Kong West Cluster (No UW 15-626). The clinic manager of each site coordinated the recruitment of physiotherapists, who then invited their patients selectively to take part in the study. Inclusion criteria for patient recruitment were as follows: (i) at least 18 years of age, and (ii) exercise therapy was part of the existing treatment plan (no intervention was introduced by the research team). Exclusion criteria: (i) not being able to follow instructions, and (ii) not willing to be video-recorded. Scheduling for the recording was planned by the practice sites, and the research team was informed when a consultation had been scheduled. All participants received written information about the study including the aims and the means of data collection (i.e., video recording). Informed consent was sought from patients and therapists prior to the first recording. Even though one member of the research team was present during all recordings, there was no communication with participants during the consultations. The setup for the recording included a camcorder positioned about one to two meters away from the participants, and a small wireless microphone clipped to the physiotherapist. During the recording, the researcher adjusted the camcorder and followed the participants as they moved to different exercise stations.

A total of six physiotherapists and sixteen patients participated in the study, all of whom except four patients were Cantonese native speakers (Table 8.1). Each patient was scheduled to be filmed for three consecutive visits, which allowed a greater variety of exercise to be captured. One patient (RC01) dropped out after one

Table 8.1 Participants' demographic information and patients' medical diagnosis

Patient code	Age	Gender	Diagnosis	Clinic	Physiotherapist code	Gender
RC01	61	F	Carpal tunnel syndrome	Private	PTa	M
RC02	53	M	Back pain	Private	PTa	M
RC03[*]	46	M	Left Middle Cerebral Artery infarct	Private	PTb	F
RC04	50	F	Right arm pain	Private	PTc	F
RC05[**]	27	F	Ankle sprain	Private	PTd	F
ML01	64	F	Left rotator cuff repair	Public	PTe	F
ML02	71	F	Bilateral knee osteoarthritis	Public	PTe	F
ML03	77	F	Right lower limb pain	Public	PTe	F
ML04[*]	35	M	Left ACL reconstruction	Public	PTe	F
ML05	23	F	Left knee arthroscopy	Public	PTe	F
ML06	59	F	Right knee pain; spinal stenosis	Public	PTe	F
ML07	61	F	Right knee osteoarthritis	Public	PTf	F
ML08	53	M	Left supraspinatus partial thickness cuff tear	Public	PTf	F
ML09	64	F	Right rotator cuff repair	Public	PTf	F
ML10	67	F	Right shoulder rotator cuff repair	Public	PTf	F
ML11[*]	32	M	Arthroscopic Bankart repair	Public	PTf	F

Note [*]communicates in English; [**]communicates in Mandarin consultation session, and one patient (RC05) was filmed four times because the initial visit was only an assessment rather than exercise therapy. The entire corpus comprised of forty-seven consultations of about 18 h of video-recordings, each consultation lasting between 30 and 60 min. While there was no prerequisite regarding a patient's treatment stage, most patients were in the middle to later stages of their rehabilitation.

The analytical approach of this study drew on the inductive methodology of Conversation Analysis (CA), which views conversation as naturally occurring interaction (Maynard & Heritage, 2005). While ethnomethodology has been described as the intellectual framework of CA (ten Have, 2004), it is particularly the applied CA that can bring to light the workings of an institution and the possible ways to improve professional practice (Antaki, 2011). This method, therefore, enables the features of interactions in relation to physiotherapists' instructions for exercise initiation to be delineated. Upon completion of data collection, both verbal and nonverbal components during exercise therapy were transcribed based on Jefferson's (2004) conventions. Balancing the richness of the video-recorded data and the focus in this article, the transcripts are presented here in a basic and easy-to-read manner by adopting a simplified version of transcription (Appendix A). The software ELAN (Brugman & Russel, 2004) was used for the transcription process to organize multimodal communication. For consultations conducted in Cantonese or Mandarin, an idiomatic English translation was provided in a second line to display the interactional meaning. All transcripts were first prepared by the second author (a linguist and native Cantonese speaker), who also identified all instances of physiotherapists' questions in the initial phase and coded the collection of such sequences. These preliminary observations were then discussed extensively with the first author (a sociologist and health professional with expertise in health communication and physiotherapy) as well as during various data sessions with other CA researchers. Such collaborative viewing is seen as a means to neutralize the authors' preconceived notions (Jordan & Henderson, 1995).

A primary focus when examining the transcripts was on turn design. Drew, Chatwin, and Collins (2001) illustrated how this fundamental building block in CA reveals the actions performed by each utterance, the ways actions are connected and dependent upon each other, and the overall sequential patterns emerge from the data as the interaction develops. Here is an example:

01 Physiotherapist: Have I taught you this one?
02 Patient: No.
03 Physiotherapist: No. Alright. I will teach you this time.

It is clear in this example that turn designs have sequential consequences: the patient's response (line 2) is not random but orients to the physiotherapist's turn design (line 1), and the subsequent turn by the physiotherapist (line 3) is also designed according to patient's turn. Moreover, the use of "question-answer" adjacency pair (Schegloff & Sacks, 1973) is evident here: the first pair part being the question asked by the physiotherapist and the second pair part being the answer given by the patient (lines 1–2). Additionally, as Maynard and Heritage (2005) noted, every detail in the interaction is orderly and a part of its organization, therefore other interactional features including vocabulary, grammar, overlapping speech, silence, gaze, and gesture were also examined. All these different aspects of interlocutors' speech influence the uptake by subsequent speakers. Through accumulating collections of various practices, the selections made by physiotherapists when initiating exercises and how they were responded by patients were unfolded.

3   Results

The results will be presented as follows: first, the type of questions physiotherapists used to have patients initiate the exercises, followed by the detailed analysis of (a) resources used by physiotherapists (verbal—embodied), and (b) patients' responses and the outcome of the interaction.

A total of 98 questions were initiated by physiotherapists during the initial phase of exercise. Questions were categorized into five groups according to the functions they served (Table 8.2). First, invitation was used to solicit an embodied action, which was often but not always exercise-related. Second, memory check was an instance of checking if the patient remembered a previously taught exercise. It could be a general question about the exercise or more specific details regarding body movements and positions. Third, information seeking referred to a question that solicited input from a patient regarding information of which physiotherapist had no knowledge (excluding information about patient's adherence to exercise, which was classified as "adherence check"). While it could be non-exercise-related or small talk, it was usually about patient's movement, symptom, and competence regarding a specific exercise. Fourth, understanding check was a question that confirmed patient's understanding about physiotherapist's preceding utterance, which was usually related to exercise instruction, correction of movement or exercise prescription. Very often it was formed by adding a tag (e.g., ok, right) to an

Table 8.2 Categorization of questions initiated by physiotherapists

Question function	Definition	Example
Invitation	Ask patient to perform a bodily action	"Can you come forward?"
Memory check	Ask patient about a previously taught exercise	"Remember the knees?"
Information seeking	Ask patient about their movement, symptom, and competence	"Was it still quite tight?"
Understanding check	Ask patient to confirm their understanding	"Open the chest, ok?"
Adherence check	Ask patient about exercise adherence	"What exercises are you doing at home?"

instruction formulated as a declarative. Fifth, adherence check was used to ask patients to report whether they performed the exercise learnt during previous consultations, and how their progress was.

As detailed in Tables 8.3, 8.4 and 8.5, physiotherapists' questions led to a variety of embodied and verbal outcomes. Embodied outcomes were defined as bodily actions that patients performed following therapists' initiation. Verbal outcomes indicated how patients responded in words to the initial questions. While it was acknowledged that they existed alongside each other and were highly interdependent, the distinction is important here for facilitating the discussion and enhancing our understanding of how the two modes of communication were

Table 8.3 The use of questions by physiotherapists for exercise initiation

Question type	Patient's verbal response			
	Conforming	Partial conforming	Nonconforming	Total
Memory	4	7	4	15
Invitation	0	0	6	6
Information-seeking	6	3	3	12
Understanding check	2	0	4	6
Adherence	2	0	0	2
Total	14	10	17	41

Table 8.4 The use of questions by physiotherapists for preparation of exercise initiation

Question type	Patient's verbal response			
	Conforming	Partial conforming	Nonconforming	Total
Memory	0	1	1	2
Invitation	3	4	3	10
Information-seeking	0	0	2	2
Understanding check	1	0	1	2
Adherence	1	0	0	1
Total	5	5	7	17

Table 8.5 The use of questions by physiotherapists for exercise-related discussions

Question type	Patient's verbal response			
	Conforming	Partial conforming	Nonconforming	Total
Memory	0	1	1	2
Invitation	1	1	3	5
Information-seeking	12	2	3	17
Understanding check	3	2	9	14
Adherence	2	0	0	2
Total	18	6	16	40

mobilized by physiotherapists and patients respectively during exercise therapy. Let us first consider the three embodied outcomes (numbers in brackets represent the number of questions leading to that embodied outcome out of the 98 questions initiated by physiotherapists):

(i)   exercise initiation (41/98): patient started an exercise;
(ii) preparation initiation (17/98): patient produced an embodied response prior to an exercise, including body positioning, equipment set-up, and other preparation;
(iii) exercise-related discussion (40/98): there was no observable change in phase —patient maintained their position or their ongoing bodily orientations/ movements.

About 40% of the questions used by therapists had the effect of the patient starting the exercise (yet mainly unrelated to the question function), while in about 40% there was no observable change. The remainder included a preparation before starting the exercise.

As for patients' verbal responses, an examination of both their grammatical structure and content indicated that patients were found to either conform (37/98), partially conform (21/98), or not conform (40/98) to the questions. A conforming response oriented to the grammatical structure (a "yes" or "no" response to a "yes-no question") and content of a question. A partially conforming response oriented to the question content but not its grammatical form, whereas a non-conforming response oriented to neither. These three types of responses are exemplified below:

Question: Can you show me the exercise I taught you last time?

(i)   Yes, I can. (conforming)
(ii) The exercise last time? (partially-conforming)
(iii) It's a bit painful here. (non-conforming)

In achieving each of the three embodied outcomes, physiotherapists utilized a combination of different categories of questions. They also employed various other resources, both verbal and embodied, in addition to questions. Extracts 1 to 3 illustrate the ways physiotherapists' questions led to the observed outcomes. Let's look at each of the outcomes separately followed by an example.

3.1   Question Types for Achieving "Exercise Initiation"

First, for exercise initiation, the most frequently used question types were "memory check" and "information seeking" (Table 8.3). Majority of these questions were followed either by nonconforming or partially conforming responses. It is also interesting to note that invitations (e.g., "can you do twenty more repetitions?") always received nonconforming verbal responses, a majority of which included absence of any verbal utterances. Instead, patients prefer to reply with only an embodied response, which is demonstrated in the extract 1 below.

Extract 1 illustrates how physiotherapist introduced the revision of an arm raise exercise through the use of a "memory check" type of question. Prior to the sequence, PTe revised another exercise with ML03.

Extract 1 (ML03 PTe Rx1a)—Arm raise exercise

1	*((ML03 lies on plinth; PTe stands next to the plinth on the side.))*
2 PTe	哼 (.) 第二個 (.) 記唔記得呀?
	look (.) the second one (.) remember?
3	(0.8)
4	*((ML03 initiates an exercise by moving her right leg up and down.))*
5 ML03	er: [呢度]
	er: [here]
6	*((PTe moves towards the upper body of ML03 and looks at her.))*
7 PTe	[第]二個運動
	[the] second exercise
8 ML03	呢度
	here
9 PTe	第二個運動囉
	the second exercise
10	(0.2)
11 PTe	遮手嗰個呢
	the arm raising one
12	*((PTe raises her arms over her head and back down.))*
13	*((ML03 follows and raises her arms over her head.))*

(PTe: physiotherapist, female; ML03: patient, female)

In line 2, PTe induced the transition from the previous exercise by the discourse marker "*look*" and asked whether ML03 remembered "*the second one*" without describing the exercise further. ML03 initiated a leg exercise (embodied outcome) after a short pause (line 4) and signaled her movement verbally with "here" (line 5). The verbal response here, as a second pair part of the question-answer adjacency pair, was considered partially conforming as it oriented to the question content but did not indicate whether she "remembered". However, the patient's response was not taken up by PTe, whose gaze was directed towards the upper body/head of ML03 (line 6). PTe then repeated 'the second exercise' twice (lines 7 and 9) before adding further specificity about the exercise (line 11) and demonstrating the arm movements briefly (line 12). It was only then when ML03 was able to perform the exercise intended by PTe (line 13). In this extract, while the physiotherapist's choice of question led to an embodied outcome, the patient did not perform the desired exercise and produced a partially conforming verbal response. Additional resources including specific exercise description and demonstration were required for achieving the intended outcome.

3.2 Question Types Achieving "Preparation of Initiation"

Second, for preparation initiation, the most frequently used question type was formulated as an "invitation", majority of which received a nonconforming or partially conforming verbal response.

Extract 2 shows how the physiotherapist prepared the patient's positioning for learning a new exercise.

Extract 2 (ML08 PTf Rx1)—Hand bar exercise

1 PTf	教多 個吖 (.) 今日 (.) 好唔好呀
	teach one more (.) today (.) is it okay
2	((ML08 nods.))
3 ML08	[(好呀)]
	[(okay)]
4 PTf	[ok (.)] <我地就唔如-> 我地左手係唔係?
	[ok (.)] <why don't we-> it's the left arm right?
5 ML08	係呀 (.) 左手呀
	yes (.) left arm
6 PTf	我地打側瞓 (0.2) 噉樣瞓 (0.4) [好唔好?]
	we lie down on the side (.) lie down like this (.) [alright?]
7	((PTf demonstrates by lying on her right on the plinth))
8 ML08	[打側]
	[on the side]
9 PTf	係喇 (0.2) 你好似我噉瞓 (.) 無錯 (.) 上返嚟
	yes (0.2) you lie down like me (.) that's right (.) come back up
10	((PTf stands up from the plinth.))
11	(3.7)
12	((ML08 lies on his left on the plinth.))
13 ML08	( )
14 PTf	左手吖嘛
	it's the left arm
15	(2.4)
16	((ML08 turns to lie on his right; PTf gestures the turning-around motion with her hands and nods after ML08 starts turning.))
17 PTf	係喇 (.) ok
	yes (.) ok

(PTf: physiotherapist, female; ML08: patient, male)

It began with PTf's suggestion of teaching a new exercise, to which ML08 expressed his agreement bodily and verbally (lines 2–3). After confirming with ML08 that they should work on his left arm (lines 4–5), PTf invited him to prepare for the exercise by lying down on the plinth (line 6). Although she did not specify on which side ML08 should lie, she demonstrated briefly by lying on her right (lines 7, 9). In response, ML08 gave a partially conforming verbal response by repeating the invitation "*on the side*" (line 8) and proceeded to the starting position (line 12). He corrected his starting position after PTf pointed out his mistake (lines 14–16). This extract illustrates how a physiotherapist's invitation successfully led to the embodied outcome of preparation initiation. Unlike Extract 1, the question was accompanied by a more specific instruction, alongside the bodily resource of demonstration provided by the physiotherapist. While these additional resources supported understanding, the desired embodied outcome was still not fully attained at first.

3.3 Question Types During "Exercise-Related Discussion"

Third, as far as exercise-related discussion was concerned, the most frequently used question types were "information seeking" and "understanding check". Typically, understanding checks were instructional statements ending with the tag "ok?", and they largely received a nonconforming or partially conforming verbal response. On the other hand, a majority of information-seeking questions received conforming verbal responses.

Extract 3 illustrates an exercise-related discussion initiated by physiotherapist with the use of an information-seeking question. Prior to the sequence, PTe asked ML05 to perform a plank exercise that she had learnt previously.

Extract 3 (ML05 PTe Rx2b)—Plank exercise

1 PTe	( ) posture ( ) 我睇一睇先
	( ) posture ( ) let me take a look first
2	(0.4)
3 ML05	ha ouch [( )]
4	((ML05 is in a push-up position and presses up a little before lowering back down quickly))
5 PTe	[你hold]到幾耐呀而家 (.) plank
	how long can you hold now (.) plank
6 ML05	我而家: (一般-)l
	I now: (usually-)
7	(0.3)
8 PTe	[一分鐘]
	[one minute]
9 ML05	[一分十]秒啦::
	[one minute and ten] seconds::
10 PTe	ok (.) 好好喎
	ok (.) very good
11 ML05	可以呀 (.) 我 [side] plank多咗好多喎 [( )]
	I can (.) I can hold for a lot longer for side plank [( )]
12 PTe	[good]
13 PTe	[oh (.) then it's very good]

(PTf: physiotherapist, female; ML05: patient, female)

ML05 was about to start the exercise when PTe inquired about her progress (lines 4–5). ML05 delayed the exercise initiation and answered with a conforming response. After obtaining the information, PTe produced positive evaluations with which ML05 concurred (lines 10–13). This extract exemplifies how the physiotherapist achieved the initiation of an exercise-related discussion (which primarily manifested verbally) that was followed by a verbally conforming response.

4 Discussion

The aim of this study was to identify physiotherapists' questions to achieve patients' initiations of exercises and to analyze patients' verbal and embodied responses to these questions. Streeck, Goodwin, and Le Baron (2011) argued that "talk and embodied behavior co-occur as interdependent phenomena, not separable modes of communication and action" (p. 7) and that embodied interaction means that the body is "conceived in its concrete, unique, pre-verbal, skilled, and practical coupling" (p. 6) with the world. The findings of this study are analyzed within this framework by examining embodied interactions to show how participants interactively draw on multiple resources to negotiate their social lives. Embodied interaction can be understood as the study of "ways in which several bodily «channels» are coordinated in social interaction to show how environmental sources of meaning are drawn into the production of inter-subjective understanding" (p. 9, Streeck et al., 2011). In view of this concept, physiotherapists designed their questions as invitations, memory check, information-seeking, understanding check or adherence check, and used embodied resources to complement verbal resources. The detailed analyses highlighted the importance of the often discounted nonverbal means of communication, and enabled us to shed light on the relationship between patients' embodied outcome and the verbal conformity to questions. This section discusses these findings within the wider literature on question design, multimodal resources in exercise instruction, patient participation, and ends with implications.

4.1 Question Types and Responses

Physiotherapists used various question types to achieve patients' initiation of exercise. Studies in Conversation Analysis have detected that certain question types lead to specific outcomes, for example, requests are responded to or invitations are accepted (Schegloff, 2007). In this study, different question types used by physiotherapists—verbal resources as one modality of communication—achieved embodied responses. As shown in the first extract, the most frequent question types accomplishing the communicative goal of having patients start the exercises were memory check and information-seeking questions. A question *"remember that one?"* (memory check) was sufficient for the patient to start the exercise. Often, the patient's response was only embodied without verbally conforming to the question. What we note is that questions are not treated by patients as to be responded to verbally but that embodied responses are oriented to by both participants as sufficient. In order to achieve exercise initiation, physiotherapists use question types such as information-seeking, memory check, and invitations, requiring no verbal response from patients.

This use of question also applied to the second outcome—preparation for initiation of exercises. The predominant question was formulated as an invitation, which mostly received a nonconforming or partially conforming verbal response. However, the bodily component (i.e., demonstration) accompanying the question seems to be important to achieve this outcome.

As for the last outcome, the exercise-related discussion, physiotherapists did not aim to invite patients to deliver a bodily performance immediately but have them provide information or listen to further instructions. The most frequently used question types were "information seeking" and "understanding check". The former question type indicated that there was a gap in physiotherapist's knowledge that needed to be filled with patient's input. Given this steep epistemic gradient (Heritage, 2010) between the unknowing physiotherapist and the knowledgeable patient, it is not surprising that conforming verbal responses were the majority of produced responses. Conversely, understanding checks were largely informative or instructional, with tags such as "ok?" which mostly received nonconforming or partially conforming verbal responses.

These findings are quite novel as in the health care literature verbal communication is often analyzed with much detail, while embodied communication is overlooked. In addition, current communication models (e.g., Cambridge-Calgary model; Kurtz, Draper & Silverman, 2016) are based on medical interactions, which do not represent all health care practices. Yet, in physiotherapy, touch is indeed an important communication resource (Hiller, Delany & Guillemin, 2015a). Furthermore, Heritage (2010) has shown that questions in medical interviews are designed to incorporate preferences, set agenda, embody presuppositions, and convey epistemic stance. In our examples, however, questions from a physiotherapy context are designed to achieve the intended outcome by considering various modalities, including verbal and nonverbal dimensions. It can, therefore, be an expansion of the current literature by including the embodied interactional resources (e.g., physiotherapists' demonstration).

Type-conforming responses to yes-no interrogatives (Raymond, 2003) have been examined in studies of ordinary (mundane) interactions, yet have so far received limited attention in institutional settings. Our findings suggest that verbal type-conforming responses are not needed in order for patients and therapists to interact during exercise therapy. Patients' non-conforming or partially conforming responses are not oriented to by participants as problematic. As shown in our extracts, the embodied response is weighted more importantly than the non-conforming verbal response. This is in line with findings from mundane interaction where Berger and Rae (2012) found that gestures can respond to talk and thereby accomplish sequential actions autonomously.

4.2 Multimodal Resources in Exercise Instruction

As discussed previously, questions as "invitation" and "memory check" might require multiple modalities from physiotherapists in order to achieve the intended outcome: the use of touch in combination with talk seems to be more effective for achieving a response. It is argued here that while information seeking or adherence questions were less often accompanied by non-verbal resources, question types such as "memory check" and "invitation" were more often used in conjunction with touch, pointing, or demonstration. These findings aligned with a study on instructions-in-interaction in the context of learning how to knit (Lindwall & Ekström, 2012). The authors argue that the instructions in form of corrections build upon the teacher's assessment of the action so that the learner's mistakes observed by the teacher are corrected with talk and gestures. In the current context, physiotherapists use their own body both for instructional purposes (demonstration, pointing, etc.) as well as for providing therapeutic interventions (e.g., mobilization, lymphatic drainage).

Despite the importance of multimodal resources for physiotherapists, there is only limited research on touch as a means of communication and interaction. Bjorbaekmo and Mengshoel (2016) observed that physiotherapists invite patients to co-construct therapy through touch, non-touch and movements, insisting on a dialogue through touch and movement (p. 10). The authors further argue that touch is also dependent on the physiotherapist's embodied skills as these skills need to be cultivated and explored before physiotherapists being able to use embodied resources for exercise instruction. In another study from an Australian context, Hiller et al. (2015b) argued that "touch occurred in conjunction with extensive use of other non-verbal communication skills" (p. 1225) in order to engage with and demonstrate their interest in the patient as an individual person. In our study, physiotherapists' non-verbal resources, however, seemed to be more targeted toward achieving their objective of exercise instruction, rather than "a pat or stroke on a patient's leg" (p. 1225) as described by Hiller et al. (2015a, b). Our findings, therefore, extend the current literature by identifying how physiotherapists use verbal and embodied resources to initiate and have patients start their exercises. This is a first step in understanding embodied communication in the physiotherapy context.

4.3 Patient Participation

The concept of "patient participation" in the literature has various definitions. Collins, Britten, Ruusuvuori, and Thompson (2007) used a wide-reaching conceptualisation stating that "participation includes all forms of action or omission of action in which an interactant is involved" (p. 122). Considering this, Peräkylä, Ruusuvuori, and Lindfors (2007) argued that it is impossible not to participate and patients do participate even if there is silence. This is the approach chosen in this article, as we considered patient participation here as a patient responding to physiotherapist's questions verbally or non-verbally. As shown with our detailed analysis, patients did participate and initiate exercises when being invited, reminded, or inquired about what happened at home.

Our findings revealed that certain question types achieved not only a verbal response from the patient but also the exercise performance that they were intended to. Also, physiotherapists used embodied resources, and they clearly showed their understanding of the nature of their work: verbal communication is only one part of the picture, especially if the work is about the body, its functions, or troubles with the body. That patient acts on a physiotherapist's question and/or bodily activity suggests that there are alternatives to more direct instructional statements. The rationale behind the physiotherapist's choice of communicative resource, and the patient's perception of and reaction to it are beyond the scope of this chapter. It is possible that physiotherapists try to create a more welcoming environment for patients by being less confrontational and more polite. Meanwhile, over time, the patient could become more familiar with the physiotherapist's communicative behaviors and participate through exercise performance more readily. A longitudinal comparison involving patients at different stages might shed light on this assumption. Based on the current interactional analysis, what we can conclude in terms of patient participation is that it is less a "script-like type of question" that engages patients in exercises; question design seems less important as the focus is on achieving the outcome of patients initiating the exercise (patient participation). Physiotherapists can use their own body as a means of instruction for patients to respond and initiate/learn their exercises more proficiently.

It also has to be noted that even though health care communication in a Chinese context is considered less patient-centered than in a Western context (Anderson, 2001), our data indicated that physiotherapists' integrated use of verbal and non-verbal resources helped to achieve patients' active participation during exercise therapy. Even though some studies suggested that Chinese patients weighed the importance of a harmonious relationship with health professionals higher than their own right to ask questions (Ting, Yong, Yin & Mi, 2016; Kwok & Koo, 2017), our own data did not confirm this argument, maybe due to a different health care context (physiotherapy instead of medical interaction) or the continuous collaboration over several weeks as it is common in physiotherapy.

In summary, we were able to demonstrate that patients orient to physiotherapists' questions in ways that indicate they are not merely "passive recipients". This was evident in examples when patients did not respond to a memory check question by responding verbally with "yes" or "no" but by initiating the exercise. Meanwhile, in relation to the professionals, we suggest that physiotherapists mobilize various types of questions that are more "participation-friendly" and less restrictive than giving a direct order (which has not been recorded in our data). Ultimately, with a categorization of question types to engage patients in exercise, physiotherapists can now have a better understanding of how to use multiple resources available to them. At the end of the day, therapists need to achieve active patient participation by providing an environment in which patients can become proficient and independent with their entire exercise program.

5 Implications

The multimodal analysis of exercise instruction in a physiotherapeutic setting demonstrates that initiations of exercises are situated in task-relevant actions. Instructional sequences in the praxeological context of exercise therapy are often manifested as questions. Therefore, studying question design seems important as physiotherapists and patients often "cooperate and struggle with one another over what matters" (Heritage, 2010). Second, physiotherapists presuppose with memory check that patients are able to remember the exercise they practiced in a previous session, and their question design prefers a positive response. It seems that patients are eager to represent themselves as "good patients" who adhere to the exercise at home—they often give "yes" responses, even when they fail to demonstrate their knowledge afterwards. Third, both physiotherapists and patients orient to not only verbal but also nonverbal resources, and the former does not always take precedence over the latter. Embodied resources provide probably a more direct and intersubjectively clear instruction of what action the physiotherapist would like to achieve.

One limitation to the findings of this study concerns the small sample size. While our participants might not be representative of the range of practices across various rehabilitation settings in this context, our goal is to draw attention to the importance of utilizing a multimodal perspective in examining patient–physiotherapist interactions. Although it is unlikely that there is a definitive, universal "communicative manual", physiotherapists should be more aware of the communicative resources alternative to verbal means and the sequential implications of their turn designs. Furthermore, a detailed representation of physiotherapy interactions through recordings and transcripts can enhance the reliability of results (Peräkylä, 2004). Even though these interactions do not represent *all* practices of physiotherapists, practices described here are descriptions of what any *professional can do* in these situations (Peräkylä, 2004). While qualitative results cannot be generalizable to a wider population, the detailed description of data production and analyses allow for the transferability of findings (Murphy, Dingwall, Greatbatch, Parker, & Watson, 1998). Further studies in different contexts would help validate the findings of this study.

Acknowledgements This study was funded by the Department of Rehabilitation Sciences, The Hong Kong Polytechnic University (Grant No 1-ZE4F).

References

Anderson, C. M. (2001). Communication in the medical interview team: An analysis of patients' stories in the United States and Hong Kong. *Howard Journal of Communication, 12*, 61–72.

Antaki, C. (2011). Six kinds of applied conversation analysis. In C. Antaki (Ed.), *Applied conversation analysis: Intervention and change in institutional talk* (pp. 1–14). Basingstoke: Palgrave Macmillan.

Berger, I., & Rae, J. (2012). Some uses of gestural responsive actions. *Journal of Pragmatics, 44* (13), 1821–1835.

Bjorbækmo, W. S., & Mengshoel, A. M. (2016). "A touch of physiotherapy"—The significance and meaning of touch in the practice of physiotherapy. *Physiotherapy Theory and Practice, 32* (1), 10–19.

Brugman, H. & Russel, A. (2004). Annotating multi-media/multi-modal resources with ELAN. In *Proceedings of the 4th International Conference on Language Resources and Language Evaluation (LREC)*, pp. 2065–2068.

Collins, S., Britten, N., Ruusuvuori, J., & Thompson, A. (2007). *Patient participation in health care consultations: Qualitative perspectives.* Maidenhead: Open University Press.

Drew, P., Chatwin, J., & Collins, S. (2001). Conversation analysis: A method for research into interactions between patients and health-care professionals. *Health Expectations, 4*(1), 58–70.

Essery, R., Geraghty, A. W. A., Kirby, S., & Yardley, L. (2017). Predictors of adherence to home-based physical therapies: A systematic review. *Disability and Rehabilitation, 39*(6), 519–534.

Heritage, J. (2010). Questioning in medicine. In A. F. Freed & S. Ehrlich (Eds.), *"Why do you ask?": The function of questions in institutional discourse.* New York: Oxford University Press.

Hiller, A., Delany, C., & Guillemin, M. (2015a). The communicative power of touch in the patient–physiotherapist interaction. *Physiotherapy, 101*, e565–e566.

Hiller, A., Guillemin, M., & Delany, C. (2015b). Exploring healthcare communication models in private physiotherapy practice. *Patient Education and Counseling, 98*(10), 1222–1228.

Jefferson, G. (2004). Glossary of transcript symbols with an introduction. In G. H. Lerner (Ed.), *Conversation analysis: Studies from the first generation.* Amsterdam: John Benjamins.

Jordan, B., & Henderson, A. (1995). Interaction analysis: Foundations and practice. *Journal of the Learning Sciences, 4*(1), 39–103.

Kurtz, S., Draper, J., & Silverman, J. (2016). *Skills for communicating with patients* (3rd ed.). Boca Raton: CRC Press.

Kwok, C., & Koo, F. K. (2017). Participation in treatment decision-making among Chinese-Australian women with breast cancer. *Supportive Care in Cancer, 25*(3), 957–963. https://doi.org/10.1007/s00520-016-3487-5.

Lewthwaite, R., & Wulf, G. (2010). Social-comparative feedback affects motor skill learning. *Quarterly Journal of Experimental Psychology, 63*(4), 738–749.

Liddle, S. D., Baxter, G. D., & Gracey, J. H. (2007). Chronic low back pain: Patients' experiences, opinions and expectations for clinical management. *Disability and Rehabilitation, 29*(24), 1899–1909.

Lindwall, O., & Ekström, A. (2012). Instruction-in-interaction: The teaching and learning of a manual skill. *Human Studies, 35*(1), 27–49.

Martin, C. (2004). *From other to self. Learning as interactional change.* Ph.D. Thesis, University of Uppsala, Sweden.

Maynard, D. W., & Heritage, J. (2005). Conversation analysis, doctor–patient interaction and medical communication. *Medical Education, 39*(4), 428–435. https://doi.org/10.1111/j.1365-2929.2005.02111.x.

Murphy, E., Dingwall, R., Greatbatch, D., Parker, S., & Watson, P. (1998). *Qualitative research methods in health technology assessment: A review of the literature.* Southampton: Health

Technology Assessment, NHS R&D HTA Programme, NCCHTA, University of Southampton, UK.

O'Keeffe, M., Cullinane, P., Hurley, J., Leahy, I., Bunzli, S., O'sullivan, P. B., et al. (2016). What influences patient-therapist interactions in musculoskeletal physical therapy? Qualitative systematic review and meta-synthesis. *Physical Therapy, 96*(5), 609–622.

Parry, R. (2004). The interactional management of patients' physical incompetence: A conversation analytic study of physiotherapy interactions. *Sociology of Health & Illness, 26* (7), 976–1007.

Parry, R. (2005). A video analysis of how physiotherapists communicate with patients about errors of performance: Insights for practice and policy. *Physiotherapy, 91*(4), 204–214.

Peräkylä, A. (2004). Reliability and validity in research based on naturally occurring social interaction. In D. Silverman (Ed.), *Qualitative research: Theory, method and practice* (2nd ed., pp. 283–304). London, UK: Sage.

Peräkylä, A., Ruusuvuori, J., & Lindfors, P. (2007). What is patient participation? Reflections arising from the study of general practice, homeopathy and psychoanalysis. In S. Collins, et al. (Eds.), *Patient participation in health care consultations: Qualitative perspectives* (pp. 121–142). Maidenhead: Open University Press.

Physioswiss (2019). *Profil professionnel du physiothérapeute*. Retrieved from www.physioswiss. ch/fr/profession-fr/profession2-fr/berufsbild-physiotherapie-1.

Raymond, G. (2003). Grammar and social organization: Yes/no interrogatives and the structure of responding. *American Sociological Review*, 939–967.

Rhodes, R. E., & Fiala, B. (2009). Building motivation and sustainability into the prescription and recommendations for physical activity and exercise therapy: The evidence. *Physiotherapy Theory and Practice, 25*(5–6), 424–441.

Robinson, J., & Heritage, J. (2016). How patients understand physicians' solicitations of additional concerns: Implications for up-front agenda setting in primary care. *Health Communication, 31* (4), 434–444.

Schegloff, E. A., & Sacks, H. (1973). Opening up closings. *Semiotica, VIII, 4,* 289–327.

Schegloff, E. A. (2007). *Sequence organization in interaction: A primer in conversation analysis I* (Vol. 1). Cambridge: Cambridge University Press.

Slade, S. C., Patel, S., Underwood, M., & Keating, J. L. (2014). What are patient beliefs and perceptions about exercise for nonspecific chronic low back pain? A systematic review of qualitative studies. *The Clinical Journal of Pain, 30*(11), 995–1005.

Streeck, J., Goodwin, C., & Le Baron, C. (2011). *Embodied interaction: Language and body in the material world*. Cambridge: Cambridge University Press.

Stivers, T., Heritage, J., Barnes, R. K., McCabe, R., Thompson, L., & Toerien, M. (2017). Treatment recommendations as actions. *Health Communication*, 1–10.

ten Have, P. (2004). *Understanding qualitative research and ethnomethodology*. London: Sage.

Ting, X., Yong, B., Yin, L., & Mi, T. (2016). Patient perception and the barriers to practicing patient-centered communication: A survey and in-depth interview of Chinese patients and physicians. *Patient Education and Counseling, 99,* 364–369.

Shift-to-Shift Nursing Handovers at a Multi-cultural and Multi-lingual Tertiary Hospital in Singapore: An Observational Study

Phillip R. Della, Fazila Aloweni, Shin Yuh Ang, Mei Ling Lim, Thendral Uthaman, Tracey Carol Ayre, and Huaqiong Zhou

Abstract Ineffective communication, during handover, is a major factor in subsequent incidents and patient harm. There is a dearth of evidence on the quality of handovers in a multi-cultural, multi-lingual and cohort care setting, such as in Singapore. This is the first Singaporean study aimed to observe, analyse and evaluate clinical handover by nurses. Fifty shift-to-shift handovers were observed and video-recorded. Content and discourse analyses were used and focused on informational, structural and interactional dimensions of handover. Findings revealed that patient safety information was sometimes missed out. The transfer of responsibility and accountability for ongoing patient care was not explicit and poor information framework and flow during the handover process were observed. Some nurses preferred to perform physical assessments prior to handover instead of during or afterwards. Patients' background and medical history were either not mentioned at handover commencement or excluded. Some nurses appeared apprehensive to bedside handover and had poor patient engagement. Few nurses effectively involved patients or reinforced patient education. Results highlight that nurses need support and training to master some aspects of handover, focused on reducing clinical errors.

Keywords Handover · Ineffective communication · Patient harm · Patient safety · Nurses

P. R. Della (✉) · H. Zhou
School of Nursing, Midwifery & Paramedicine, Curtin University, Perth, WA 6845, Australia
e-mail: p.della@curtin.edu.au

F. Aloweni · S. Y. Ang · M. L. Lim · T. Uthaman · T. C. Ayre
Nursing Division, Singapore General Hospital, Bukit Merah, Singapore

M. L. Lim
Neuroscience Research Australia, University of New South Wales, Sydney, NSW, Australia

© Springer Nature Singapore Pte Ltd. 2020   179
B. Watson and J. Krieger (eds.), *Expanding Horizons in Health Communication*,
The Humanities in Asia 6, https://doi.org/10.1007/978-981-15-4389-0_9

1 Background

Singapore is a multi-cultural island country in Southeast Asia. While Malay, Mandarin Chinese and Tamil are commonly spoken, English remains the working language and primary mode of communication among Singaporeans (Tenzer, Terjesen, & Harzing, 2017). There is also a local colloquial variety of English used in Singapore (i.e. 'Singlish'), which has its unique slang and syntax. Singlish is a mixture of English, Mandarin, Tamil, Malay and other local dialects such as Hokkien, Cantonese and Teochew. Singlish is commonly used during a casual conversation between locals. While the official language used in the Singapore clinical environment is English, this study demonstrated that nurses do use Singlish and Malay during handover and their communication with patients and other staff. The use of this colloquial variety of English is despite Singapore's language policy which states that there is no place for Singlish (Wee, 2009).

Importantly, the healthcare workforce in Singapore is comprised of professionals from different races as well as nationalities. Particularly in Singapore, the nursing workforce relies increasingly on international nurses who may have a good command of English, but they may not understand Singlish. This may lead to communication difficulties especially during handovers. While clinical communication and handovers have been studied in numerous settings there, there have been limited studies in the nature and efficacy of communication in healthcare conversations in multi-cultural and multi-lingual societies such as Singapore.

During shift handover, the outgoing and receiving nurses transfer accountability by exchanging information about the patients under their charge (Mayor, Bangerter, & Aribot, 2012). An effective handover is the transfer of critical information that allows for continuity of care, whereas poor communication can cause serious breakdowns in the continuity of care, inappropriate treatment and potential harm to the patient (Mayor et al., 2012). It has been reported that about 50% of adverse events result from ineffective communication among healthcare providers. The international research evidence acknowledged that improvements in clinical handover are as a priority area for action (Australian Commission on Safety and Quality in Health Care, 2012).

In recent years, scholars have advocated for handovers to be conducted at the patient's bedside, as it provides an opportunity to involve patients and promote patient-centred care and safety (Spinks, Chaboyer, Bucknall, Tobiano, & Whitty, 2015). While this is a positive improvement in patient-centred care, it is only one aspect and the whole handover process must be examined to improve clinical safety.

Table 9.1 Frequency of the location during the shift handovers

Location	Count
Bedside the patient's bed (Fig. 9.1)	11
In front of the patient's bed (Fig. 9.2)	6
In the room, along the aisle	32

Table 9.2 Frequency of each position during the shift handovers

Position	Count
Independent	21
Sandwich	13
Buddy	14

It is critical to gain an understanding of the process, information exchanged, patient engagement during shift handovers and the quality of clinical handovers among nurses. There are only two papers published on nursing communication and handovers in Singapore focused on compliance with the best practices in nursing shift-to-shift handover and nurses' perceptions of bedside clinical handovers (Poh, Parasuram, & Kannusamy, 2013; Roslan & Lim, 2017). This chapter describes the first study in Singapore that aimed to observe, analyse and evaluate nursing shift handover.

Hospital nurses in Singapore are centrally employed by the hospital and deployed to work in specific units/wards. Most ward nurses perform rotating shifts (i.e. morning, evening and night shifts). In a typical shift, there are two nurses looking after six to eight patients in a general ward setting. The nurse-in-charge is involved in administering medication, coordinating care documentation and handing over. Therefore, at each handover, there is a minimum of three nurses: one outgoing nurse-in-charge and two incoming nurses.

1.1   Nursing Shift-to-Shift Handovers—iSBAR

Nursing shift-to-shift handover is a critical factor in ensuring the safety of patient care as it includes essential clinical information, clinical care requirements and the transfer of care responsibility. Increasingly there has been a research focus on how to improve the information exchange and the process of handover. One overarching improvement strategy has been to standardise the handover process and introduce mnemonics such as iSBAR. The iSBAR (Identify, Situation, Background, Assessment and Recommendation) has a focus on improving patient safety in the transfer of critical clinical information.

1.2   Communication Theories and Shift-to-Shift Handovers

Numerous communication theories have been explored for use in healthcare communication; two of which have informed this study.

1.2.1 The Linear Model of Communication

Communication flows in one direction, i.e. from sender to the receiver without feedback or response in the linear model of communication (Mohorek & Webb, 2015). Thus, the sender plays a more prominent role than the receiver, which is typical of a nursing handover. Linear communication model has also been identified as the most appropriate conceptual framework for healthcare handoffs (Mohorek & Webb, 2015). However, as with any communication, linear communication is susceptible to internal and external noises that can corrupt the information at any time point between the sender and the receiver. Internal noise such as physiological, psychological and semantic noise can corrupt the understanding of the messages. For example, if the outgoing nurse is stressed or in a hurry, the information transmitted may be missing some critical information. External noise such as interruption, which is common in the clinical setting, will also have an impact on both the transmitter (sender) and receiver of the message.

1.2.2 Facework and Politeness Theory

The concept of 'face' is long-standing in Asian societies and exerts a significant impact on human behaviours. 'Face' has been defined as the positive social value or image of oneself, as imposed by society or self (Goffman, 1967). According to Goffman, the information given during an interaction that leads to a better face than one has assumed will result in positive feelings (Goffman, 1967). On the contrary, disconfirming information in front of others implies one's weak points that are revealed publicly, and thus will harm one's feeling of the face (Han, 2016). This theory was considered in the observations during the clinical handovers.

Given the multi-lingual nurses from different ethnicities and nationalities in Singapore, it is essential to understand how language and culture play a role in the communication process particularly during the shift handovers among the nurses from the different nationalities. Thus, the current study addresses the following research questions:

1. Do nurses use all the components of iSBAR during their shift handovers?
2. What is the crucial information that is present in all the shift handovers?
3. How do nurses connect with the patients and with the next shift nurses?
4. What are the unique characteristics of the handovers among nurses in Singapore?

2   Methodology

This study was conducted in one of the largest publicly funded teaching hospitals (1700-bedded) in Singapore. Using an ethnographical approach, the research team observed and video-recorded nurses during their shift-to-shift clinical handovers. Field notes were also taken to capture the related activities during the handover. The research team randomly selected two medical and two general surgical wards to participate in this study. Ethics approval was sought and obtained from the SingHealth Centralised Institutional Review Board before conducting this study. Informed consent from the nurses involved in the clinical handovers was also obtained. Handover audio and video recordings were transcribed verbatim, which included actual spoken words in English, Singlish or Malay, and analysed independently by two research team members and verified by the principal investigator.

2.1   Data Analysis

Analysis of the quality of the clinical handovers was structured according to

1. **Informational dimension**, i.e. *what was said,* e.g. communicating clearly and concisely the relevant clinical information that accurately portrays the patients' situation (Eggins, Slade, & Geddes, 2016). The iSBAR framework was used to inform the analyses of the informational dimension. Studies have shown that using iSBAR has improved the quality and safety of the physician handover of patient information in various clinical areas (Alolayan et al., 2017; Ramasubbu, Stewart, & Spiritoso, 2017). Example of iSBAR is seen below.

Identify (i)	• Identify patients with two identifiers (e.g. patient's unique identifier, name or date of birth) • Introduce the name and title/role of the staff handing over
Situation (S)	• Reason for admission • Diagnosis if known • Operation and date
Background (B)	• Relevant previous history (e.g. emergency tracheostomy) • Any allergies • Any social issues of note • Any special precautions
Assessment (A)	• Latest clinical assessment, clinical and investigations
Recommendation (R)	• Actions required after handover (e.g. call surgeon for an urgent consult—specify the level of urgency with a timeframe) • Risks—falls, pressure injury • Assign individual responsibility for conducting any task

2. **Structural dimension** referred to the sequence of information used to transmit the information. Using iSBAR as a tool to convey information provides structure to the information being transferred. As the tool had previously been validated by (Eggins & Slade, 2015), the tool used in this study was subjected to face validity using a panel of five Singapore nurses considered to have expertise in clinical communication. The panel of experts has found the tool to be appropriate for this study. Each transcript was analysed by two trained nurses (part of the research team) on the sequence of iSBAR during each handover dialogue.

3. **Interactional dimension** referred to assessing how the nurses communicate, e.g. whether there was the active involvement of the healthcare team and patients during the handover. Research has shown that the interactional dimension goes beyond the information that is being transferred. In fact, it offers clarifications and that messages have been understood (Eggins & Slade, 2015). The 'Connect, Ask, Respond, Empathize' (CARE) framework was used to analyse the interactional dimension (Eggins et al., 2016). Using the CARE framework, we examined how do nurses in Singapore interact during their shift handovers, i.e. how do they connect, ask, respond and empathise.

3 Results

Fifty shift-to-shift nursing handovers were observed and video-recorded. One was eliminated due to poor audio quality. Results are organised around three themes: Informational Dimension—identifying the right patient, Informational Dimension—telling a clear and consistent patient's story, and Unclear and missing information. Nurses participated in this study often used local Singlish, a colloquial variety of English terms, to communicate with colleagues and patients. The Singlish terms and the Malay terms are identified and an explanation of the term is provided in the first instance. Refer to Annexe 1 for the transcription conventions and Singlish and Malay terms explanation.

3.1 Informational Dimension—Identifying the Right Patient

Forty shift handovers identified patients' names, but out of these, only six outgoing nurses identified patient's name together with the patient's unique identification number. Nine shift handovers had used both patients' identifiers and introduced the nurses who were taking over the care of the patients (receiving nurse). There were eight shift handovers that did not identify the patients at all. In this study, using the patient's name is the most commonly used identifier, but it is not recommended to only use patients' name because there might be two patients with the same name.

Therefore, using an additional identifier such as date of birth or unique identification number is recommended. Below is the example of a shift handover that only identified the patient's name with no additional identifier.

	Transcript	iSBAR Code
Outgoing nurse 2.1	*Ok. So* **\<patient name\>** *went for left wing middle finger base fracture (inaudible) fracture site, open reduction, (inaudible) under GA. (inaudible) he complained pain score of 5 but he said pain is bearable lah* (Singlish - *places emphasis on the sentence before).. *nurse pointing at surgical chart**	(i), (A)
Receiving nurse	**looking at the chart and nodding**	
Outgoing nurse 2.1	*Other than that paracetamol given last at 3. No blood test. (inaudible) due at 1.30 pm*	(R)
Receiving nurse	*1.30 pm right? *checking the orders on post-operation document**	
Outgoing nurse 2.1	**showing the receiving nurse, the orders on the document**	

Compared to the above, the excerpt below is a better example of the use of two patient's identifiers. The identity of the patient was initiated by the receiving nurse as she was verifying the patient's wrist tag at the beginning of the handover.

	Transcript	iSBAR code
Receiving nurse 20.1	*Patient's* **\<NRIC number\>** *(national registration identification card) *while checking patient's wrist tag**	(i)
Outgoing nurse	*Uh-huh?* (Singlish—*signalling to repeat*)	
Receiving nurse 201.1	**\<NRIC number\>** *(repeat patient's NRIC number)*	(i)
Outgoing nurse	*Okay. Ya* (Singlish—*yes, it is so*). *Correct. *nodding head in approval** **\<patient name\>** *B2 class under* **\<doctor name\>** *Came in for acute appendicitis. Then uhh..* (Slang—*Interjection used to express thought*) *history of asthma lah* (Singlish) *Childhood asthma*	(i), (S), (B)

3.2 Informational Dimension—Telling a Clear and Consistent Patient's Story

The iSBAR framework allows for information to be transmitted in an organised and consistent manner. However, it is commonly observed that nurses do not handover all the information according to the iSBAR sequence but instead using only iBS or iSAB or iAR. Thus, the handovers were short due to the omission of information that may or may not be known by the receiving nurses. Thirteen shift handovers went straight to recommendation after identifying the patient. Below is an example, where the outgoing nurse provided a very brief background of the patient and proceeded to assessment and recommendation. It is not known if the receiving nurse had prior knowledge of the patient's situation.

	Transcript	iSBAR code
Outgoing nurse N78.2	So yesterday *flipped the paper records* they did an operation for this patient ah (Singlish) They did ah (Singlish).. left neck ah (Singlish) excision and biopsy *looking at the post-operation notes*	(B)
Outgoing nurse N78.1	First POD? (post-operation day)	Clarification
Outgoing nurse N78.2	Today is the first POD. Okay, medication *looking at the computer screen* The patient is on IV (intravenous) co-amoxiclav (antibiotics) 1.2 g (dosage) 8 h (frequency). So, I gave at around 1245 am due your time around eight o' clock. The patient is on per oral Paracetamol (analgesia) only. So, you, it's only a PRN (when necessary) dose only. If the patient complaining of pain. The plug (peripheral intravenous catheter) is over the left (hand?)	(A), (R)

The observed handovers displayed an element of 'efficiency' by the nurses, which was not documented in other literature. The outgoing nurse would begin the handover by querying the receiving nurse-in-charge familiarity with the patient. An abridged version typically skipped the identification, situation, background component of the iSBAR and proceeded to the recommendation. An abridged version of the handover was conducted as shown below:

	Transcript	iSBAR code
Outgoing nurse 23.1:	So.. and then this patient, you don't know? *looking at the receiving nurse* You know this patient or not?	(i)
Receiving nurse:	*looking at case note and nodding*	
Outgoing nurse 23.1:	You know this patient, ah?(Singlish)	(i)
Outgoing nurse 23.1:	Oh you know ah (Singlish). Under <Doctor name> and then she is at *flipping the case note* patient came from ACC (Anti-coagulation clinic) So many ACC, DM (diabetes mellitus), aah (Singlish). then trauma 30 years and then ahh (Singlish).. ostomy. So many lah (Singlish) (medical conditions?), a lot. This one also *pointing to case note* (medical conditions?) This one is the chemo drug *pointing to computer*, they say	(R)

The above practice is risky because the rest of the receiving care team might not be familiar with the patient, and the receiving nurse might not be prompted to query and request for more information. In the context of face and politeness theory, the other receiving nurses might not speak up even if they do not know the patient or have forgotten about the patient's background so as not to lose 'face'.

3.3   Unclear and Missing Information

Ineffective communication at clinical handover has been associated with irrelevant, missing or repetitive information, which can result in nurses wasting time attempting to retrieve relevant and correct information (Manias, Gerdtz, Williams, & Dooley, 2015). An example of a shift handover in a surgical ward is presented below. The outgoing nurse started the handover by identifying the patient using the patient's name and the NRIC number, in addition to his nationality and age. Next, the situation and background were provided, i.e. reason for admission and/or procedure. Under assessment, the outgoing nurse only provided the medication information. There was a lack of assessment on the latest clinical findings, vital signs or clinical investigations that were done for the patient. The outgoing nurse then proceeded to the recommendation, i.e. actions/tasks to be carried out by the receiving nurse. There was no information provided on risk alerts, past medical, surgical history or social history.

	Transcript	iSBAR Code
Outgoing nurse 3.1:	Ms *look at computer screen* <patient name> in 31 bed 2 under <Doctor name> , came in under General Surgery. The patient is from Indonesia, 25 years old. The NRIC number is <NRIC number>	(i)
Receiving nurse:	Mmm…*nodding*	
Outgoing nurse 3.1:	The patient came in because of this left neck abscess	(S)
	So yesterday *flipped the case note* they did an operation for this patient. They did a left neck excision and biopsy	(B)
Receiving nurse:	So, first POD (post-operation day)?	Clarification
Outgoing nurse 3.1:	Today is the first POD. Okay, medication *went back to computer screen*. The patient is on IV co-amoxiclav (antibiotic). 1.2 g 8 h. So, I've given at around 12.45 am	(A)
	IV (intravenous) co-amoxiclav (antibiotic) 1.2 g (dosage) 8 h (frequency) is due your time around 8 am The patient is on per oral Paracetamol (a type of medication) only. It's only a PRN (when necessary) dose only so to give if the patient complaining of pain	(R)

Doctor's orders were also not communicated consistently between shifts. For example, we observed four shift handovers on the same patient, but only one out of four handovers communicated that the patient requires strict monitoring on how much fluid was consumed or given intravenously and how much was the total fluid output. Such omission of vital information is an example of ineffective communication that could lead to incomplete observation or even delay escalation of care. Ineffective communication is recognised as one of the contributors to patient harm in hospitals (Joint Commission on Accreditation of Healthcare Organizations, 2005; Lingard et al., 2004).

Under the patient's **assessment**, information such as the need for monitoring of vital signs, pain assessment, wound assessment and laboratory tests were frequently handed over, but there was often a lack of clarity on the information. For example:

	Transcript
Outgoing nurse 3.2:	CRA VRA (a type of investigation to check for infectious status) this one yesterday dispatched already Okay. So. Flowsheet *looking at computer*. Okay, no hypocount (blood glucose monitoring) for this patient I/O (intake/output) charting. BO (bowel open) chart only. So yesterday she already passed (motion) already
Receiving nurse 3:	Okay
Outgoing nurse 3.2:	Vital signs for hourly parameters plus SpO^2 (oxygen saturation) so after about my time is okay 100–99% room air. Hourly parameters times 6 (six times) temporarily then 4 hourly, so now 4 hourly. So already taking the diet
Receiving nurse 3:	Okay

In the above scenario, Nurse 3.2 was stating the activities during her shift but did not provide further information such as availability of test results, fluid balance status, vital signs readings or appetite/tolerance. There was a lack of information on the outcome of assessment, of which the receiving nurse also did not clarify nor ask for more details which depicted the linear model of communication.

In other shift handovers, vital information such as allergies and infection status were missed out. Below is an example of two shift handovers on the same patient by different nurses. Nurse 1 identified the patient and provided some situation information before proceeding to the recommendation. In contrast, Nurse 2 alluded that patient was allergic to contrast and was Methicillin-resistant Staphylococcus aureus (MRSA) positive. This information was missed by Nurse 1. Transferring the right medication information is critical to patient safety in any handover because of its increased risk in the discontinuity between shift handovers (Eggins & Slade, 2015).

Nurse 1

	Transcript	iSBAR code
Nurse 16.2:	*Okay, so today in bed four **<patient name>** under DIM (department of internal medicine). So, she comes for this polycystic kidney and liver disease lah (Singlish). And then sepsis also. So, for her normal saline drip last put up at 330 (pm) so next due at 930 (pm) your time*	(i), (S), (R)

Nurse 2

	Transcript	iSBAR Code
Nurse 16.3:	*31/4 (room and bed number) ah (Singlish).. is under DIM, **<Doctor name>*** *Came in for this adult ah.. polycystic kidney plus liver disease. She came in for query sepsis. Then they did a blood culture on the 16th then there's a growth ah (Singlish). They didn't say what growth lah (Singlish). The full report will be out tomorrow. Then allergic to contrast media (patient is allergic). MRSA positive (patient's infection status)*	(S), (B), (A)

In general, nurses did not use all the components and sequence of iSBAR, but at its minimum, nurses would identify the patient using at least one identifier and handed over the list of recommendations to continue care.

3.4 Conflicting Information

We also observed conflicting information being handed over. For example, the patient had an abdominal tap done, and orders were given for a maximum of 10 litres of fluids to be drained out daily in three consecutive volumes of three to four litres each time. However, this information was communicated as 'to drain 10 litres a day' by the outgoing nurse, with no details of drainage volume at each time.

	Transcript
Outgoing nurse 63.15	*Urine hourly, yes. Also, need to monitor the abdominal tap lah (Singlish)*
Receiving nurse 63.20	*If more than 10 l clamp?(clamp the tubing to stop the flow)*
Outgoing nurse 63.15	*Yes. More than*
Receiving nurse 63.20	*Currently is 2.4 l?*
Receiving nurse 63.21	*So dia ada dua (translated from Malay: he got two) bag ah?* **looking at the outgoing nurse**

(continued)

(continued)

	Transcript
Outgoing nurse 63.15	*nodding* ada dua bag (translated from Malay: got two bags) ah *If more than* 10 1 *for today only you need to clamp. If less, it's okay lah* (Malay/Singlish). *So right now, my time is* 2 1 *lah* (Malay/Singlish). *The patient doesn't have hypocount. Okay, the medication this one (inaudible) during your time.* *pointing at order on the computer screen*

The below transcript illustrated the same patient's information being handed over by a different nurse on the next shift. At this handover, the instructions were more concise and accurate.

	Transcript
Outgoing nurse 63.18	*To sign all this ya* (Singlish). *You were the one, right? For the insertion of the (inaudible) Ya* (Singlish)? *Okay then*
Receiving nurse	*looking at the form and nodding*
Outgoing nurse 63.18	*So (patient is monitored?) for fall precaution reinforced. IDC (indwelling catheter)* insitu *for urine. Plug (peripheral intravenous catheter)* insitu *over (left hand?) at 250* mcg *per hour at 2 mls per hour lah* (Singlish) *infusing well. So, IV (drip?) in progress also Hourly urine output monitoring. (my shift?) is 1.9 litres lah* (Singlish). *So the whole, the whole day should drain* 10 1 *but must 3, 3, 4 1. Ya* (Singlish).. *don't drain um.. ya* (Singlish) *straightaway So, for ultrasound Doppler, I don't know if they still want to do this one at 10 am. But that's the initial um... the initial plan*

3.5 Assuming Responsibilities and Delegation of Roles

One of the key elements during clinical shift handover is to transfer professional responsibility and accountability on all the aspects of patient care to the nurse who is assuming responsibility for the patient we found that the delegation of responsibilities was not clear, i.e. who will be carrying out the orders. For example, in one communication as detailed below; initially, the outgoing nurse (78.10) reported 'later we will take from her' when referring to the urine specimen that was ordered but at the end of the handover, she reported, 'so later to collect'. It is not clear who exactly (outgoing or receiving nurse) will collect the urine specimen. See transcript in blue. Nevertheless, the injection in the tone of the voice indicates that the receiving nurse will carry out the responsibilities. This colloquial way of speaking will only be understood if one is when both nurses are part of the nursing culture in Singapore.

	Transcript
Outgoing nurse 78.10	*Mm.. still hourly. Still hourly. She got urine ah (?)*(Singlish). *Later we will take from her. Ya* (Singlish). *Then you got blood to take from her today morning. Ultrasound abdo (abdomen) is pending*
Receiving nurses 78.11	*(inaudible) handwriting nice. *looking at case note* (commenting at the Doctor's handwriting)*
Outgoing nurse 78.10	*Their handwriting nicer. Correct. Ya* (Singlish). *nodding in agreement* *So, this one is the CTSP (blood products?) ah for. They bolus her two times still low. So HO4 (house officer team 4) say bolus her another time lah* (Singlish) *So, for her, today is seen by the team already ah. Continue Rocephine, Flagyl (antibiotics). Trace cultures (laboratory results). Then urine for UFEME and culture (urine investigations). So later to collect lah* (Singlish) *All these bloods this coming morning (next day). So originally, they wanted to send for dengue (blood test for dengue), but after that, they confirm with the boss (consultant in-charge) say don't need lah* (Singlish). *Then uh. abdo (abdomen) exam (examination) with increased pain and deterioration for KIV (keep in view) urgent CT (computed tomography) scan but I think now they want to change plan, send her for abdo (abdomen) ultrasound first ah* (Singlish)

Nurses consistently communicated actions, i.e. recommendations that the receiving nurse needs to do. However, the instructions are not always communicated clearly. For example, when we compared two consecutive handovers, the night nurse handed over to the morning nurse to keep the patient's oxygen saturation more than 95%. But when the morning nurse handed over to the next shift, she had simply reported that the patient is on oxygen saturation monitoring but did not specify the targeted value to be achieved or maintained.

3.6 Structural Dimension—Forming the Complete Patient's Story

It was observed that the nurses do not use the iSBAR in its sequence but would go back and forth or jump between elements during the shift handover. As shown in the handover below, after identifying patients, the nurse went straight to handing over the medication that the receiving nurse needed to administer during her shift. The sequence was not in order, and there were a few times that the nurse needed to go back and forth between *Recommendation* and *Assessment*. As such, an important alert such as 'do not take blood pressure or blood taking on patient's left hand' was only triggered at the end when the receiving nurse asked about the peripheral intravenous catheter. If the patient's past medical and surgical history (background) had been handed over using the iSBAR sequence, this information would not have been missed out.

	Transcript	iSBAR code
Outgoing nurse 17.1:	*Okay 24/1 (room and bed number) patient <**patient name**> Patient under DIM Dr <**Doctor name**>. The patient came in for hyponatremia (low blood sodium). Secondary to the medication infamap (a type of medication)*	(i), (S)
Receiving nurse:	*mmm...*nodding**	
Outgoing nurse 17.1:	*So, for him they already—for her they already off the drips lah (Singlish) Then the patient has this Teriparatide (name of drug) injection. This injection is currently in our fridge. And not to be served by us lah (Singlish). We just give the box to the patient (the box containing the injection)*	(R)
	The patient knows how to do it by herself. She has been doing it by herself. So just give her the box at 10 o'clock	(B)
Receiving nurse:	*Okay *nodding**	
Outgoing nurse 17.1:	*Okay then other than that all oral meds (medication) to serve as per normal. He has PRN (when necessary), Paracetamol (a type of medication) Orders for her. She doesn't have any pending orders. She's not on insulin (a type of medication used to regulate blood sugar) Okay, intake and output. She just on I/O (intake and output) charting lah (Singlish). I/O monitoring Okay, so 4 hourly para (parameters). So far my time stable (patient's condition was stable)*	(B), (A)
Receiving nurse	*Hmmm..ok *nodding**	
Outgoing nurse 17.1:	*Okay. Nursing assessment. Moderate fall risk lah (Singlish). Okay so today seen by the team. To please see spine and X-ray report for the myeloma panel. Then lactulose (a type of medication).*	(A)
Receiving nurse	*The X-ray was done a few days ago ya?*	(B)
Outgoing nurse 17.1:	*Mm yes, correct*	
Outgoing nurse 17.1:	*Okay. So. Uh..home coming morning (next day) as per patient's request. Then this one is all the TCUs (outpatients' appointments) ortho (orthopaedic), endo (endocrinology) and also onco (oncology). All follow old dates ah (Singlish). Then this is a Memo to OPS (outpatient services)*	(R)
Receiving nurse	*Any plug on her? (peripheral intravenous catheter)*	(A)
Outgoing nurse 17.1:	*Ya, she has right dorsum plug. Then no BP (blood pressure) and blood taking on the left hand*	(A)
Receiving nurse	*Because of what?*	Clarification

(continued)

(continued)

	Transcript	iSBAR code
Outgoing nurse 17.1:	Because of this wait ah.*searching the case note for information* Forget they told me. Left breast CA (cancer)	(A)
Receiving nurse	Mastec (mastectomy) done?	(B)
Outgoing nurse 17.1:	Yes, correct	(B)

3.7   Location of Handover

Although beside handover was advocated, only 12 shift handovers were conducted at patient's bedsides. Among the handovers that were carried out in the room, the location where the nurses would hold the handovers varies from *beside the patient's bed* (Fig. 9.1), *in front of patient's bed* (Fig. 9.2) or *in the patients' room along the aisle*. Among these locations, the most commonly observed handover location is in the patient's room along the corridor.

3.8   The Position of Nurses During Handover

We also recorded how nurses position themselves during the shift handovers and observed three different types of position as illustrated in the figure below. The sandwich position is when the outgoing nurse is in between the two incoming nurses. The independent position is when one of the incoming nurses will check the documentation on the computer on her own while the outgoing nurse hand over the patient's information to the incoming nurse-in-charge. Lastly, the buddy position is

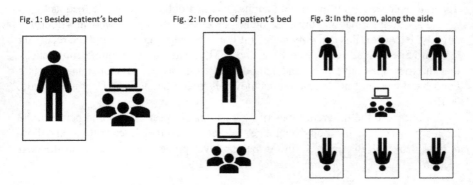

Fig. 1: Beside patient's bed   Fig. 2: In front of patient's bed   Fig. 3: In the room, along the aisle

Fig. 9.1 Location where shift handover occurred

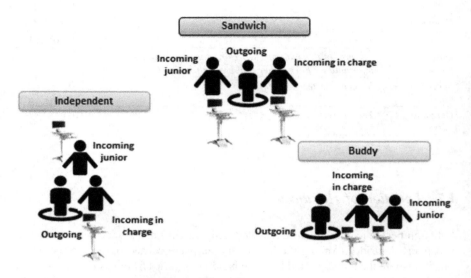

Fig. 9.2 Position of shift handover

when both incoming nurses will stand beside each other throughout the handover process. The sandwich position is preferred as it allowed both incoming nurses to interact with the outgoing nurse. This position also gives 'face' or recognition to the incoming junior nurse that she is a vital member of the incoming team.

3.9 Interactional Dimension—Going Beyond Words

An effective handover is a combination of two dimensions: the interactional and the informational aspect; however, most studies on handover concentrate mainly on the informational content. The value of the interactional component in a handover is imperative because only when interacting, one can obtain immediate feedback and exchange of information; thus, problems or errors can be noticed and rectified quickly. However, this can only happen if both the outgoing nurse and the receiving team are encouraged to ask questions and clarify. The outgoing nurse could check that the messages have been understood. Thus, the saying, 'a short handover is a good handover, but an interactive handover is a safe handover' (Eggins & Slade, 2015).

We observed the different types of interactions between nurses and patients, the language used and the body language. We also recorded interruptions and how nurse's deal with disruptions during the handover process as discussed in the next section.

3.10 Interaction Between Nurses

Although the iSBAR framework is being advocated in the institute, many of the handovers were not presented in the iSBAR framework. Most of the nurses readily accepted the shift handovers without the iSBAR structure, especially when they have prior knowledge of the patient's situation and background. Interaction between nurses was mostly in the context of clarifying whether the orders had been carried out and if they need to follow-up on the matter. It is observed that the receiving nurse would connect by asking questions to confirm what she has heard or when the medical team ordered something out of ordinary or expectation. For example:

	Transcript	iSBAR code
Outgoing nurse N75.3	... So, otherwise, he slept fairly lah (Singlish) Make sure (inaudible) left-hand lah (Singlish). Then, nil paracetamol (analgesia) given ah (Singlish).. IV cannula over the right forearm ah (Singlish).. nil phlebitis seen Antibiotics to give on the left hand. Dressing dry. Intact. No bleeding was seen lah (Singlish), so there's no (inaudible) over the left finger. KIV (keep in view) home today lah (Singlish) And for the team to review by today. That's all lah (Singlish)	(R)
Receiving nurse N75.2	Ok	
Receiving nurse N75.2	Eh, wait. No blood to take ah (Singlish)?	(R)
Outgoing nurse N75.3	No bloods right now (blood-taking). I didn't see anything. Ok, lah (Singlish)	(R)
Outgoing nurse N75.3	Ok ah (Singlish). Thank you	
Receiving nurse N75.2	Welcome	

One notable best practice that was observed involved the outgoing nurses checking with the receiving nurses if they needed more information before the handover ended. However, not all outgoing nurses provided a chance for the receiving nurse to ask additional questions at the end of the handover process. By asking 'Is there anything else?' before ending the handover process, it gives the receiving nurse time a chance to think and ask questions or clarify before taking over the care of the patient. As illustrated below:

	Transcript
Outgoing nurse N75.4	During my shift ah (Singlish).. the patient slept very late IV plug over the right hand insitu, nil redness seen. (antibiotics?) done, so I disconnect the IV drip already Left hand dressing dry and intact with mini vac drain times 1 insitu (1 drainage bottle). On active suction draining hemoserous fluid. SMD (save measurement drainage) is 20 ml

(continued)

(continued)

	Transcript
	Then KIV (keep in view) home today if well then renal panel dispatched (blood test). And ADL (activities of daily living) attended. Nil complains of pain
Receiving nurse N75.5	*Ok*
Outgoing nurse N75.4	**Anything else?**
Receiving nurse N75.5	*Hmm.. (shaking head left to right)*
Outgoing nurse N75.4	*If there's anything, just call me*
Receiving nurse N75.5	*Ok*

Throughout the handover process, the receiving nurses were often seen asking and clarifying questions to the outgoing nurses; however; there were also instances when some of the questions were being ignored. Such situations occurred when the receiving staff was a new graduate or new to the ward. For instance, as detailed below, the new nurse tried to enquire on the medication being transfused but was not provided with more details.

	Transcripts
Outgoing nurse 63.16	*So, 21/7 (room and bed number) Mr <patient name> lah (Singlish). He's under Gastro (Gastroenterology department)*
Receiving nurse 63.15	*Okay*
Outgoing nurse 63.16	*Okay his*
Receiving nurse 63.15	*Got pending orders?*
Outgoing nurse 63.16	*No pending orders and*
Receiving nurse 63.15	*Blood was taken already ah?*
Outgoing nurse 63.16	*Ya. The bloods were taken and dispatched lah (Singlish). This morning. I just dispatch. So, no hypocount, vital hourly still hourly* *On nasal prong 2 1 lah (Singlish). They order just now the MO8 (house officer team 8) lah (Singlish). They order Frusemide (a type of medication) IV bolus stat (immediately). They give already lah (Singlish). Then he was on IV somatostatin (a type of medication)*
Receiving nurse 63.15	*Somatostatin? *looking at the computer screen for order**
Outgoing nurse 63.16	*IV continuous lah (Singlish)*

(continued)

(continued)

	Transcripts
New nurse 63.19	**What is that?**
Receiving nurse 63.15	Somatostatin *continue to look at the computer screen*
Outgoing nurse 63.16	He's on continuous somatostatin

We also observed that some of the nurses tend to 'switch' to their native languages when transmitting information that was perceived to reflect poorly on the person. It is probable that switching of languages was an attempt to save one's face. An example of one of the transcripts of nurses speaking in Malay is provided below. The receiving nurse N63.20 asked the outgoing nurse if she had transferred the patient to a different doctor, which she predicted was not done yet.

Outgoing nurse N63.15	Trace this one what ah (Singlish)?
Receiving nurse N63.20	Trace culture (laboratory result) when need
Outgoing nurse N63.15	Trace culture when need then KIV (keep in view) assist ...
Receiving nurse N63.20	To transfer under doctor **<Doctor name>** *Da transfer belum?*(Translated from Malay: transfer already?) I don't think so *speaking to self* And then ECG done? (electrocardiogram)
Outgoing nurse N63.15	ECG here *pointing to the slip of paper*
Receiving nurse N63.20	Ask them to order (ask Doctor to order)
Outgoing nurse N63.15	KK—(Informal exclamation)

3.11 Interaction Between Nurses and Patients

When assessing the interactions using the CARE framework, it was observed that some nurses appeared apprehensive to bedside handover and had poor patient engagement. However, others could effectively engage patients.

	Transcript	CARE code
Receiving nurse 58.2	**<patient's name>** ah? Right? What's your IC number ah?	Connect
Patient	*tells NRIC number*	
Receiving nurse	Ok. We are the afternoon nurses' lah (Singlish). Me, **<nurse name 1>** and **<nurse name 2>** there. *pointing and looking at the nurse*	Connect

(continued)

(continued)

	Transcript	CARE code
	Ok if anything you just call us lah hor (Singlish—*lah* a suffix used to place emphasis, *hor* seeks out consensus and agreement *(ok?)*	
Patient	*Ah, hungry now, ah*	Ask
Receiving nurse	*Ah? Hungry ah? *laughs* bo pian (no choice) lah* (Singlish). *(as) you going for the procedure*	Respond
Patient	*Ten hours you know. *looking exasperated**	
Receiving nurse	*Ok, later I give a call for the Angio (angiography nurse?). See when your appointment is. Ok, can* (Singlish—Sure, this means "able to"),*?(A way of asking if something is possible/ can be achieved)*trying to coax the patient**	Empathise
Receiving nurse	*Sir, later we call Angio for you lah hor* (Singlish) *Then after that we see because we got need. We need to give you some medication because you got asthma and for the pain medication. Ok? Can* (Singlish—Sure, this means "able to")	Connect

Empathise, as part of the CARE framework, involves acknowledging patient's personal needs for reassurance. For example, in the communication above, the receiving nurse respected the patient's feeling of hunger due to long period of fasting. The nurse reassured the patient that he would check the estimated time for the procedure. Effective interactional practices build a good rapport and facilitate the exchange of important clinical information about the patient (Eggins et al., 2016). In this study, not many interactions were seen between nurses and patients during the handovers except during patient identification and when the nurses introduced themselves at the start of the handover. Most of the nurses' interactions were in the form of connecting with the receiving nurses by asking if they were familiar with the patient and if they were ready to take over. Connections were also created when looking at the e-documentation and laboratory orders and result on the computer while handing over.

Nurses' body language during the handover was also observed. In some instances, the receiving nurse appeared disinterested and was not facing the patient throughout the handover process. In such scenarios, the potential to create a rapport between the patient and the nurse is lost. However, there may be a possibility that the connection or rapport was made immediately after the handover. However, this was not observed in the video.

Empathising encourages nurses to develop collegial respect and at the same time recognise the colleagues' professional abilities and interpersonal needs (Eggins et al., 2016). However, none of the nurses observed in this study showed empathy towards the receiving nurses or vice versa. It could indicate the nurses' lack of awareness and training on how to show compassion during a shift handover and could be a valuable learning point for the hospital's educator to improve in the future.

3.12   Interruptions During Handover

Interruption during handovers is often cited as one of the factors contributing to errors and is identified as a significant barrier to the delivery of effective handovers (Spooner, Corley, Chaboyer, Hammond, & Fraser, 2015). According to the linear model of communication, interruption is noise that affects the quality of the message (Mohorek & Webb, 2015). In this study, we also recorded the frequency and type of interruptions that occurred. Seventeen interruptions were by other nursing, medical and ancillary staffs and only one handover was interrupted by a patient who was enquiring about his care. At every interruption, both receiving and outgoing nurses would stop and attend to the queries. In general, it is the norm for nurses to stop their handover whenever interrupted. Most of the time, the interruption only took less than 3 min and usually involved taking messages or orders that needed to be done after the shift handover. Culturally, it is deemed impolite to ignore colleagues, especially those who are more senior in rank or age when they talk to junior colleagues, which is aligned with politeness theory (Goffman, 1967). Professionally, it is not acceptable to ignore patients when they speak to nurses even though they were interrupting the handover process. This is especially true in Singapore, where the nursing profession is viewed as service provider. Thus, nurses must always put their patients first.

4   Discussion

This study aimed to observe, analyse and evaluate clinical shift handover by nurses in Singapore. Although shift handover is mandatory for care continuity, it is not taught formally in nursing schools (Lally, 1999). Nurses learn to perform handovers from their peers or experienced nurses in the clinical area; hence, it seems to work very differently depending on the ward and the person who is doing it. Such differences were well observed in this study. Some ward nurses performed the shift handovers by the patient's bedside; some performed along the corridor while some performed outside of the patient's room. Most of the shift handovers were conducted away from the patient's bedside; therefore, there is a lack of patient involvement and interaction during the handover process. By bringing the handover process to the patient's bedside, nurses can empower patients to become involved in their care, which improves patient safety and patient satisfaction ratings (Mardis et al., 2016). While the literature on patient safety has advocated for bedside shift handover (Maxson, Derby, Wrobleski, & Foss, 2012), sustaining this practice in real-world settings has been challenging and not fully implemented.

Common barriers to effective communication during shift handovers are too little or too much information, inconsistent quality, limited opportunity to ask questions and interruptions (Welsh, Flanagan, & Ebright, 2010). These barriers were all observed in this study, too. Despite implementing the iSBAR framework for the nurses to use during shift handovers, most of the shift handovers observed were still unstructured and disorganised. The lack of systematic structure during handovers can lead to failure to hand over all relevant and important content, such as medications, risk alerts and significant laboratory results (Schifano et al., 2010). In this study, we observed an abridged version of shift handover process which may be a unique practice in Singapore as nurses generally work in the same unit for an extended period; hence, it is expected that they would know their patients' background well.

The CARE framework is rather new to the current hospital; hence, nurses may not be familiar with how to apply it in practice (Eggins et al., 2016). Generally, it was observed that nurses and patients connect during the identification process. The Ask and Respond component in the CARE framework were observed in practice; however, some questions were ignored (e.g. the student nurse example). Nevertheless, there is a lack of empathy observed between nurses. Empathy was more commonly seen during the interactions between the nurses and the patients.

Lack of knowledge or education is associated with poor communication during handovers (Fryman, Hamo, Raghavan, & Goolsarran, 2017). The interaction between nurses in this study was merely in the form of acknowledgement, with little clarification, challenge and empathy. Therefore, mentoring and guidance on how to communicate effectively during shift handovers is vital, especially among new graduate nurses. More importantly, there is the need to change the perceptions of nurses towards handover to view it as a component of patients' safety rather than merely a handing over of existing tasks. We recommend teaching best practices in clinical handovers early, so that good communication skills during handovers will continue in the clinical settings.

Ineffective communication during clinical handover has been associated with irrelevant, missing or repetitive information, which can result in nurses wasting time attempting to retrieve relevant and correct information (Manias et al., 2015). We observed that the iSBAR framework was not used in its original sequence. The assessment was one of the most commonly missed out components of the iSBAR. Nurses were very good at handing over the list of recommendations, but sometimes the information was not consistent and accurate. Given this finding, it is recommended that a patient handover should contain information on current clinical issues. The clinical issues should include the patients current clinical status, care plans and future anticipated care needs and contingency plans (Meth, Bass, & Hoke, 2013).

This study also observed the lack of patients' involvement during the shift handover; hence, it is recommended that patients are educated on the benefits of participating during shift handovers. Additionally, there is the need to develop strategies to improve patient's participation in handovers, such as including information on 'participating in shift handovers' during patient orientation to the ward during admission. Perhaps, when designing smart wards in the future, we can leverage technology to improve the quality of information being transferred between the healthcare team and patients.

Finally, this study did not examine the level of education, expertise and comprehension of the registered nurses who were involved in the shift handovers. Future research can consider these factors. For example, it is possible that novice nurses differ in the type and amount of information they need during handovers and the way the information is being transferred and used.

5 Conclusions/Implications

This study provides an understanding of current nursing shift-to-shift handover practice in Singapore. Similar to previous studies' findings, there is a lack of clarity in the transfer of responsibility and accountability (Anderson, Malone, Shanahan, & Manning, 2015), there were variations in the order of the information presented and patient participation was rare (Johnson, Jefferies, & Nicholls, 2012). Adoption of the iSBAR framework was evident during the shift handovers, but was not used consistently. Interestingly, an abridged version of the handover was commonly observed and practiced by nurses who were familiar with the patients. Nurses connect with each other and the patients by using their native and colloquial language. Asking and Responding were observed at times during the shift handovers. Our results highlighted the need to educate nurses on the CARE framework, especially on empathising.

Funding This study was funded by the SingHealth Research Foundation Grant (SHF/HSR076/ 2014).

Appendix

Transcription conventions

(inaudible)	Used when the audio recording could not be heard
< >	Confidential information
comment	Indicate non-verbal action
(..)	Two dots are indicative of using fillers during the conversation
[comments in square brackets]	Relevant contextual information
[comments with questions mark?]	Transcriber's contextual inference

Singlish Terms

Ah	An exclamation used at the end of sentences
bo pian	No choice
Can	Sure, this means 'able to'
Lah	Places emphasis on the sentence before
Uh-huh	Signalling to repeat
Ya	Yes, it is so

Malay Translations

Da transfer belum	Translated from Malay: transfer already
dia ada dua	Translated from Malay: he got two
Lah	Places emphasis on the sentence before (shared with Singlish)

References

Alolayan, A., Alkaiyat, M., Ali, Y., Alshami, M., Al-Surimi, K., & Jazieh, A.-R. (2017). Improving physician's hand over among oncology staff using standardized communication tool. *BMJ Quality Improvement Reports, 6*(1). https://doi.org/10.1136/bmjquality.u211844. w6141.

Anderson, J., Malone, L., Shanahan, K., & Manning, J. (2015). Nursing bedside clinical handover —An integrated review of issues and tools. *Journal of Clinical Nursing, 24*(5–6), 662–671. https://doi.org/10.1111/jocn.12706.

Australian Commission on Safety and Quality in Health Care. (2012). Safety and quality improvement guide standard 6: Clinical handover. Retrieved from https://www. safetyandquality.gov.au/sites/default/files/migrated/Standard6_Oct_2012_WEB.pdf.

Eggins, S., & Slade, D. (2015). Communication in clinical handover: Improving the safety and quality of the patient experience. *Journal of Public Health Research, 4*(3), 666–666. https://doi.org/10.4081/jphr.2015.666.

Eggins, S., Slade, D., & Geddes, F. (2016). *Effective communication in clinical handover: From research to practice* (Vol. 15). Germany: De Gruyter.

Fryman, C., Hamo, C., Raghavan, S., & Goolsarran, N. (2017). A quality improvement approach to standardization and sustainability of the hand-off process. *BMJ Quality Improvement Reports, 6*(1). https://doi.org/10.1136/bmjquality.u222156.w8291.

Goffman, E. (1967). *Interaction ritual: Essays on face-to-face behavior.* New York: Doubleday Anchor.

Han, K.-H. (2016). The feeling of "face" in confucian society: From a perspective of psychosocial equilibrium. *Frontiers in Psychology, 7,* 1055–1055. https://doi.org/10.3389/fpsyg.2016.01055 .

Johnson, M., Jefferies, D., & Nicholls, D. (2012). Exploring the structure and organization of information within nursing clinical handovers. *International Journal of Nursing Practice, 18* (5), 462–470. https://doi.org/10.1111/j.1440-172X.2012.02059.x.

Joint Commission on Accreditation of Healthcare Organizations. (2005). National Patient Safety Goals. *Joint Commission.* Retrieved from http://www.hcpro.com/ACC-40751-851/Check-out-the-2005-National-Patient-Safety-Goals.html.

Lally, S. (1999). An investigation into the functions of nurses' communication at the inter-shift handover. *Journal of Nursing Management, 7*(1), 29–36.

Lingard, L., Espin, S., Whyte, S., Regehr, G., Baker, G. R., Reznick, R., et al. (2004). Communication failures in the operating room: An observational classification of recurrent types and effects. *Quality & Safety in Health Care, 13*(5), 330–334. https://doi.org/10.1136/qhc.13.5.330.

Manias, E., Gerdtz, M., Williams, A., & Dooley, M. (2015). Complexities of medicines safety: Communicating about managing medicines at transition points of care across emergency departments and medical wards. *Journal of Clinical Nursing, 24*(1–2), 69–80. https://doi.org/10.1111/jocn.12685.

Mardis, T., Mardis, M., Davis, J., Justice, E. M., Riley Holdinsky, S., Donnelly, J., et al. (2016). Bedside shift-to-shift handoffs: A systematic review of the literature. *Journal of Nursing Care Quality, 31*(1), 54–60. https://doi.org/10.1097/ncq.0000000000000142.

Maxson, P. M., Derby, K. M., Wrobleski, D. M., & Foss, D. M. (2012). Bedside nurse-to-nurse handoff promotes patient safety. *Medsurg Nursing, 21*(3), 140–144; quiz 145.

Mayor, E., Bangerter, A., & Aribot, M. (2012). Task uncertainty and communication during nursing shift handovers. *Journal of Advanced Nursing, 68*(9), 1956–1966. https://doi.org/10.1111/j.1365-2648.2011.05880.x.

Meth, S., Bass, E. J., & Hoke, G. (2013). Considering factors of and knowledge about patients in handover assessment. *IEEE Transactions on Human-Machine Systems, 43*(5), 494–498. https://doi.org/10.1109/THMS.2013.2274595.

Mohorek, M., & Webb, T. P. (2015). Establishing a conceptual framework for handoffs using communication theory. *Journal of Surgical Education, 72*(3), 402–409. https://doi.org/10.1016/j.jsurg.2014.11.002.

Poh, C. L., Parasuram, R., & Kannusamy, P. (2013). Nursing inter-shift handover process in mental health settings: A best practice implementation project. *Int J Evid Based Healthc, 11*(1), 26–32. https://doi.org/10.1111/j.1744-1609.2012.00293.x.

Ramasubbu, B., Stewart, E., & Spiritoso, R. (2017). Introduction of the identification, situation, background, assessment, recommendations tool to improve the quality of information transfer during medical handover in intensive care. *Journal of the Intensive Care Society, 18*(1), 17–23. https://doi.org/10.1177/1751143716660982.

Roslan, S. B., & Lim, M. L. (2017). Nurses' perceptions of bedside clinical handover in a medical-surgical unit: An interpretive descriptive study. *Proceedings of Singapore Healthcare, 26*(3), 150–157. https://doi.org/10.1177/2010105816678423.

Schifano, F., Dhillon, S., Pezzolesi, C., Pickles, J., Randell, W., Hussain, Z., et al. (2010). Clinical handover incident reporting in one UK general hospital. *International Journal for Quality in Health Care, 22*(5), 396–401. https://doi.org/10.1093/intqhc/mzq048.

Spinks, J., Chaboyer, W., Bucknall, T., Tobiano, G., & Whitty, J. A. (2015). Patient and nurse preferences for nurse handover—Using preferences to inform policy:A discrete choice experiment protocol. *British Medical Journal Open, 5*(11), e008941. https://doi.org/10.1136/bmjopen-2015-008941.

Spooner, A. J., Corley, A., Chaboyer, W., Hammond, N. E., & Fraser, J. F. (2015). Measurement of the frequency and source of interruptions occurring during bedside nursing handover in the intensive care unit: An observational study. *Australian Critical Care, 28*(1), 19–23. https://doi.org/10.1016/j.aucc.2014.04.002.

Tenzer, H., Terjesen, S., & Harzing, A.-W. (2017). Language in international business: A review and agenda for future research. *Management International Review, 57*(6), 815–854. https://doi.org/10.1007/s11575-017-0319-x.

Wee, L. (2009). 'Burdens' and 'handicaps' in Singapore's language policy: On the limits of language management. *Language Policy, 9*(2), 97–114. https://doi.org/10.1007/s10993-009-9159-2.

Welsh, C. A., Flanagan, M. E., & Ebright, P. (2010). Barriers and facilitators to nursing handoffs: Recommendations for redesign. *Nursing Outlook, 58*(3), 148–154. https://doi.org/10.1016/j.outlook.2009.10.005.

Part III
Health Communication in Organizational, Campaign and Information Contexts

Assessment of Safety Culture: A Singapore Residential Aged Care Cross-Sectional Study

Phillip R. Della, Lina Ma, Pamela A. Roberts, Huaqiong Zhou, Rene Michael, and Satvinder S. Dhaliwal

Abstract Background: Despite a significant amount of attention towards the safety and quality of acute care, little focus has been paid to the residential aged care sector, especially in the Asian region. This research aimed to assess the safety and quality culture within two nursing homes in Singapore. **Methods**: A cross-sectional study used a validated 42-item Nursing Home Survey on Patient Safety Culture (NHSPSC) tool. Minor linguistic adjustments were made to the tool, and its internal reliability was assessed using Cronbach's alpha. **Results**: The Cronbach's alpha values for the 12 PSC Composites ranged from 0.519 to 0.781, nine PSC Composites were >0.6 (adequate), indicating NHSPSC had acceptable internal reliability in the Singapore context. Of the 12 PSC Composites calculated for the two Singapore nursing homes, six were >90th percentile, four were >75th percentile and two >50th percentile. **Conclusion**: The NHSPSC tool provided an assessment of residential aged care safety and quality culture of the two nursing homes in Singapore. In general, the staff at the nursing homes in Singapore perceived a higher percentile residential safety culture compared to the US Comparative Database. The findings of this study demonstrated the importance of communication openness in residential safety culture.

Keywords Patient safety · Quality culture · Singapore aged care · Cross-sectional · Communication openness

P. R. Della (✉) · P. A. Roberts · H. Zhou · R. Michael
School of Nursing, Midwifery & Paramedicine, Curtin University, GOP Box U 1987, Perth, WA 6845, Australia
e-mail: p.della@curtin.edu.au

L. Ma
Clinical/Aged Care Services, Lions Home for the Elders, Singapore, Singapore

Curtin University, Perth, WA 6845, Australia

S. S. Dhaliwal
School of Public Health, Curtin University, Perth, WA 6845, Australia

© Springer Nature Singapore Pte Ltd. 2020
B. Watson and J. Krieger (eds.), *Expanding Horizons in Health Communication*,
The Humanities in Asia 6, https://doi.org/10.1007/978-981-15-4389-0_10

List of Abbreviations

PSC   Patient Safety Culture
NHSPSC Nursing Home Survey on Patient Safety Culture
AHRQ   Agency for Healthcare Research Quality

1   Background

Globally, there is increasing growth in residential aged care facilities, which is directly related to the ageing phenomena (O'Keeffe, 2016). Patient safety culture (PSC) is increasingly a critical factor in the delivery of safe and quality residential aged care, especially with a decreased incidence of falls (El-Jardali, Dimassi, Jamal, Jaafar, & Hemadeh, 2011; Thomas et al., 2012). Open communication is considered a foundation of safe care. While there has been a significant amount of attention towards the safety and quality of acute care (see Della, Aloweni, Ang et al., this edition), little focus has been paid to the residential aged care sector, especially in the Asian region. Previous studies have demonstrated that PSC in nursing homes is poorly developed (Thomas et al., 2012). This paucity of attention indicates the necessity of this research to expand our understanding of safety and quality at residential aged care settings of Singapore. This research contributed to the implementation of research-based practice, which ultimately results in improved residential care (Castle, Wagner, Perera, Ferguson, & Handler, 2011).

The twenty-first century has been labelled as one of ageing by McDonald (2015). While this is a global phenomenon, there are specific localised regional aspects that need to be considered when it comes to the provision of residential aged care. Within the Asian region, the social impact of ageing is also related to increasing life expectancy and decreasing fertility rates, all of which are occurring simultaneously. The combined effect of ageing and the decline in fertility rates in Asian regions has a double impact on the residential aged care sector resulting in an unprecedented demand for residential aged care placements coinciding with a reduction in the available local healthcare workforce. Specifically, the Singapore population continues to age. In 2015, 13.1% of the population were aged over 65 years, with decreasing numbers of citizens in the working-age band of 20–64 years (National Population and Talent Division, Prime Minister's Office, Singapore Department of Statistics, Ministry of Home Affairs, & Immigration & Checkpoints Authority, 2015). This decline in the local working-age group band reduces the pool and supply of individuals entering the health professions, and eventually the supply of well-educated/trained health workforce.

Singapore has an ageing policy in place that focuses on healthy ageing, living fulfilled lives and the provision of good health care (Nieva & Sorra, 2003). To enable implementation of this policy, Singapore relies on international recruitment of nurses and other care professionals to meet the workforce demand for the provision of high-quality health care. Recruitment in the aged care sector has focussed predominantly on attracting nurses from nearby Asian countries such as China, India, Malaysia, Myanmar, Philippines and Sri Lanka. While international recruitment has, in part, assisted in the provision of the workforce, other issues arise that impact and require consideration and attention. These include differences in health and educational preparation of international workforce, cultural and linguistic contexts, including perceptions of what constitutes residential aged care safety and quality. It is acknowledged that while English is the official language used in the Singapore healthcare setting, there is variation in vocabulary, pronunciation and meaning of words among international nurses working at the nursing homes (O'Keeffe, 2016). This can lead to difficulties in clinical communication, handovers and residents communication engagement and understanding.

To address residential aged care safety and quality, there is a need to appraise the concept. While this field is still developing, Nieva and Sorra (2003) identified the concept as the group and personal values, positions, perceptions, competencies and behaviour that related to patient safety. Patient safety culture is an important measurement metric as it closely relates to the safety and quality of residential aged care delivery and patient outcomes (Ausserhofer et al., 2013). When there is a high focus on PSC in aged care facilities, patient outcomes improve as safety is a guiding factor in patient care delivery (Halligan & Zecevic, 2011). A number of studies using the NHSPSC tool have been undertaken in recent years focusing on the culture of patient safety in residential aged care settings mainly in the US (Arnetz et al., 2011; Handler et al., 2006; Thomas et al., 2012) and Europe (Zúñiga, Schwappach, De Geest, & Schwendimann, 2013). Limited evidence exists with regard to previously conducted studies in Asia using the NHSPSC tool in the aged care setting. As a result, the tool has not been assessed for the internal and external validities of the 12 PSC Composites in Asian residential aged care settings. More specifically, the tool has not been validated in relation to their association with two overall questions regarding 'rating' and 'referral' of the nursing home.

This research assessed the safety and quality culture within two residential nursing homes in Singapore using the Nursing Home Survey on Patient Safety Culture (NHSPSC) tool consisting of 12 PSC Composites. The researchers then tested the validity and internal reliability of the NHSPSC tool. The predictive validity of the 12 PSC Composites was also evaluated against the two overall questions on the nursing home rating and referral using logistic regression.

2   Methods

2.1   Study Design

A cross-sectional study was conducted using the validated NHSPSC tool.

2.2   Setting, Sample and Procedure

The study involved two Voluntary Welfare Organisation residential nursing homes in Singapore with a total of 354 nursing home beds and 165 administrative, nursing and care assistant staff, allied health professional and support staff. Both residential nursing homes are branches, under the same executive management. All staff were included in the study and approval was obtained from the Human Research Ethics Committees at Curtin University, Western Australia and the Management Committee of the two residential nursing homes. Staff were recruited to complete the NHSPSC with a turnaround time of 1 week. The survey package was explained to the staff by one of the co-investigators and distributed to all employees through the managers of their respective departments. Each package contained an information sheet describing the study, a copy of the survey and a reply envelope for confidential return. Following the completion of the survey, participants placed it in the provided envelope in a box marked Curtin University Research Project placed in each department of the homes. One of the co-investigators subsequently collected boxes. All 165 staff responded to the survey.

2.3   Survey Instrument

Respondents were surveyed using the NHSPSC tool developed specifically for nursing homes by the Agency for Healthcare Research Quality (AHRQ) in the United States of America context (2016) to measure the culture of patient safety from the nursing home staff perspective. The NHSPSC survey was developed by Westat and is described in detail on their website: http://www.ahrq.gov/professionals/quality-patient-safety/patientsafetyculture/nursing-home/index.html.
This study examined the opinions, perspectives, attitudes and beliefs of nursing home staff and providers in relation to PSC in their nursing home. The NHSPSC has 42 items, which are structured based on four areas: working in the nursing home, communication, your supervisor and your nursing home. Response options were in the form of a 5-point Likert scale of agreement ('strongly disagree to agree strongly') or frequency ('never to always'). The questionnaire also includes two overall rating questions: I would tell my friends that this is a safe nursing home for their family (Yes, Maybe No) and please give this nursing home an overall rating

on patient safety (Poor, Fair, Good, Very good, Excellent). The 42 items in the questionnaire are grouped into 12 PSC Composites: Overall Perceptions of Resident Safety (three items); Feedback and Communications About Incidents (four items); Supervisor Expectations and Actions Promoting Resident Safety (three items); Organisational Learning (four items); Management Support for Resident Safety (three items); Training and Skills (three items); Compliance With Procedures (three items); Teamwork (four items); Handoffs (four items); Communication Openness (three items); Non-punitive Response to Mistakes (four items); Staffing (four items). The survey was pilot-tested in 40 nursing homes across the US in 2007 with 3,698 respondents. The Cronbach's α values for the Composites ranged from 0.71 to 0.86 (Agency for Healthcare Research and Quality, 2016).

The NHSPSC tool with minor modification used in this study was subjected to face validity by a panel of three Singaporean senior health professionals of aged care to ensure the questions were context appropriate to Singapore aged care and measured the Composites (Turner, 1979). For this research, a minor linguistic adjustment was made to change the word 'Handoffs' to 'Handover'. Demographic and other background questions were added to the questionnaire as Singapore is a multicultural society and has recruited and relied on global healthcare worker for its residential aged care workforce. The added items include age, gender, country of origin, highest education qualification, period worked in this nursing home, hours per week worked in this nursing home, job in this nursing home and whether respondents has direct contact with residents most of the time.

2.4 Data Analysis

Item and composite scores were computed using AHRQ's data entry and analysis tool for Microsoft Excel (Agency for Healthcare Research and Quality, 2016). The proportion of NHSPSC positive scores was calculated for all items in each of the 12 Composites. Scores were classified as positive if respondents strongly agree or agree with items on the agreement scale or most of the time or always for items on the frequency scale as per the NHSPSC 2016 User Comparative Database Report in the USA (Agency for Healthcare Research and Quality, 2016). The summary score for each Composite is the average proportion of positive scores for all items in the Composites.

This study divided the respondents based on their primary role at the nursing home (direct contact versus no direct contact with patients) and this allowed comparison between clinical caregivers and administrative staff (Agency for Healthcare Research and Quality, 2016). Licensed nurses, nursing aides/healthcare assistants, direct care staff and other providers (i.e. advanced practice nurse, clinical nurse specialist) were classified as having 'direct contact' with residents. Administrator/manager, administrative staff and support staff were grouped as 'no direct contact'.

Internal consistency of the questionnaire was assessed using Cronbach's alpha, for each group of items of each of the 12 PSC Composites. Reliability of the questionnaire was considered adequate if the alpha values were >0.60 and good if the alpha values were >0.70 (Manser, 2014).

Logistic regression was used in this study to establish if the 12 Patient Safety Culture Composites are valid predictors of the overall questions of 'I would tell friends that this is a safe nursing home for their family' and 'Please give this nursing home an overall rating on patient safety' (Portney & Watkins, 2009). Logistic regression is an established statistical technique, and we utilised this technique to assess which of the Composites were significant predictors of the two overall questions. Odds ratio and associated 95% confidence intervals represent a 10% change in the positive response. Univariate analysis was undertaken by considering each patient safety culture Composite individually, and multivariable analysis was used to identify Composites that were collectively and independently associated with the outcome. All statistical analyses were conducted using SPSS version 22 and p-values less than 5% were considered statistically significant.

3   Results

A total of 165 surveys were distributed and returned. Missing information for each survey item ranged between 0 and 4%. According to Schafer (1999), less than 5% missing data will not bias results. Given that the missing data for each item fell below this threshold, no statistical adjustments to account for missing data were needed. The majority of the respondents were female (65.9%), staff were generally working more than 40 h per week (88.4%), and about 73% had a degree qualification. The sample had a mean ± standard deviation age of 34.3 ± 10.6 years, and the majority of the workforce (81.1%) did not originate from Singapore. Approximately, 80% of the staff worked for more than 1 year in the nursing home. The characteristics of respondents are presented in Table 1.

Cronbach's alpha, a measure of internal consistency of the items, was calculated using the questionnaire items in each PSC Composites (Table 2). The Cronbach's alpha values for the 12 PSC Composites ranged from 0.519 to 0.781. Three PSC Composites had Cronbach's alpha between 0.5 and 0.6, five PSC Composites >0.6 and four Composites >0.7, indicating that the questionnaire had acceptable internal validity. The four PSC Composites with Cronbach's alpha values >0.7 were Overall Perceptions of Resident Safety, Management Support for Resident Safety, Handovers, and Communication Openness.

The mean percentage positive response for the 12 PSC Composite score is presented in Table 3. The mean percentage positive responses were greater than 80% for 9 out of the 12 Composites, with Communication Openness, Non-punitive Response to Mistakes and Staffing scoring ranged from 59.9 to 65.6%. Of the 12 PSC Composites, six were greater than the 90th percentile for the positive

Table 1 Characteristics of respondents stratified by direct contact with residents

Demographics	No direct contact	Direct contact	Total
Number of respondents	28 (17.0%)	137 (83.0%)	165 (100%)
Age (years)	49.3 ± 10.9	31.3 ± 7.6	34.3 ± 10.6
Branch			
Bedok	5 (17.9%)	55 (40.1%)	60 (36.4%)
Toa Payoh	23 (82.1%)	82 (59.9%)	105 (63.6%)
Gender			
Female	19 (67.9%)	89 (65.4%)	108 (65.9%)
Male	9 (32.1%)	47 (34.6%)	56 (34.1%)
Country of origin			
China	1 (3.6%)	4 (2.9%)	5 (3%)
India	1 (3.6%)	15 (11%)	16 (9.8%)
Malaysia	1 (3.6%)	2 (1.5%)	3 (1.8%)
Myanmar	1 (3.6%)	39 (28.7%)	40 (24.4%)
Philippines	2 (7.1%)	61 (44.9%)	63 (38.4%)
Singapore	22 (78.6%)	9 (6.6%)	31 (18.9%)
Sri Lanka	0 (0%)	6 (4.4%)	6 (3.7%)
Highest education qualification			
Sec 2/3 vocational level	3 (10.7%)	8 (6.2%)	11 (7%)
GCE 'O' level	8 (28.6%)	11 (8.5%)	19 (12%)
GCE 'A' level	5 (17.9%)	23 (17.7%)	28 (17.7%)
Degree (non-nursing)	8 (28.6%)	0 (0%)	8 (5.1%)
Degree (nursing)	3 (10.7%)	87 (66.9%)	90 (57%)
Masters	0 (0%)	1 (0.8%)	1 (0.6%)
Ph.D.	1 (3.6%)	0 (0%)	1 (0.6%)
Period worked in this nursing home			
Less than 2 months	0 (0%)	9 (6.7%)	9 (5.5%)
2–11 months	3 (10.7%)	21 (15.6%)	24 (14.7%)
1–2 years	4 (14.3%)	37 (27.4%)	41 (25.2%)
3–5 years	7 (25%)	33 (24.4%)	40 (24.5%)
6–10 years	6 (21.4%)	27 (20%)	33 (20.2%)
11 years or more	8 (28.6%)	8 (5.9%)	16 (9.8%)
Hours per week worked in this nursing home			
15 or fewer hours per week	1 (3.6%)	8 (5.9%)	9 (5.5%)
16–24 h per week	0 (0%)	1 (0.7%)	1 (0.6%)
25 to less than 40 h per week	4 (14.3%)	5 (3.7%)	9 (5.5%)
Greater than or equal to 40 h per week	23 (82.1%)	122 (89.7%)	145 (88.4%)

*n.s. Categorical measurements are represented as n (%), and continuous measurements are represented as mean ± SD

Table 2 Cronbach's alpha within each of the 12 PSC composites

Composites	Cronbach's alpha	Number of items
Overall perceptions of resident safety	0.781	3
Feedback and communications about incidents	0.673	4
Supervisor expectations and actions promoting resident safety	0.646	3
Organisational learning	0.549	4
Management support for resident safety	0.723	3
Training and skills	0.617	3
Compliance with procedures	0.519	3
Teamwork	0.697	4
Handovers	0.706	4
Communication openness	0.732	3
Non-punitive response to mistakes	0.553	4
Staffing	0.638	4

Table 3 Mean percent positive response and percentiles of the 12 PSC Composites at the two nursing homes in Singapore

Composites	No direct contact (%)	Direct contact (%)	Overall
Overall perceptions of resident safety	98.8	95.8	96.3% (>75%ile)
Feedback and communications about incidents	91.1	91.2	91.2% (>75%ile)
Supervisor expectations and actions promoting Resident safety	90.1	93.4	92.9% (>75%ile)
Organisational learning	86.6	90.1	89.5% (>90%ile)
Management support for resident safety	85.7	84.8	85.0% (>90%ile)
Training and skills	92.9	91.1	91.4% (>90%ile)
Compliance with procedures	72.6	83.7	81.8% (>90%ile)
Teamwork	84.2	91.1	89.9% (>90%ile)
Handovers	91.1	92.2	92.0% (>90%ile)
Communication openness	71.4	64.4	65.6% (>50%ile)
Non-punitive response to mistakes	51.8	61.6	59.9% (>75%ile)
Staffing	66.4	61.4	62.3% (>50%ile)

responses, four were greater than the 75th percentile and two greater than the 50th percentile (Communication Openness and Staffing).

When the respondents were asked the two overall questions, the mean percentage positive agreement of the two Singapore nursing homes for the question 'I would tell my friends that this is a safe nursing home for their family' (Yes vs. Maybe, No) was 84.8%. The corresponding result for the question on the overall rating of nursing home (Excellent; Very good versus Good, Fair; Poor) was 77.4%.

In univariate analysis, 10 out of the 12 Composites were significant predictors of the outcome that staff responded 'yes', to the question 'I would tell friends that this is a safe nursing home for their family' (Table 4). The only two Composites that were not significantly associated with the outcome were Feedback and communications about incidents, and Training and skills. With every 10% change in the positive score in Overall Perceptions of Resident Safety, staff were 1.42 times more likely to recommend the nursing home as safe to their family and friends. In multivariable logistic regression, only 2 of the ten significant Composite were found to be independently associated with the outcome. Staff, who had 10% higher overall positive perceptions of resident safety scores, were 33% more likely and 10% higher positive. Communication openness scores were 19% more likely to recommend the nursing home as safe to their family and friends.

All 12 Composites were significant predictors of the overall rating of the nursing home, using univariate analysis. In multivariable logistic regression, only 2 of the

Table 4 Association between patient safety culture composite scores and staff response to 'I would tell friends that this is a safe nursing home for their family'

Association between 12 PSC Composites with staff response to 'I would tell friends that this is a safe nursing home for their family' (Yes vs. No and Maybe)

Composites	Univariate	Multivariable
Overall perceptions of resident safety	1.42 (1.11–1.82); p-value = 0.005	1.33 (1.03–1.72); p-value = 0.031
Feedback and communications about incidents	1.08 (0.90–1.30); p-value = 0.399	n.s.
Supervisor expectations and actions promoting resident safety	1.19 (1.00–1.42); p-value = 0.048	n.s.
Organisational learning	1.31 (1.09–1.56); p-value = 0.004	n.s.
Management support for resident safety	1.20 (1.06–1.36); p-value = 0.005	n.s.
Training and skills	1.14 (0.96–1.34); p-value = 0.134	n.s.
Compliance with procedures	1.24 (1.08–1.44); p-value = 0.003	n.s.
Teamwork	1.31 (1.12–1.54); p-value = 0.001	n.s.
Handovers	1.16 (0.97–1.38); p-value = 0.106	n.s.
Communication openness	1.22 (1.09–1.37); p-value = 0.001	1.19 (1.05–1.34); p-value = 0.004
Non-punitive response to mistakes	1.23 (1.07–1.41); p-value = 0.004	n.s.
Staffing	1.24 (1.08–1.43); p-value = 0.002	n.s.

(continued)

Table 4 (continued)

Association between 12 PSC Composites with staff response to 'I would tell friends that this is a safe nursing home for their family' (Yes vs. No and Maybe)

Composites	Univariate	Multivariable

Association between 12 PSC Composites with staff response to 'Please give this nursing home an overall rating on patient safety' (Very good and Excellent versus Poor, Fair and Good)

Composites	Univariate	Multivariable
Overall perceptions of resident safety	1.78 (1.19–2.65); p-value = 0.005	n.s.*
Feedback and communications about incidents	1.20 (1.02–1.41); p-value = 0.030	n.s.
Supervisor expectations and actions promoting resident safety	1.33 (1.11–1.57); p-value = 0.002	n.s.
Organisational learning	1.51 (1.24–1.84); p-value < 0.0005	1.34 (1.06–1.69); p-value = 0.015
Management support for resident safety	1.45 (1.27–1.67); p-value < 0.0005	1.38 (1.20–1.60); p-value < 0.0005
Training and skills	1.41 (1.18–1.68); p-value < 0.0005	n.s.
Compliance with procedures	1.15 (1.01–1.31); p-value = 0.033	n.s.
Teamwork	1.24 (1.06–1.44); p-value = 0.006	n.s.
Handovers	1.28 (1.08–1.51); p-value = 0.004	n.s.
Communication openness	1.26 (1.14–1.39); p-value < 0.0005	n.s.
Non-punitive response to mistakes	1.22 (1.08–1.38); p-value = 0.001	n.s.
Staffing	1.23 (1.09–1.38); p-value = 0.002	n.s.

*n.s. represents non-significant effect using multivariable logistic regression (p > 0.05)

12 significant Composites were found to be independently associated with the outcome. Staff who had 10% higher overall mean percentage positive agreement were 34% more likely and 10% higher positive Management Support for Resident Safety were 38% more likely to rate the nursing home as very good and excellent.

Odds ratio and associated 95% confidence intervals represent a 10% change in the positive response. Univariate analysis was undertaken by considering each patient safety culture Composite individually, and multivariable analysis identifies those that are independently associated with the outcome, using logistic regression.

4 Discussion

This research examined the patient safety culture at two residential nursing homes in Singapore. The survey results of this study were compared to the NHSPSC *Nursing Home Survey 2014 US Comparative Database Report* (Agency for Healthcare Research and Quality, 2016; Goh, Welborn, & Dhaliwal, 2014). The Comparative Database consists of data from 263 nursing homes and 18,969 nursing home staff respondents who completed the survey from January 2009 to May 2014. Singapore nursing homes' mean percentage positive scores were greater than the comparative database on all 12 PSC Composites, ranging from 7.2 to 29%. The difference in the mean percentage positive scores, relative to the scores from the comparative database, was greater than 20% for Training and Skills, Teamwork and Handoff. In terms of the two overall questions, the mean percentage positive agreement of the two Singapore nursing homes 'I would tell my friends that this is a safe nursing home for their family' was 84.8%, and greater than the 50th percentile of the comparative database. The corresponding result for the question on the overall rating of the nursing home was 77.4%, which is similar to the 75th percentile of the comparative database.

This study confirmed the face validity of the modified NHSPSC tool via a panel of experts. The minor modifications included demographics to align with the Singapore nursing classifications and the linguistic adjustment of *handoff to handovers*, which is used in Singapore to hand on the responsibility of resident care between shifts. The finding of the tool's validity is of importance, as with many developed countries, Singapore has relied on a multi-international nursing workforce for residential aged care. However, the internal consistency of the modified NHSPSC tool used in this research ranged from 0.519 to 0.781, compared to the Cronbach's α values for the 12 PSC Composites from 0.71 to 0.86. Thus, further work on developing a residential aged care assessment tool for safety and quality is required for the Asian context is needed.

The findings of this study were similar to a Taiwanese research undertaken in the acute care setting by Chen and Li (2010) using the HSPSC tool developed for use in the hospital environment by AHRQ found that hospital staff were positive towards the culture of patient safety. Modifications to the translated tool were made following an initial pilot test, and construct validity was undertaken. These changes included demographic and linguistic to localise the questionnaire to the Taiwanese health setting. In this study, the 12 Composites of the tool demonstrated influence in the patient safety culture with 'teamwork within units' the most positive and 'staffing' the least positive. Although the setting was different, the results are similar to those of this study, particularly about 'staffing', which was one of the least positive identified. Previous studies using the NHSPSC tool in the residential aged care setting (Arnetz et al., 2011; Buljac-Samardzic, van Wijngaarden, & Dekker–van Doorn, 2015; Handler et al., 2006) had similar findings, suggesting that differing staffing profiles between the aged care and the acute sectors and different ratios of licensed staff may influence the safety and quality.

Variations between the NHSPSC results from Taiwan and this study suggest that cultural diversity must be considered when using the model in settings where cultural and linguistic challenges can potentially influence the provision of care. Chen and Li (2010) suggested that variations could partly be due to differences in behaviours between cultural settings. Overall, they were of the view that diversity in cultural settings must be considered when undertaking research. This view was acknowledged by Johnstone and Kanistsaki (2006) who suggested in 2006 that despite progress with regard to awareness of patient safety and quality, the issue of the impact of culture and its link to patient safety outcomes required further research. In a recent Australian study, O'Keeffe (2016) found that failure to recognise the link between culture and language and safety standards in the provision of care exposes patients to preventable adverse patient outcomes. It can be equally surmised that failure to localise the questionnaire tool to settings may influence the validity of the tool and the usefulness of presenting the culture of safety and quality results.

With the acknowledged changes to the population demographics in Singapore now and for the future, nursing recruitment remains a high priority for Singapore. In this survey, more than half of the respondents were employed less than 3 years, suggesting a high turnover of staff. International recruitment of staff for residential aged care will continue to remain an essential requirement in the future. Survey findings indicate the global nursing workforce originated from China, India, Malaysia, Myanmar, Philippines and Sri Lanka. About 90% work full time, reflecting the nature of Singapore work contracts. While English is the universal language of the nursing workforce, there are many variations with a blending of phrases borrowed from other languages posing difficulties with the administration of standard collection surveys and tools. There is thus the potential for misunderstanding and miscommunication resulting in an adverse event for a patient is significant (Nichols, Horner, & Fyfe, 2015; O'Keeffe, 2016).

This research also examined the prediction of the 12 PSC Composites to the two overall questions on referral and rating of the nursing homes. The two Composites found to independently predict staff's recommendation were Overall Perception of Resident Safety and Communication Openness. Chen and Li (2010) found in the acute setting that overall perception of patient safety related to the perception of staff that there were adequate procedures and systems in place preventing errors. Communication has been identified as an important factor in the failure or success of organisations and aged care and is critical to residential safety and quality (Verma, 2013). Communication openness in which the individuals are encouraged to express their feelings and concerns regarding residential care creates a positive safety culture (Bonner, Castle, Perera, & Handler, 2008). Communication openness also improves employee participation which allows information to flow upwards to inform senior management (Schiller & Cui, 2010) and in residential aged, this will enable managers to make changes to organisation policies and procedures that affect the safety and quality of residential care delivery and whether staff would recommend the facility.

Management support for safety is critical to the foundation and development of a culture of safety (Johnstone & Kanitsaki, 2006; O'Keeffe, 2016). Zúñiga et al. (2013) in their study suggested a high degree of correlation between organisational learning and the overall perception of resident safety. Both of which they suggested measure management support for resident safety. Although communication openness and non-punitive response to mistakes were not significantly different between the different staff demographics (direct contact, degree qualification or full-time work) in this study, these composite variables were individually significant predictors of 'I would tell friends that this is a safe nursing home for their family'. Being able to speak up is a characteristic of a positive relationship between management, supervisor and staff, in which direct care staff are able to raise concerns that may negatively affect residential care in a culture that is supportive and where organisational learning is about improving resident safety (Bonner et al., 2008). This finding was significant and may not be the case in other contexts in the Asian community where individuals are not encouraged to speak up (Wagner, Smits, Sorra, & Huang, 2013). Supporting this finding, the elements of staff training, feedback and communication about incidents and teamwork are foundations, and the findings in these areas while not significant are higher than the comparative database.

5   Conclusions

Conducting research into safety culture is critical for improved residential aged care. This research has provided valuable and useful insight into the measurement of patient safety culture in the Singapore setting. The results have been compared to the international comparative database highlighting a higher PSC in Singapore. This difference while important may also reflect the cultural aspects of Singaporeans and the global nursing workforce. Caution, therefore, should be exercised in generalising these research findings.

This study has demonstrated that the NHSPSC tool had an acceptable level of reliability with minor linguistic adjustment to the Singapore Residential Aged Care Sector. The Singapore nursing home sector composite patient safety culture means percentages were higher than the US comparative database. While English is the universal language of the nursing workforce, there are many variations with a blending of phrases borrowed from other languages posing difficulties with the administration of standard collection surveys and tools. This study has found that with minor adjustments to wording, the AHRQ-NHSPSC Patient Safety Tool can be utilised satisfactorily with an international workforce who has demonstrated a positive attitude to patient safety. The finding indicating the questionnaire was valid in this context was important as Singapore, like many developed countries, have relied on a multi-international nursing workforce for residential aged care. However, further modifications to the tool to improve the internal validity within each of the PSC Composites are recommended to suit the international workforce within the Asian setting. These modifications to the NHSPSC will have to be assessed against a larger sample to ensure validity.

Acknowledgements The Lions Home for the Elders, Singapore provided in-kind support for this study.

Funding No external funding.

Ethics Approval

Ethics approval was obtained from the Human Research Ethics Committees of Curtin University, Western Australia, and permission was granted by the Management Committee of the two residential nursing homes in Singapore.

Availability of Data and Materials

The datasets generated during and/or analysed during the current study are not publicly available but summary data as tables can be made available from the corresponding author on reasonable request.

Competing Interests

The authors declare that they have no competing interests.

References

Agency for Healthcare Research and Quality. (2016). *Nursing home survey on patient safety culture*. Retrieved, from http://www.ahrq.gov/professionals/quality-patient-safety/patientsafetyculture/nursing-home/resources/nhsurvey.html, http://www.ahrq.gov/professionals/quality-patient-safety/patientsafetyculture/nursing-home/index.html.

Arnetz, J. E., Zhdamova, L. S., Elsouhag, D., Lichtenberg, P., Luborsky, M. R., & Arnetz, B. B. (2011). Organizational climate determinants of resident safety culture in nursing homes. *Gerontologist, 51*(6), 739–749. https://doi.org/10.1093/geront/gnr053.

Ausserhofer, D., Schubert, M., Desmedt, M., Blegen, M. A., De Geest, S., & Schwendimann, R. (2013). The association of patient safety climate and nurse-related organizational factors with selected patient outcomes: a cross-sectional survey. *International Journal of Nursing Studies, 50*, 240–252. https://doi.org/10.1016/j.ijnurstu.2012.04.007.

Bonner, A. F., Castle, N. G., Perera, S., & Handler, S. M. (2008). Patient safety culture: A review of the nursing home literature and recommendations for practice. *The Annals of Long-term Care: The Official Journal of the American Medical Directors Association, 16*(3), 18–22.

Buljac-Samardzic, M., van Wijngaarden, J. D., & Dekker–van Doorn, C. M. (2015). Safety culture in long-term care: a cross-sectional analysis of the Safety Attitudes Questionnaire in nursing and residential homes in the Netherlands. *BMJ Quality & Safety*. https://doi.org/10.1136/bmjqs-2014-003397.

Castle, N. G., Wagner, L. M., Perera, S., Ferguson, J. C., & Handler, S. M. (2011). Comparing the safety culture of nursing homes and hospitals. *Journal of Applied Gerontology, 30*, 22–43. https://doi.org/10.1177/0733464809353603.

Chen, I., & Li, H. (2010). Measuring patient safety culture in Taiwan using the hospital survey on patient safety culture (HSOPSC). *BMC Health Services Research, 10*, 152. https://doi.org/10.1186/1472-6963-10-152.

El-Jardali, F., Dimassi, H., Jamal, D., Jaafar, M., & Hemadeh, N. (2011). Predictors and outcomes of patient safety culture in hospitals. *BMC Health Services Research, 11*, 45. https://doi.org/10.1186/1472-6963-11-45.

Goh, L. G. H., Welborn, T. A., & Dhaliwal, S. S. (2014). Independent external validation of cardiovascular disease mortality in women utilising Framingham and SCORE risk models: a mortality follow-up study. *BMC Womens Health, 14*(1), 118. https://doi.org/10.1186/1472-6874-14-118.

Halligan, M., & Zecevic, A. (2011). Safety culture in healthcare: a review of concepts, dimensions, measures and progress. *BMJ Quality & Safety, 20*, 338–343. https://doi.org/10.1136/bmjqs.2010.040964.

Handler, S. M., Castle, N. G., Perera, S., Fridsma, D. B., Nace, D. A., & Hanlon, J. T. (2006). Patient safety culture assessment in the nursing home. *Quality & Safety in Health Care, 15*, 400–404. https://doi.org/10.1136/qshc.2006.018408.

Johnstone, M., & Kanitsaki, O. (2006). Culture, language, and patient safety: making the link. *International Journal for Quality in Health Care, 18*(5), 383–388.

Manser, A. (2014). *The use of the hospital survey on patient safety culture in Europe. Patient safety culture-theory, methods and application (W* (P ed.). Wey Court East, Union Road, Farnham: Ashgate Publishing Limited.

McDonald, P. (2015). Growing older before growing rich in Asia. In *East Asia Forum: Economics, Politics and Public Policy in East Asia and the Pacific.* http://www.eastasiaforum.org/2015/12/08/growing-old-before-growing-rich-in-asia/.

National Population and Talent Division, Prime Minister's Office, Singapore Department of Statistics, Ministry of Home Affaires, & Immigration & Checkpoints Authority. (2015). *Population in brief.* Singapore. http://population.sg/population-in-brief/files/population-in-brief-2015.pdf.

Nichols, P., Horner, B., & Fyfe, K. (2015). Understanding and improving communication processes in an increasingly multicultural aged care workforce. *Journal of Aging Studies, 32*, 23–31. https://doi.org/10.1016/j.jaging.2014.12.003.

Nieva, V. F., & Sorra, J. (2003). Safety culture assessment: a tool for improving patient safety in healthcare organizations. *Quality & Safety in Health Care, 12*, ii17–ii23.

O'Keeffe, V. (2016). Saying and doing: CALD workers' experience of communicating safety in aged care. *Safety Science, 84*, 131–139. https://doi.org/10.1016/j.ssci.2015.12.011.

Portney, L. G., & Watkins, M. P. (2009). *Foundations of clinical research: applications to practice* (Vol. 892). Upper Saddle River, NJ: Pearson/Prentice Hall.

Schafer, J. L. (1999). Multiple imputation: A primer. *Statistical Methods in Medical Research, 8*, 3–15.

Schiller, S. Z., & Cui, J. (2010). Communication openness in the workplace: the effects of medium (F2F and IM) and culture (U.S. and China). *Journal of Global Information Technology Management, 13*, 37–75.

Thomas, K. S., Hyer, K., Castle, N. G., Branch, L. G., Andel, R., & Weech-Maldonado, R. (2012). Patient safety culture and the association with safe resident care in nursing homes. *Gerontologist, 52*, 802–811. https://doi.org/10.1093/geront/gns007.

Turner, S. P. (1979). The concept of face validity. *Quality & Quantity, 12*, 85–90.

Verma, P. (2013). Relationship between organizational communication flow and communication climate. *International Journal of Pharmaceutical Sciences and Business Management, 1*, 63–71.

Wagner, C., Smits, M., Sorra, J., & Huang, C. C. (2013). Assessing patient safety culture in hospitals across countries. *The International Journal for Quality in Health Care, 25*, 213–221. https://doi.org/10.1093/intqhc/mzt024.

Zúñiga, F., Schwappach, D., De Geest, S., & Schwendimann, R. (2013). Psychometric properties of the Swiss version of the nursing home survey on patient safety culture. *Safety Science, 55*, 88–118. https://doi.org/10.1016/j.ssci.2012.12.010.

A Systematic Scoping Review of Cancer Communication About Prevention and Detection in Bangladesh

Aantaki Raisa, Carma Bylund, Sabrina Islam, and Janice Krieger

Abstract While most cancer deaths occur in Low-to-Middle-Income countries (LMICs), little is known about cancer prevention in such places. Empirical research shows that culturally appropriate and theory-driven communication interventions for cancer prevention can produce expected health outcomes, but how it is done in LMICs like Bangladesh has not been scientifically studied. In this chapter, we conducted a systematic scoping review to reduce that knowledge gap. Out of 985 articles on cancer prevention in Bangladesh, 35 were selected for review based on the selection criteria of covering at least one concept of the transactional model of communication. These articles were coded for the four constructs of the Extended Parallel Process Model (EPPM): perceived severity and susceptibility of cancer, and perceived response and self-efficacy of cancer screening. Such a limited number of studies demonstrate the lack of research focused on Bangladesh. Only four articles mentioned the need for cultural appropriateness and none included theory. Thematic summary of the articles found that perceived susceptibility of cancer and self-efficacy of cancer screening are low among Bangladeshis. Future cancer prevention campaigns should address these two key factors in message design to improve effectiveness and integrate a sociocultural context that considers its target population.

Keywords Awareness raising · Cancer · Bangladesh

A. Raisa (✉) · C. Bylund · J. Krieger
STEM Translational Communication Center, University of Florida, Florida, USA
e-mail: a.raisa@ufl.edu

S. Islam
School of Public Health, University of California, Berkeley, USA

Prevention Research Center, Pacific Institute for Research and Evaluation, Beltsville, USA

© Springer Nature Singapore Pte Ltd. 2020
B. Watson and J. Krieger (eds.), *Expanding Horizons in Health Communication*, The Humanities in Asia 6, https://doi.org/10.1007/978-981-15-4389-0_11

1   Introduction

Cancer is the second leading cause of mortality worldwide, with 70% of cancer deaths occurring in Low-to-Middle-Income countries (LMICs) (Cancer, 2018). The public health focus in many LMICs has historically been centered on the prevention of communicable diseases and the success of these programs has resulted in longer life expectancy in many countries. However, an inevitable consequence of longer life spans is an increase in the prevalence of chronic diseases such as cancer.

Like many other LMICs, cancer care in Bangladesh is hindered by an inadequate healthcare infrastructure, a lack of national cancer registry, and limited cancer literacy among the general population (Hussain & Sullivan, 2013). Cancer communication research and interventions are poised to play an important role in the coming years as Bangladesh works toward meeting the needs of its nearly 1.5 million patients (Uddin et al., 2013). As a first step, this chapter seeks to understand the current state of the cancer communication research conducted in Bangladesh. Specifically, we conducted a systematic scoping review to synthesize the existing scientific knowledge in the area of cancer prevention and detection.

1.1   Country Overview

With an area of 56,000 miles^2 and a population of 160 million, Bangladesh is the tenth most densely populated country in the world (The World Bank, 2016). Unfortunately, many people in Bangladesh are diagnosed with cancer at later stages because they lack adequate access to quality healthcare (Blankart 2012). This is partially due to a dearth in healthcare providers qualified to provide care. There are only four active physicians per 100,000 people in Bangladesh (Hussain & Sullivan, 2013). Of these, most healthcare providers are concentrated in urban hospitals, despite the fact that 70% of the population lives in rural areas (Hussain & Sullivan, 2013). Although there are more physicians in urban areas, cities are plagued with socioeconomic disparities. As such, the urban poor also have inadequate access to healthcare (Banarjee et al., 2012). Given that geographic and socioeconomic disparities are part of the overall landscape of cancer continuum in Bangladesh, the current review sought to identify how and when studies included vulnerable populations.

1.2   Theoretical Underpinnings

It is well-established that there are significant benefits to using theory to guide health communication intervention development, implementation, and evaluation (Fishbein & Cappella, 2006). However, most (if not all) theory development has occurred in Western contexts; at present, it is unclear how theories developed in the West are being used to guide health communication practice in the East. Understanding how theories are being applied in a given cultural context is a first step toward improving the cultural appropriateness of our conceptual choices.

Fortunately, health communication, health education, and public health research often rely on similar theories and constructs to guide intervention research and evaluation. In order to capture the diversity of health communication research and interventions being conducted in Bangladesh, we focused on three overarching frameworks that contain the most common constructs utilized for evaluating interventions in the literature: (1) the source credibility model (Hovland & Weiss, 1951), (2) the Extended Parallel Process Model (EPPM, Witte, 1992), and (3) the Theory of Planned Behavior (TPB, Ajzen, 1991). Drawing on the source credibility model, we focused on the perceived expertise and trustworthiness of cancer communication sources (e.g., physicians, community health workers).

We also examined five key constructs from the EPPM: susceptibility (i.e., likelihood of a cancer diagnosis), severity (i.e., seriousness of cancer diagnosis), response efficacy (i.e., value of a recommended behavior for alleviating the threat of cancer), self-efficacy (i.e., personal ability to enact the recommended behavior), and behavioral intentions (i.e., plans to enact a recommended behavior). The EPPM is especially useful to examine because of its ability to guide every aspect of a health campaign, including message design, implementation, and evaluation (Popova, 2012). We coded for two additional constructs from Ajzen's (1991) Theory of Planned Behavior (TPB): attitude toward a health topic (e.g., cancer screening) and subjective norms (e.g., societal acceptance of cancer screening). Perceived behavioral control (e.g., perception of the ease or difficulty of getting screened for cancer) and behavioral intentions were not coded given the conceptual overlap with response efficacy and behavioral intentions in the EPPM. As such, we posed the following research question:

RQ: How is theory being used to enhance cancer communication in the context of prevention and screening research in Bangladesh?

2 Method

To answer our research question, we conducted a systematic scoping review. A systematic scoping review is a type of systematic review that is limited in time and resource, requires narrow breadth, little depth, and/or other restrictions to achieve speed of review (Gough et al., 2017). The review was conducted based on the Preferred Reporting Items for Systematic review and Meta-Analysis protocols (PRISMA-P). Articles were included in the review if they met the following criteria: (1) Qualitative or quantitative research published in peer-reviewed journal, (2) written in English, (3) focus on prevention and detection of cancer (e.g., tobacco control, diet, uptake of human papillomavirus vaccine, screening), (4) mention at least one aspect of the transaction model of communication (e.g., message, source, receiver), and (5) conducted (at least in part) in Bangladesh. Publications from any year, meeting these criteria were included. Given that the goal of the review was to examine health communication efforts among Bangladeshis living in their home country, studies with population samples of non-Bangladeshis (e.g., Rohingya refugees, foreigners in Bangladesh temporarily) and migrant Bangladeshis living in other countries were excluded (Tables 1 and 2).

Articles were identified by searching PubMed, PsycINFO, and Academic Search Premier using the MeSH terms: "Bangladesh," "Cancer," and "Communication" (see Appendix 1 for more information). This resulted in identification of 985 potential articles. Article titles and abstracts were imported to the software

Table 1 Journal impact factor

Journal	Impact factor/Scimago Journal & Country Rank
Bangladesh Medical Journal	0.09
Mymensingh Medical Journal	0.85*
Indian Journal of Community Medicine	0.39*
South Asian Journal of Cancer	0.58
Journal of Family and Reproductive Health	0.61*
BioResearch Open Access	0.76*
Healthcare for Women International	0.85
International Journal of Breast Cancer	1.04*
Cancer Epidemiology	1.33*
Journal of Cancer Education	1.547
PLoS ONE	1.95
Journal of Family Planning and Reproductive Health Care	2.027
Tobacco-Induced Diseases	2.092
BMC Medical Ethics	2.106
Japanese Journal of Clinical Oncology	2.140
BMC Women's Health	2.151
Transactions of the Royal Society and Tropical Medicine and Hygiene	2.184
Asian Pacific Journal of Cancer Prevention	2.52
International Journal of Environmental Research and Public Health	2.608
Addictive Behaviors	2.686
Vaccine	3.285
Maturitas	3.315
Tobacco Control	4.151
Oncologist	5.306
Global Health Research and Policy	N/A

*denotes SJR scores

Table 2 Articles about Breast Cancer prevention and detection

Title	Authors	Publication year	Journal published in	Study sample	Key findings
Feasibility Study of Case-Finding for Breast Cancer by Community Health Workers in Rural Bangladesh	Chowdhury et al.	2015	Asian Pacific Journal of Cancer Prevention	Rural women (n = 4649)	Cellphones can be an effective way to find breast cancer patients; culturally appropriate video can motivate patients with symptoms to seek care
An mHealth Model to Increase Clinic Attendance for Breast Symptoms in Rural Bangladesh: Can Bridging the Digital Divide Help Close the Cancer Divide?	Ginsburg et al.	2014	The Oncologist	Rural women (n = 22337)	Every woman with symptoms wanted CBE. Participants were more likely to seek care if CHWs helped them with the navigation to get help from a near-by clinic
Knowledge, Attitude and Practice of Breast Self-examination Among Female University Students from 24 Low, Middle Income and Emerging Economy Countries	Pengpid and Peltzer	2014	Asian Pacific Journal of Cancer Prevention	Female college students (n = 344)	64% of the participants never performed BSE, 46% knew of BSE, importance of BSE was rated 7.1
Knowledge, Attitude and Practice of Bangladeshi Women towards Breast Cancer: A Cross Sectional Study	Begum et al.	2019	Mymensingh Medical Journal	Adult female patients at hospital (n = 500)	Expenditure problem was the biggest reason for not seeking prevention for BCa
Awareness on Breast Cancer among the Women of Reproductive Age	Chowdhury & Sultana	2011	Journal of Family and Reproductive Health	Population representative adult females (n = 175)	94% mentioned BCa does not occur in old age, 54% thought it's not inherited, 52% told cancer is caused by evil spirit, 54% told BCa cannot be cured. 65% had no knowledge of symptoms and signs of BCa
Improving Outcomes from Breast Cancer in a Low-Income Country: Lessons from Bangladesh	Story et al.	2012	International Journal of Breast Cancer	Rural women (n = 12, interviews, n = 25 community meetings, n = 100 FGD)	No word for breast cancer in local language, talking about female body is not permissible in the public sphere, most participants believed they had no access to breast care, reasons not to seek care included, mistrust in physicians, lack of female physicians, preference for alternative medicine, family burden, fear of being a social outcast

(continued)

Table 2 (continued)

Title	Authors	Publication year	Journal published in	Study sample	Key findings
Effect of Educational Level on Knowledge and Use of Breast Cancer Screening Practices in Bangladeshi Women	Rasu et al.	2010	Health Care for Women International	Urban working women at a university (n = 152)	12+ years of education is significantly associated with knowledge about BCa, most common source of knowledge about BCa is news media, while 89% of the participants knew about BCa
Breast Cancer in South Asia: A Bangladeshi Perspective	Hossain et al.	2014	Cancer Epidemiology	N/A	None of the breast cancer cases is detected by organized screening in Bangladesh. Almost all breast cancer cases are detected clinically. Most of the patients (more than 90%) seek medical attention at advanced stages: i.e., stages III and IV
Awareness of Breast Cancer and Barriers to Breast Screening Uptake in Bangladesh: A Population Based Survey	Islam et al.	2016	Maturitas	(N = 1590)	High perceived severity of cancer (81.9%), high perceived response efficacy of screening (64.2%). However, low screening rate (29.1%), alluding to low perceived self-efficacy of screening

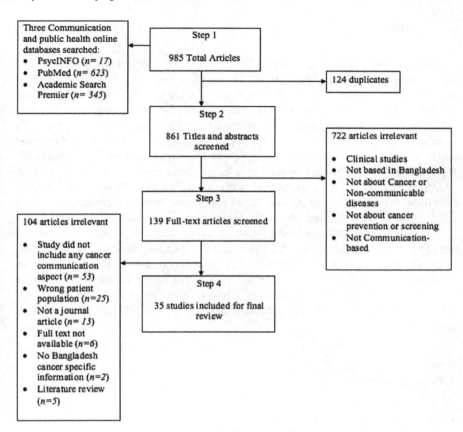

Fig. 1 Flowchart of systematic scoping review process

"Covidence." The first author and a trained assistant utilized Covidence to establish intercoder reliability for screening. The coders screened 10% of the data ($n = 100$) with 82% agreement. The remainder were screened and coded by the first author. An overview of steps used to select the final set of articles is described in Fig. 1.

Thirty-five articles were selected for review after the full-text screening. Twelve of these articles were reviewed extensively in order to develop a data charting guide (see Appendix 2). The data charting guide informed the systematic collection of information about study methods, study population, cancer type, and prevention type for all of the articles. The results section of each article was further analyzed using a thematic summary technique to extract additional information (Thomas et al., 2017).

3 Results

All articles were published between 2008 and 2019. Studies addressed diverse cancer types, including breast ($n = 11$), cervical ($n = 10$), oral ($n = 1$), lung ($n = 1$), testicular ($n = 1$), generic ($n = 2$), and cervical/breast ($n = 1$); or the studies addressed certain preventive mechanisms for tobacco-induced cancers, which were termed as tobacco control studies ($n = 8$). Out of the 35 studies, 25 were primary research, six used secondary data analysis, and four did not mention any specific methodology. Twenty-six articles were exclusively about the Bangladeshi population. Seven were conducted under the umbrella of developing countries or LMIC, with Bangladeshi participants included. Twenty articles were quantitative, three were mixed-method, and twelve were qualitative studies. Thirty articles included at least one Bangladeshi co-author.

The results are organized into two sections. First, we present a general description of the existing health communication literature in terms of the participants (or samples) studied, the communication channels used, and a description of messages tested (if applicable). Second, we summarize the available literature in relation to the theoretical constructs of interest, including source credibility, perceived threat, perceived efficacy, and subjective norms. See Tables 3, 4 and 5 for a summary.

3.1 Participants

The existing health communication literature is diverse in terms of the populations and cancers being studied. Articles reported participant ages ranging from 13 to 69 years. The number of participants in a given study ranged from 100 (Ahmad et al., 2017) to 135,735 (Basu et al., 2010). Studies that included participants under age 18 were related to tobacco cessation or breast/cervical cancer prevention. Nearly half of the articles focused on females only ($n = 16$, 45.71%) and focused on breast cancer ($n = 9$), cervical cancer ($n = 5$), breast/cervical ($n = 1$), and human papillomavirus (HPV) infection ($n = 1$). Only two (5.7%) focused only on males and addressed testicular self-examination (TSE; $n = 1$) and tobacco cessation ($n = 1$). The remainder focused either on males and females (or did not specify) and focused on tobacco cessation ($n = 7$), breast cancer ($n = 2$), cervical ($n = 1$), oral ($n = 1$), and lung cancer ($n = 1$). No studies reported the sexual orientation of the participants.

The literature reflects geographic diversity, but limited socioeconomic diversity. Eleven articles (31.4%) focused exclusively on urban populations, while three focused on rural only. The remainder included both rural and urban participants ($n = 13$) or did not specify ($n = 8$). Few articles addressed vulnerable urban populations, with only one article including garments workers and housemaids.

Table 3 Articles about cervical cancer prevention and detection

Title	Authors	Year of publication	Journal published	Study sample	Key findings
Knowledge and Acceptance of Human Papillomavirus Vaccine for Cervical Cancer Prevention Among Urban Professional Women in Bangladesh: A Mixed Method Study	Bhuiyan et al.	2018	BioResearch Open Access	High educated urban adult women (n = 160)	Most common source of information about cervical cancer is newspaper or magazines. Knowledge of prevention was poor. Reasons to not get HPV vaccines were not knowing enough about the vaccine, not being recommended by their doctors, worries about the safety of the vaccine, and perceiving themselves as too old for vaccination
Attitude and Practice of Cervical Cancer Screening among the Female Doctors of Bangabandhu Sheikh Mujib Medical University	Ferdous et al.	2016	Bangladesh Medical Journal	Female doctors (n = 401)	Knowledge was significantly associated with age. Participants aged 30–40 years had poorer knowledge score (24.2%) than the participants between 41–50 years age group (4.9%) and between 50–60 years age group (6.7%). Most common reason for not getting screened was not being referred by a doctor
Knowledge of Cervical Cancer and HPV Vaccine in Bangladeshi Women: a Population-Based, Cross-Sectional Study	Islam et al.	2018	BMC Women's Health	Population representative adult females (n = 2037)	In the sample, rural women heard of cervical cancer significantly more than urban women. But, there were significantly more urban women who underwent cervical cancer screening compared to their rural counterpart. Top perceived causes of cervical cancer: urban women- sexual intercourse; rural women- poor hygiene during menstruation. Most common source of knowledge was neighbors, relatives, and television

(continued)

Table 3 (continued)

Title	Authors	Year of publication	Journal published	Study sample	Key findings
Lack of Understanding of Cervical Cancer and Screening Is the Leading Barrier to Screening Uptake in Women at Midlife in Bangladesh: Population-Based Cross-Sectional Survey	Islam et al.	2015	The Oncologist	Population representative adult females (n = 1590)	The reasons given for not undergoing screening included having no symptoms (86.1%), not knowing screening was needed (37.5%), and possible expense associated with screening (11.5%)
Ethical Issues Related to Human Papillomavirus Vaccination Programs: an Example from Bangladesh	Salwa and Abdullah Al-Munim	2018	BMC Medical Ethics	Adolescent girls, parents, policymakers	To make vaccination communication culturally sensitive, risk of sexual intercourse is not talked about. However, this strategy has worked well for LMICs
Genital Human Papillomavirus Infection among Women in Bangladesh: Findings from a Population-Based Survey	Nahar et al.	2014	PLOS One	Rural and urban adult women (n = 1902)	While no effect of education was seen on HPV awareness in urban women, education significantly decreased the risk of any HPV infection in rural women, by increasing knowledge of the infection
Role of Print and Audiovisual Media in Cervical Cancer Prevention in Bangladesh	Nessa et al.	2013	Asian Pacific Journal of Cancer Prevention	Rural and semi-urban adult men and women (n = 176)	Knowledge about the benefits of early detection quadrupled post intervention, but increase in knowledge was low among men. Besides the media used in the intervention, people learned about it through family members and neighbors. Women said people can be informed about VIA by television (drama serials, advertisement through cable line), mike announcement and health education/discussion sessions at Uthan Baithaks/EPI meetings/community clinics

(continued)

Table 3 (continued)

Title	Authors	Year of publication	Journal published	Study sample	Key findings
Evaluation of the National Cervical Cancer Screening Programme of Bangladesh and the formulation of quality assurance guidelines	Basu et al.	2010	Journal of Family Planning & Reproductive Health	Adult women (n = 135735)	Screening was predominantly opportunistic. Only 8.6% women who got VIA did so spontaneously in the facilities evaluated. 28% of the women in the centers evaluated were under the recommended age
Cervical Cancer in Bangladesh: Community Perceptions of Cervical Cancer and Cervical Cancer Screening	Ansink et al.	2008	Transactions of the Royal Society of Tropical Medicine and Hygiene	Rural and semi-urban adult men and women (n = 220)	Strong preference for privacy and female doctors. Burden to get screened was put on women by the men, despite women's difficulties to take independent decisions about their health. Perceived consequence of getting cervical cancer differed among men and women. While women perceived being abandoned by family, men perceived the inconvenience it would cause in the family due to the physical inability of the affected women to perform her duties

Table 4 Articles about tobacco control and prevention

Title	Authors	Publication year	Journal published in	Study sample	Key findings
A Cross-Country Comparison of Knowledge, Attitudes and Practices about Tobacco Use: Findings from the Global Adult Tobacco Survey	Gupta and Kumar	2014	Asian Pacific Journal of Cancer Prevention	Population representative (n = 9619)	Awareness about the harmful effects of tobacco consumption was significantly high among Bangladeshis compared to other countries; rural Bangladeshis were also highly aware of the harmful effects
The role of negative affect and message credibility in perceived effectiveness of smokeless tobacco health warning labels in Navi Mumbai, India and Dhaka, Bangladesh: A moderated-mediation analysis	Mutti-Packer et al.	2017	Addictive Behaviors	Urban adult men and women (n = 1081)	Message effectiveness was influenced by the personal relevance and identity of the participants. Identity (age, gender, ethnicity) concordance increased effectiveness of the cessation message. Pictorial warnings on cigarette packaging were more effective than text-only warnings
Patterns of Use and Perceptions of Harm of Smokeless Tobacco in Navi Mumbai, India and Dhaka, Bangladesh	Mutti et al.	2016	Indian Journal of Community Medicine	Urban men and women both young and adult (n = 1081)	Despite knowledge of the harmful effects of smokeless tobacco, 94% of the participants used it daily. Respondents with low level of education were more likely to have a positive attitude toward smokeless tobacco
Influence of Health Warnings on Beliefs about the Health Effects of Cigarette Smoking, in the Context of an Experimental Study in Four Asian Countries	Reid et al.	2017	International Journal of Environmental Research and Public Health	Urban young and adult men, urban young women (n = 1018)	Adults who viewed the health warnings for impotence were more likely to say that smoking caused impotence, there was no effect on youth. In contrast, Bangladeshi youth who viewed the health warnings for aging were more likely to say that smoking caused aging of the skin while there was no effect on adults
Smokers' Responses to Television Advertisements about the Serious Harms of Tobacco Use: Pre-Testing Results from 10 Low- to Middle-Income Countries	Wakefield et al.	2013	Tobacco Control	Adult males urban, rural and semi-urban (n = 192)	The portrayals of external visible damage as a result of smoking and serious damage to internal organs were considered powerful and motivating. Some ads were perceived targeted toward females since the characters in the ad were females. Use of Jargon in the ad such as emphysema was a barrier to comprehension

(continued)

Table 4 (continued)

Title	Authors	Publication year	Journal published in	Study sample	Key findings
Determinants of Intentions to Quit Smoking among Adult Smokers in Bangladesh: Findings from the International Tobacco Control (ITC) Bangladesh Wave 2 Survey	Driezen et al.	2016a, b	Global Health Research and Policy	Urban, rural and semi-urban men and women from age of 15 years and above (n = 2982)	Smokers employed in indoor areas where smoking is banned had 2.0 times higher odds of plans to quit compared to smokers who worked outdoors. Smokers living in homes with children aged 5 or younger had significantly higher odds of planning to quit compared to smokers having no children in the home. Awareness of the harmful effects of smoking on one's own health was not associated with intentions to quit
Awareness of Tobacco-Related Health Harms among Vulnerable Populations in Bangladesh: Findings from the International Tobacco Control (ITC) Bangladesh Survey	Driezen et al.	2016a, b	International Journal of Environmental Research and Public Health	Population representative of young and adult men and women (n = 5278)	Illiterate Bangladeshis had significantly lower odds of being aware of the harms than Bangladeshis having nine or more years of formal education. Interestingly, significantly higher percentage of slum residents knew that smokeless tobacco causes mouth cancer compared to non-slum residents. This result might be due to the higher prevalence of smokeless tobacco use among slum residents
Predictors of Smoking Cessation Behavior among Bangladeshi Adults: Findings from ITC Bangladesh Survey	Abdullah et al.	2015	Tobacco-Induced Diseases	Population representative of young and adult men and women (n = 1861)	One point increase in self-efficacy increased the odds of successful cessation by 80%. Attempts to quit were significantly related to: residing outside of Dhaka, aged 40 or older, having a household monthly income > 10,000 taka, having intention to quit smoking in the future, working indoors

Table 5 Articles on prevention and detection of other types of Cancers

Title	Authors	Publication year	Journal published	Study sample	Key findings
Score based risk assessment of Lung Cancer and its evaluation for Bangladeshi people	Mukti et al.	2014	Asian Pacific Journal of Cancer Prevention	Urban and rural adult men and women ($n = 104$)	The socio-demographic conditions, such as annual income, residential area, occupation, and their educational level, were correlated to risk of lung cancer
Knowledge, attitudes and practice of testicular self-examination among male university students from Bangladesh, Madagascar, Singapore, South Africa and Turkey	Peltzer and Pengpid	2015	Asian Pacific Journal of Cancer Prevention	Urban college students ($n = 448$)	20% aware of TSE, 84% never conducted TSE in 12 months, 16.3% conducted more than 10 times in 12 months, importance rating 6.3. Knowledge proportion more than 20%
Bangladeshi dental students' knowledge, attitudes and behaviour regarding tobacco control and oral Cancer	Chowdhury et al.	2010	Journal of Cancer Education	Urban college students ($n = 186$)	Female respondents were significantly more likely to support receiving specific tobacco cessation training and routinely advising their patients to quit tobacco use. Nearly all (97.3%) would support the dentist having a role in giving advice on tobacco cessation, but 73.7% felt their advice would increase a patient's chances of quitting

The only articles to include residents of urban slums focused on tobacco cessation. Finally, no articles mentioned the hill tracts where many tribal Bangladeshis reside.

3.2 Cancer Communication Channels

Findings regarding preferred cancer communication channels were mixed. Four of the 35 articles reported on the participants' preferred and common channels of information about cancer and screening. Interpersonal channels were identified as being the most effective for breast and cervical cancer. Chowdhury & Sultana (2011) reported that 43% of their sample had heard of breast cancer from their relatives. Similarly, Islam et al. (2018) reported that 66% of their population heard of cervical cancer from neighbors, 45% from relatives, 16% from doctors and other health professionals (participants could select more than one response), and 14% from television.

Slightly different results were obtained by Rasu et al. (2010), who reported that most of their urban participants learned about breast cancer through the news media, more so than physicians, friends, or family. Bhuiyan et al. (2018) reported that 52% of the urban participants had heard of cervical cancer from newspapers or magazine, followed by 36% from friends or family, and 29% from television. Fewer than one-fifth of the 157 respondents had heard of cervical cancer from their doctors. More than half of the women in the study recommended reaching out to women through mass media such as television commercials, and house-to-house visit, or mass campaigns by healthcare workers.

Nessa et al. (2013) specifically tested the role of media in cervical cancer prevention and evaluated how their target population heard about a VIA test program in their vicinity. They found that 25.5% of those who came to the program camp heard about it from cable television, 21.4% from mike announcements (a common way of announcements in rural Bangladesh where an announcer travels around a community on a van with a microphone and a megaphone and reads out loud an announcement), 20.4% from front-yard meetings/focus group discussions, and 18.8% from neighbors. Women preferred discussion settings where they could ask questions. Both men and women preferred door-to-door health workers over going to the doctor. Participants recommended disseminating cervical cancer-related information through announcements and posters in school, college, mosques, temples, incorporation of cervical cancer prevention program in education curriculum, placement of billboard at important places, and hospitals.

Media were also a recommended approach for tobacco cessation. Reid et al. (2017) found that urban participants wanted more information on cigarette packages about the dangers of tobacco. Interestingly, Driezen, Abdullah, and Nargis, et al. (2016a) found that tobacco users living in the urban slums thought that all forms of tobacco packaging should contain more health information. The authors also recommended making such warnings pictorial, to reduce barriers associated with illiteracy.

Two articles investigated implementing mHealth technology to screen for breast cancer in rural Bangladesh (Ginsburg et al., 2014; Chowdhury et al., 2015). Ginsburg et al. (2014) found that cellphones act as an effective medium to collect breast cancer-related (e.g., symptoms, other health information) messages from rural women while also providing them with pre-cancer diagnosis, recommendations, and navigation information to get treatment in nearby healthcare facilities. Chowdhury et al. (2015) also found that cellphones were effective in raising awareness about breast cancer by showing relevant videos to the participants.

3.3   Cancer Communication Message Design

Surprisingly, only seven studies reported on message design interventions to disseminate information about cancer and prevention. Two breast cancer studies involved developing, implementing, and assessing culturally appropriate, communication-based interventions. Ginsburg et al. (2014) developed an mHealth model to increase clinic attendance for breast symptoms among rural Bangladeshis. The other study (Chowdhury et al., 2015) was a feasibility test of case finding for breast cancer by community health workers (CHWs) in rural Bangladesh. It was conducted in the same locality as the other study and used mHealth technology. Both studies included some components of being culturally appropriate such as including community leaders and health workers in the development phase of the intervention, making them in colloquial language, and portraying demographically concordant characters.

One cervical cancer study (Nessa et al., 2013) developed, implemented, and evaluated the effectiveness of an intervention. The only detail about the message content provided was "cervical cancer is a common cause of death of Bangladeshi women." Another study (Basu et al., 2010) evaluated the effectiveness of a national program to increase cervical cancer screening in Bangladesh. How the information about the program was disseminated among the public was not reported in the study. The study found that the uptake of the program after four years was low (target of 20 million screening in three years vs. achieved 135,735 screening in four years). Non-compliance and non-adherence were also found to be predominant among those who were screened and diagnosed with symptoms.

Two experimental articles were conducted to test the effectiveness of health warnings on tobacco packaging. Reid et al. (2017) conducted an experiment to test the influence of health warnings on beliefs about the health effects of cigarette smoking. The health warnings on cigarette packaging included both text-only and pictorial messages; texts were in Bangla, and the images were tailored to Bengali ethnicity. Mutti-Packer et al. (2017) examined the potential mediating role of negative emotions and the moderating role of message credibility in perceived effectiveness of smokeless tobacco warnings on 1081 urban men and women in Bangladesh. The study found that message credibility moderated the perceived effectiveness among the adults but not among the minors. The authors attributed this lack of effect to the fact that pictorial warnings using graphics and personal testimonials included older looking people and the minor participants did not relate to them.

Wakefield et al.'s (2013) article used a mixed-method study to assess the comprehension, acceptability, and potential effectiveness of five television advertisement in communicating anti-smoking message and motivating cessation. The study found that portrayals of visible external damage as a result of smoking and serious internal damage were perceived powerful and motivating. Some of the ads portrayed females and the male participants perceived those were for women, and the issues discussed in the advertisements did not concern them.

3.4 Trust in Message Sources

Although trust is an important component of effective health communication, only five articles reported data related to trust. Studies that did address trust focused on identifying the least and most trusted sources of health information. Physicians were the least trusted source of information (Ansink et al., 2008; Hossain et al., 2014; Story et al., 2012). Story et al. (2012) found that rural and suburban participants reported mistrust in physicians due to having personally or vicariously experienced poor treatment. The authors also reported that patients who screened positive for breast cancer are often manipulated by brokers in the hospitals who suggest seeing another doctor for 'better' results. These brokers, in return, get commissions from other doctors.

Similarly, Ansink et al. (2008) reported being referred for wrong and unnecessary tests as a primary reason for lack of trust in physicians. Hossain et al. (2014) found that a lack of trust in existing healthcare systems as a barrier to seeking medical care. Although few studies suggested alternatives, the authors of two articles found that community health workers were the most trusted source of information among rural women (Chowdhury et al., 2015; Ginsburg et al., 2014).

3.5 Perceived Threat of Cancer

To address perceived threat, articles were coded for constructs related to perceived severity and susceptibility. Severity was measured in the majority of the articles reviewed and was most frequently assessed by asking participants if they believe cancer is a deadly or serious disease. Overall, articles reported that Bangladeshis perceived that cancer was a severe illness (e.g., Begum et al., 2019; Bhuiyan et al., 2018; Chowdhury & Sultana 2011). For instance, one article reported that both men and women believed cervical cancer has lethal consequences if left untreated (Ansink et al., 2008). Another article reported 54% of its participants believed breast cancer is not a curable disease (Chowdhury & Sultana 2011).

Susceptibility was measured by asking participants how likely it was that they would develop cancer. The few articles that examined perceived susceptibility focused on breast and cervical cancer among women. For example, one study reported that only 11% of the participants in that study perceived being at risk of breast cancer (Rasu et al., 2010). Although participants in these studies reported high levels of perceiving cancer as a severe illness, most reported not being at risk of developing cancer. The exception to this was participants who felt highly susceptible to cancer because they had a family member with that particular type of cancer.

3.6 Perceived Efficacy of Cancer Screening

While many of the articles reported that Bangladeshis agreed that screening was an effective way to prevent cancer and detect it in early stages, there were significant barriers to enacting cancer screening behavior. Common barriers included a lack of healthcare facilities (especially in rural areas), lack of guarantee that there will be a doctor at the facility once they arrive at the hospital, transportation problems, and expense. Female participants expressed some specific concerns, such as shyness about talking about their problems to physicians, concerns about safety while going to the hospitals unescorted, lack of permission from husbands to go to get screened, lack of financial support, and lack of female doctors in rural areas.

3.7 Subjective Norms

There were two ways subjective norms were associated with cancer screening. The first was the perception that cancer is a punishment or a bad omen (Story et al., 2012). For example, one study reported that urban women attributed cervical cancer to socially stigmatized behaviors, such as having multiple sex partners, sex out of marriage, or lack of hygiene (Islam et al., 2018). The link between cancer and non-normative behaviors is likely one reason why women report fear of being abandoned by their family if diagnosed with cancer (Story et al., 2012).

The second applied primarily to women and focused on subjective norms related to the role of women in society. Women perceived that their immediate and extended families would find it inappropriate for them to prioritize their health over their domestic responsibilities (Ahmad et al., 2017; Story et al., 2012). Given that healthcare was not perceived as a priority in their social network, urban women reported that they would not have the time required to engage in cancer screening given their other important duties, such as taking care of their children, attending to other family members, and domestic responsibilities (Ahmad et al., 2017).

4 Discussion

Given that culture is a fundamental component of health and well-being, it is imperative for scholars to examine health communication interventions in a variety of cultural contexts. The aim of this chapter was to conduct a systematic scoping review of communication-based studies for cancer prevention and detection conducted in Bangladesh from different theoretical approaches. In doing so, we aimed to start a conversation about the ways in which indigenous knowledge and Western scholarship is informing current cancer communication practice in Bangladesh. It is hoped that the findings of this review have identified gaps that will propel a new generation of scholars forward in communicating effectively regarding the burden of cancer in LMICs such as Bangladesh.

Out of the 985 search results in this scoping review, 722 were excluded in the abstract and title screening. The top criterion for exclusion was the articles being clinical research in nature. Moreover, 53 articles in the full-text screening phase were excluded because they did not include any communication-specific information about cancer prevention (i.e., sender, receiver, message). Clearly, progress in basic and clinical cancer research is outpacing research being conducted to translate that knowledge into practice by communicating effectively with the population. Indeed, only six studies reviewed focused on developing or evaluating communication-based interventions to prevent cancer or promote screening in Bangladesh.

There are several factors that make communicating about cancer in the Bangladeshi context different from the Western or high-income countries. For example, among the studies reviewed, cancer knowledge was very general, with participants having little to no knowledge about specific cancers (i.e., cervical, breast). Cancer screening was neither well understood nor practiced. Cancer fatalism was high, with cancer being perceived as a "death sentence," alongside a lack of perceived response efficacy of existing treatments. Misinformation about the causes, symptoms, and treatment of cancer can also be common. In one study, participants thought screening itself was a treatment for cancer.

Culture and language-specific barriers to knowledge exist as well. For example, there is no word for "breast cancer" in Bangla, the native language of Bangladesh. Similarly, the term for cervical cancer translates to an "ulcer in the neck of the womb." The female body is also perceived culturally inappropriate to talk about in the public. Culture likely influences perceived susceptibility of cancer, also. For example, poor menstrual hygiene and punishment for sin were both considered reasons for developing cervical cancer. Thus, if an individual perceived that they have adequate menstrual hygiene or lived a religiously righteous life, she may have low perceived susceptibility to cancer.

Culture also informed preferences about cancer communication sources. While women were relatively more open to seeing a male doctor if conditions were painful, men only agreed for their female relatives to see a male doctor if it were a life and death situation, and male doctors were the only option. In rural Bangladesh, other household issues such as child-rearing, health of a male member of the family, would often take priority over female health, which makes it difficult for women to get screened for cancer, a barrier not commonly faced by men.

Another important factor was the range of literacy levels. All the studies that included the variable, literacy, as an indicator of cancer screening found a positive association between them. In a study conducted in urban Bangladesh, women with more than 12 years of education were significantly more likely to get screened for breast cancer than women with fewer years of education. Women were also less likely to be even aware of breast cancer if they had only primary or no education. Another study found that women with greater than high school education were more likely to get Pap smear test for cervical cancer.

Importantly, the studies reviewed showed that increased knowledge did not translate into behavioral change. Despite the perceived severity of cancer as a fatal disease and the importance and benefits of cancer screening (perceived response efficacy), motivation to screen for cancer did not significantly increase in most cases. These findings are consistent with the literature on health behavioral change in Western contexts that find increased knowledge does not equate to behavioral change.

Finally, it is important to note what the articles did not include. Some vulnerable populations were notably absent from the articles reviewed, including tribal people in the hill tracts, LGBTQI people, and sex workers. Only the tobacco-related studies included city slum dwellers, and one study on HPV infection included garments workers and housemaids. Interestingly, none of the articles addressed colon cancer, a communication context that is of high importance in Eastern cultures (see Wong, this volume).

4.1 Limitations and Future Research

Like many systematic reviews, this study only included articles that were published in English in peer-reviewed academic journals. By choosing not to include non-peer-reviewed documents (e.g., white papers) in Bangla, the sample may have yielded fewer examples of health communication interventions. However, limiting article selection to peer-reviewed journals ensured an adequate level of quality in the research described.

The results of this review indicate that there is a significant opportunity to design, implement and evaluate more communication-based intervention for cancer prevention in Bangladesh, preferably targeted toward specific population groups. Moreover, similar systematic reviews need to be conducted to synthesize existing knowledge on cancer diagnosis, treatment, and palliative care, in order to inform appropriate guidelines for cancer control. Future research can include content or textual analyses of newspapers, cancer-related websites and webpages, television advertisements, leaflets, and posters. Multi-method studies using stakeholder interviews and surveys in the policy, treatment, and research levels may help inform policies.

More research in communication is needed to utilize the knowledge base to develop effective campaigns to promote awareness about cancer and screening. Only four articles reviewed mentioned cultural appropriateness of the messages. While culturally appropriate interventions have been proven to be the most effective way to reach out to the target audience, and induce behavioral change (Briant et al., 2018), none of the studies provide information about any systematic method for designing culturally appropriate interventions, neither did they provided any theoretical basis for evaluating the effect of culture in the outcome of an intervention. The lack of explicit attention to Bangladeshi and other LMIC cultures indicate a need for research in designing, implementing, and evaluating culturally appropriate cancer-preventive communication interventions.

Appendix 1: Article Search Strategy

Research question		
What is known about the preventive cancer communication interventions in Bangladesh?	**Core Databases** PsycINFO PubMed Academic Search Premier	**Limits** *Publication Types*: Scientific articles published in peer-reviewed academic journals *Dates*: Until May 21, 2019 *Language*: English

Primary Literature Searching: Databases

Database: PsycINFO

	Concept: Bangladesh	Concept: Cancer	Concept: Communication
Thesaurus terms	Bangladesh	Cancer	Prevention Intervention Treatment Program Campaign awareness

PsycINFO SEARCH STRATEGY
("Bangladesh" AND "cancer" AND ("prevention" OR "intervention" OR "Treatment" OR "program" OR "campaign" OR "awareness"))

Conditions set in search option:
Search modes: Find all my search terms, apply related words
Language: English
Publication type: Peer-reviewed journal
Population group: Human

Methodology: All
Exclude Dissertation (Checked)
No age group selected
Total Added: 17

Database: PubMed

	Concept: Bangladesh	Concept: Cancer	Concept: Communication
Thesaurus Terms	Bangladesh	Cancer	Prevention, Awareness, Communication, Intervention, Program campaign
Mesh Terms	Bangladesh	Neoplasms, cancer	Awareness, communication, methods

SEARCH STRATEGY (("Bangladesh"[MeSH Terms] OR "Bangladesh"[All Fields]) AND ("neoplasms"[MeSH Terms] OR "neoplasms"[All Fields] OR "cancer"[All Fields])) AND (("prevention and control"[Subheading] OR ("prevention"[All Fields] AND "control"[All Fields]) OR "prevention and control"[All Fields] OR "prevention"[All Fields]) OR ("awareness"[MeSH Terms] OR "awareness"[All Fields]) OR ("communication"[MeSH Terms] OR "communication"[All Fields]) OR ("methods"[MeSH Terms] OR "methods"[All Fields] OR "intervention"[All Fields]) OR program[All Fields] OR campaign[All Fields])

Total Added: 638 → 635 (in English) → 623 (Items with abstract)

Database: Academic Search Premier

	Concept: Bangladesh	Concept: Cancer	Concept: Communication
Thesaurus Terms	Bangladesh	Cancer	Prevention Intervention Treatment Program Control Strategy

SEARCH STRATEGY ((Bangladesh) AND (Cancer) AND (Prevention OR Intervention OR Treatment OR Program OR Control OR Strategy))

Conditions set in search option:
Search modes: Find all my search terms, apply related words
Language: English
Publication type: Peer-reviewed journal
Document type: Article
Total Added: 345

Appendix 2: Qualtrics Survey

Literature review cancer communication in Bangladesh

Q1 Title of the Article
Q2 Publication year
Q3 Journal published in
Q4 Authors
Q5 Type of study...
Q6 Cancer type

Breast	Cervical	Colorectal	Lung	Oral
Prostate	Stomach	Esophageal	Liver	Leukemia
Ovarian	General	Other		

Q7 Study population type

Rural (1)	Urban (2)	Suburban (3)	Mixed (4)	Not specified (5)

Q8 Study population size

Q9 Study population gender

Male (1)	Female (2)	Both (3)	Not Specified (4)

Q10 Age of the population
Q11 Study population SES
Q12 Aims of the study.
Q13 Methodology of the study
Q14 Outcome measures
Q15 Important results
Q16 Conclusions drawn by the authors
Q17 Any additional information, not coded in the questionnaire but seemed important to the coder.

References

Abdullah, A. S., Driezen, P., Quah, A. C., Nargis, N., & Fong, G. T. (2015). Predictors of smoking cessation behavior among Bangladeshi adults: findings from ITC Bangladesh survey. *Tobacco induced diseases*, *13*(1), 23. https://doi.org/10.1186/s12971-015-0050-y*

Ahmad, F., Kabir, S. F., Purno, N. H., Islam, S., & Ginsburg, O. (2017). A study with Bangladeshi women: Seeking care for breast health. *Health Care for Women International, 38*(4), 334-343. https://doi.org/10.1080/07399332.2016.1263305*

Ajzen, I. (1991). *The theory of planned behavior.* Doi:https://doi.org/10.1016/0749-5978(91) 90020-T

Ansink, A., Tolhurst, R., Haque, R., Saha, S., Datta, S., & Broek, N. (2008). Cervical cancer in Bangladesh: Community perceptions of cervical cancer and cervical cancer screening. *Transactions of the Royal Society of Tropical Medicine and Hygiene, 102*(5), 499–505 *

Banerjee, A., Bhawalkar, J. S., Jadhav, S. L., Rathod, H., & Khedkar, D. T. (2012). Access to health services among slum dwellers in an industrial township and surrounding rural areas: a rapid epidemiological assessment. *Journal of family medicine and primary care*, *1*(1), 20–26. https://doi.org/10.4103/2249-4863.94444

Basu, P., Nessa, A., Majid, M., Rahman, N., & Ahmed, T. (2010). Evaluation of the national cervical cancer screening programme of Bangladesh and the formulation of quality assurance guidelines. *Journal of Family Planning & Reproductive Health*, *36*(3), 131–134. https://doi.org/10.1783/147118910791749218 *

Begum, S. A., Mahmud, T., Rahman, T., Zannat, J., Khatun, F., Nahar, K., et al. (2019). Knowledge, Attitude and Practice of Bangladeshi Women towards Breast Cancer: A Cross Sectional Study. *Mymensingh Medical Journal: MMJ*, *28*(1), 96–104.

Bhuiyan, A., Sultana, F., Islam, J. Y., Chowdhury, M., & Nahar, Q. (2018). Knowledge and Acceptance of Human Papillomavirus Vaccine for Cervical Cancer Prevention Among Urban Professional Women in Bangladesh: A Mixed Method Study. *BioResearch open access*, *7*(1), 63–72. https://doi.org/10.1089/biores.2018.0007*

Blankart, C. R. (2012). Does healthcare infrastructure have an impact on delay in diagnosis and survival? https://doi.org/10.1016/j.healthpol.2012.01.006

Briant, K. J., Sanchez, J. I., Ibarra, G., Escareño, M., Gonzalez, N. E., Gonzalez, V. J., et al. (2018). Using a Culturally Tailored Intervention to Increase Colorectal Cancer Knowledge and Screening among Hispanics in a Rural Community. *Cancer Epidemiology Biomarkers & Prevention*, *27*(11), 1283–1288.

Cancer (2018). WHO News. Retrieved from https://www.who.int/news-room/fact-sheets/detail/cancer

Chowdhury, S., & Sultana, S. (2011). Awareness of breast cancer among the women of reproductive age. *Journal of Family and Reproductive Health*, *5(4)*.

Chowdhury, T. I., Love, R. R., Chowdhury, M. T. I., Artif, A. S., Ahsan, H., Mamun, A., & Salim, R. (2015). Feasibility Study of Case-Finding for Breast Cancer by Community Health Workers in Rural Bangladesh. *Asian Pacific Journal of Cancer Prevention*, *16*(17), 7853–7857. https://doi.org/10.7314/apjcp.2015.16.17.7853*

Driezen, P., Abdullah, A. S., Nargis, N., Hussain, A. K., Fong, G. T., Thompson, M. E., & Xu, S. (2016a). Awareness of Tobacco-Related Health Harms among Vulnerable Populations in Bangladesh: Findings from the International Tobacco Control (ITC) Bangladesh Survey. *International journal of environmental research and public health*, *13*(9), 848. https://doi.org/10.3390/ijerph13090848*

Driezen, P., Abdullah, A. S., Quah, A., Nargis, N., & Fong, G. T. (2016b). Determinants of intentions to quit smoking among adult smokers in Bangladesh: findings from the International Tobacco Control (ITC) Bangladesh wave 2 survey. *Global health research and policy*, *1*, 11. https://doi.org/10.1186/s41256-016-0012-9*

Ferdous, J., Khatun, S., Ferdous, N. E., Sharmin, F., Akhter, L., & Keya, K. A. (2016). Attitude and practice of cervical cancer screening among the female doctors of Bangabandhu Sheikh Mujib Medical University. *Bangladesh Medical Journal*, *45*(2), 66–71.

Fishbein, M., & Cappella, J.N. (2006). The role of theory in developing effective health communications. *Journal of Communication*, 56, S1-S17. https://doi.org/10.1111/j.1460-2466.2006.00280.x

Ginsburg, O. M., Chowdhury, M., Wu, W., Chowdhury, M. T., Pal, B. C., Hasan, R., & Salim, R. (2014). An mHealth model to increase clinic attendance for breast symptoms in rural Bangladesh: Can bridging the digital divide help close the cancer divide? *The Oncologist*, *19* (2), 177–185. https://doi.org/10.1634/theoncologist.2013-0314*

Gough, D, Oliver, S., & Thomas, J. (2017). *An Introduction to Systematic Reviews*. California, SAGE Publication

Gupta, B., & Kumar, N. (2014). A Cross-Country Comparison of Knowledge, Attitudes and Practices about Tobacco Use: Findings from the Global Adult Tobacco Survey. *Asian Pacific Journal of Cancer Prevention*, 15 *(12)*, 5035–5042. doi:http://dx.doi.org/10.7314/APJCP.2014.15.12.5035*

Hossain, S., Ferdous, S., & Karim-Kos, H. (2014). Breast cancer in South Asia: A Bangladeshi perspective. *Cancer Epidemiology, 38*(5), 465–470.*

Hovland, C., & Weiss, W. (1951). The Influence of Source Credibility on Communication Effectiveness. *Public Opinion Quarterly, 15(4),* 635–650, https://doi.org/10.1086/266350.

Hussain, S., & Sullivan, R. (2013). Cancer control in Bangladesh. *Japanese Journal of Clinical Oncology, 43*(12), 1159–1169. 10.1093/jjco/hyt140

Islam, J. Y., Khatun, F., Alam, A., Sultana, F., Bhuiyan, A., Alam, N., & Nahar, Q. (2018). Knowledge of cervical cancer and HPV vaccine in Bangladeshi women: a population based, cross-sectional study. *BMC women's health, 18*(1), 15. https://doi.org/10.1186/s12905-018-0510-7*

Islam, R. M., Bell, R. J., Billah, B., Hossain, M. B., & Davis, S. R. (2015). Lack of Understanding of Cervical Cancer and Screening Is the Leading Barrier to Screening Uptake in Women at Midlife in Bangladesh: Population-Based Cross-Sectional Survey. *The oncologist, 20*(12), 1386–1392. https://doi.org/10.1634/theoncologist.2015-0235*

Islam, R., Bell, J., Billah, B., Hossain, M., & Davis, S. (2016). Awareness of breast cancer and barriers to breast screening uptake in Bangladesh: A population based survey. *Maturitas, 84,* 68–74 *

Mohammad, T., Hossain, C., Allan, P., & Ray, C. (2010). Bangladeshi dental students' knowledge, attitudes and behaviour regarding tobacco control and oral cancer. *Journal of Cancer Education, 25*(3), 391–395 *

Mutti, S., Reid, J. L., Gupta, P. C., Pednekar, M. S., Dhumal, G., Nargis, N., & Hammond, D. (2016). Patterns of Use and Perceptions of Harm of Smokeless Tobacco in Navi Mumbai, India and Dhaka, Bangladesh. *Indian journal of community medicine: official publication of Indian Association of Preventive & Social Medicine, 41*(4), 280–287. https://doi.org/10.4103/0970-0218.193337*

Mutti-Packer, S., Reid, J. L., Thrasher, J. F., Romer, D., Fong, G. T., Gupta, P. C., & Hammond, D. (2017). *The role of negative affect and message credibility in perceived effectiveness of smokeless tobacco health warning labels in Navi Mumbai, India and Dhaka, Bangladesh: A moderated-mediation analysis* doi:https://doi.org/10.1016/j.addbeh.2017.04.002*

Mukti, R.F., Samaddar, P.D., Al Emran, A., Ahmed, F., Bin Imran, I, Malaker, A., & Yeasmin, S. (2014). Score based risk assessment of lung cancer and its evaluation for Bangladeshi people. *Asian Pacific Journal of Cancer Prevention, 15(17), 7021-7027,* https://doi.org/10.7314/apjcp. 2014.15.17.7021*

Nahar, Q., Sultana, F., Alam, A., Islam, J. Y., Rahman, M., Khatun, F., & Reichenbach, L. (2014). Genital human papillomavirus infection among women in Bangladesh: findings from a population-based survey. *PloS one, 9*(10), e107675. https://doi.org/10.1371/journal.pone. 0107675*

Nessa, A., Hussain, A., Rashid, H., Akhter, N., Roy, S., & Afroz, R. (2013). Role of print and audiovisual media in cervical cancer prevention in Bangladesh. *Asia Pacific Journal of Cancer Prevention, 14*(5), 3131-3137 *

Peltzer, K., & Pengpid, S. (2015). Knowledge, attitude and practice of testicular self-examination among male university students from Bangladesh, Madagascar, Singapore, South Africa and Turkey. *Asian Pacific Journal of Cancer Prevention, 16,*(11), 4741-474 https://doi.org/10. 7314/apjcp.2015.16.11.4741*

Pengpid, S., & Peltzer, K. (2014). Knowledge, attitude, and practice of breast self-examination among female university students from 24 low, middle income and emerging economy countries. *Asian Pacific Journal of Cancer Prevention, 15(20), 8637-8640,* https://doi.org/10. 7314/apjcp.2014.15.20.8637*

Popova, L. (2012). The Extended Parallel Process Model. *Health Education & Behavior, 39*(4), 455–473.

Rasu, S., Rianon, J., Shahidullah, M., Faisel, J., & Selwyn, J. (2010). Effect of educational level on knowledge and use of breast cancer screening practices in Bangladeshi women. *Health Care Women International, 32*(3), 177-189 *

Reid, J. L., Mutti-Packer, S., Gupta, P. C., Li, Q., Yuan, J., Nargis, N., & Hammond, D. (2017). Influence of Health Warnings on Beliefs about the Health Effects of Cigarette Smoking, in the Context of an Experimental Study in Four Asian Countries. *International journal of environmental research and public health*, *14*(8), 868. https://doi.org/10.3390/ijerph14080868*

Salwa, M., & Abdullah Al-Munim, T. (2018). Ethical issues related to human papillomavirus vaccination programs: an example from Bangladesh. *BMC medical ethics*, *19*(Supplement 1), 39. https://doi.org/10.1186/s12910-018-0287-0*

Story, L., Love, R., Salim, R., Roberto, A., Krieger, J., & Ginsburg, O. (2012). Improving outcomes from breast cancer in a low-income country: Lessons from Bangladesh. *International Journal of Breast Cancer, 2012* https://doi.org/10.1155/2012/423562 *

The World Bank (2016). Poverty & equity data portal: Bangladesh. Retrieved from http://povertydata.worldbank.org/poverty/country/BGD

Thomas, J., O'Mara-Eves, A., Harden, A., & Newman, M (2017). Synthesis methods for combining and configuring textual or mixed methods data. In Gough, D, Oliver, S., & Thomas, J. (Eds.), *An Introduction to Systematic Reviews* (pp 185–187). California, SAGE Publication

Uddin, A. F., Khan, Z. J., Islam, J., & Mahmud, A. (2013). Cancer care scenario in Bangladesh. *South Asian journal of cancer*, *2*(2), 102–104. https://doi.org/10.4103/2278-330x.110510

Wakefield, M.A., Bayly, M., Durkin, S.J., Cotter, T.F., Mullin, S., & Warne, C. (2013). Smokers' responses to television advertisements about the serious harms of tobacco use: pre-testing results from 10 low- to middle-income countries. Tobacco control, 22 1, 24–31 *

Witte, K. (1992). Putting the fear back into fear appeals: The extended parallel process model. *Communication Monographs, 59*(4), 329–349. https://doi.org/10.1080/03637759209376276

Convincing a Sceptical Public: The Challenge for Public Health

Louise Cummings

Abstract Public health communications are an everyday occurrence. However, compliance with them and the recommendations they contain is often limited. One reason for poor compliance is the failure on the part of experts to construct public health messages that accord with the rational resources of the public. This chapter examines how one set of rational strategies, a group of cognitive heuristics based on the informal fallacies, has the potential to facilitate decision-making about public health issues. Among the informal fallacies, the argument from ignorance plays an important role in public health communication. A comparative analysis is undertaken of the use of this argument in the public health communications issued by the Department of Health in Hong Kong and Public Health England in the UK. It is argued that there are qualitative differences in the use of the argument from ignorance across these two contexts. Specifically, the public in Hong Kong is encouraged to reflect on epistemic conditions that are integral to the rational warrant of this argument. These conditions are less often acknowledged by public health agencies in the UK. Greater rational evaluation of these conditions, it is argued, leads to better decision-making in matters relating to public health.

Keywords Argument from ignorance · Cognitive heuristic · Informal fallacy · Public health communication · Reasoning

1 Introduction

Public health information pervades our environment. Every day of our lives, we are given advice on how to lead healthier lifestyles to prevent cancers, strokes and heart disease, reduce the risk of spreading and contracting infectious diseases, and avoid behaviours such as illicit drug use, smoking and excessive alcohol consumption.

L. Cummings (✉)
Department of English, The Hong Kong Polytechnic University, Hong Kong SAR, China
e-mail: louise.cummings@polyu.edu.hk

© Springer Nature Singapore Pte Ltd. 2020
B. Watson and J. Krieger (eds.), *Expanding Horizons in Health Communication*,
The Humanities in Asia 6, https://doi.org/10.1007/978-981-15-4389-0_12

Public health messages may be all around us. Yet, public compliance with the content of these messages continues to decline. This is reflected worldwide in growing obesity rates and rates of sexually transmitted infections and increasing levels of harm associated with alcohol and tobacco consumption despite sustained public health campaigns (Ng et al., 2014; WHO, 2014; Newman et al., 2015; Arroyo-Johnson and Mincey, 2016). There are many reasons for this lack of compliance with public health recommendations. Perceived failures on the part of public health agencies to contain infectious disease outbreaks (e.g. Ebola) and to offer consistent advice on the health risks associated with certain lifestyle choices (e.g. alcohol consumption) and types of foods (e.g. salmonella in eggs) have eroded public trust in these agencies (Cummings, 2014b) (see Ward (2017) for discussion of trust in public health). Another reason for poor compliance is the perception of commercial conflicts of interest on the part of public health agencies. These agencies, it is claimed, promote the widespread use of products such as vaccines that are produced by a pharmaceutical industry motivated by profit over the health of populations (Cummings, 2005; Lenzer, 2016).

In this chapter, I argue that there is a further, and possibly more fundamental, reason why members of the public display poor compliance with public health recommendations. That reason concerns a failure on the part of public health agencies to devise health messages that accord with the rational resources of the public. To address this issue, we must develop a better appreciation of the rational resources that members of the public use to assess risks to their health. For too long, there has been a widespread belief that these resources consist exclusively of some type of deductive or inductive logic, and that improved decision-making about health is only possible when the public is versed in principles of deduction and induction. That deduction and induction can seem like the only contenders in health reasoning are evident in comments by Mosley-Jensen and Panetta (2017). These authors state that "health professionals and the public puzzle through new or controversial issues by deploying patterns of reasoning that are found in a variety of social contexts", but then go on to add that "deductive and inductive reasoning have been the most widely studied patterns in the disciplines of communication, philosophy, and psychology". It is now urgent that we move beyond the dichotomy between deduction and induction in reasoning and begin to look to other forms of reasoning to explain the rational judgements that people make when they engage in deliberation about health (see Christakos et al. (2005) for the use of different modes of reasoning in public health).

To this end, I have argued for some time that there is a group of arguments known as the informal fallacies that may prove to be beneficial for our purposes (Cummings, 2010, 2015a). These arguments include some well-recognized names such as slippery slope argument, begging the question and straw man argument as well as some lesser known examples like expert appeal and the argument from ignorance. The forms of reasoning that these arguments represent are, I believe, something of a hidden gem in logic. However, it should be emphasized that these arguments have not always been held in such high regard. Indeed, until the late twentieth century, many philosophers and logicians viewed these arguments with disdain and contempt. The standard view was that begging the question or using a straw man argument were aberrations of logic that all 'right-thinking men' should be disposed to avoid. But a more positive conception of these arguments does exist (e.g. Walton, 2008) and will be developed in this chapter. Specifically, it will be contended that the informal fallacies are an unexplored rational resource that has the potential to reveal new modes of reasoning of relevance to health.

As the term 'fallacy' suggests, informal fallacies are typically characterized as bad, weak or fallacious forms of reasoning or argument. The term 'informal' indicates that the flaw or error in each case cannot be characterized by means of formal or deductive logic. This latter point requires some expansion. When I reason that the radiator is leaking because water is on the floor, my reasoning is based on a deductively valid inference called *modus ponens*:

Modus ponens inference:

PREMISE: If water is on the floor, then the radiator is leaking.

PREMISE: Water is on the floor.

CONCLUSION: The radiator is leaking.

If I then reason that because water is not on the floor, the radiator is not leaking, I have committed a logical flaw or error called *denying the antecedent*. The rules of formal (deductive) logic prohibit this form of reasoning, relegating it to the group of arguments logicians call 'formal' fallacies:

Denying the antecedent:

PREMISE: If water is on the floor, then the radiator is leaking.

PREMISE: Water is not on the floor.

CONCLUSION: The radiator is not leaking.

However, there are no rules or principles in deductive logic that prohibit a person from using the conclusion-to-be-proved as a premise in argument (the flaw in begging the question) or using the negative consequences of an action to reject acceptance of a claim (the flaw in slippery slope argument). Because these purported errors of reasoning cannot be prohibited by the principles of *formal* logic, they are described as *informal* fallacies. But, as I will argue in this chapter, when viewed in their actual contexts of use, the informal fallacies are anything but fallacious. Instead, they are an effective rational resource that can confer many benefits on our thinking and reasoning. These contexts arise when there is a lack of knowledge or evidence on which to base a conclusion in reasoning. This is, in fact, the situation that confronts most members of the public when they are required to come to judgement on a complex health issue about which they lack knowledge.

This chapter will focus on one informal fallacy, the so-called argument from ignorance. This argument embodies the lack of knowledge that attends much health deliberation in that the arguer reasons from a lack of knowledge or evidence that X is true (false) to the conclusion that X is false (true). The logical and epistemic features of this argument are examined in two public health contexts. The contexts in question are the press releases of the Department of Health in Hong Kong and Public Health England in the UK. These releases are hosted on the websites of these agencies and were searched during October 2018 using the single search term 'no evidence'. The ten extracts from these releases examined in Sect. 3 have been chosen to exemplify certain logical points and are not intended to fulfil sampling criteria. It will be argued that by variously emphasizing and suppressing logical and epistemic features of the argument from ignorance, these agencies can lead the public to engage in systematic versus heuristic reasoning about public health issues. Qualitative differences in the use of the argument from ignorance by these public health agencies reflect two distinct approaches to public health communication and two opposing views of the role of the public in this communication. It is concluded that a form of public health communication that views the public as a rational agent is more likely to be met with compliance and improved public health outcomes.

2 Arguing from Ignorance: Logical and Epistemic Features

It might strike readers as strange, to say the least, that anyone should promote the use of ignorance in reasoning. After all, ignorance is something that we almost invariably characterize in negative terms and that we go to considerable lengths to avoid. But our dismissal of ignorance has also caused us to overlook the powerful contribution that this concept can make to cognitive deliberations such as reasoning. This is nowhere more clearly demonstrated than in the argument from ignorance. When we argue from ignorance, an absence of knowledge or evidence is used as grounds for accepting that a claim is true (or false). By way of illustration, consider the following argument from ignorance. It was used during the bovine spongiform encephalopathy (BSE) epidemic that devastated British cattle in the 1980s and 1990s (Cummings, 2010). 'Scrapie' in the premise of this argument is a brain disease in sheep:

There is *no evidence* that scrapie has transmitted to humans.
Therefore, scrapie has *not* transmitted to humans.

This is a rationally warranted use of the argument from ignorance. What makes the *lack of evidence* that scrapie had transmitted to humans strong grounds on which to conclude that scrapie had *not* transmitted to humans? The rational warrant of this argument derives from its satisfaction of two epistemic conditions. The first condition is a *closed-world assumption* (what Walton (1995), following de Cornulier (1988), calls *epistemic closure*). By the time BSE emerged in British cattle, there was already a well-developed knowledge base on scrapie, a transmissible spongiform encephalopathy (TSE) in sheep which early epidemiological studies suggested may be the cause of BSE in cattle. Public health officials were eager to use the fact that scrapie had never transmitted to humans as grounds for claiming that BSE posed no risk to human health—BSE, it was argued, would behave like scrapie and not transmit to humans. The reason that investigators could be confident that scrapie had not transmitted to humans (even if they could not be confident that BSE would behave similarly) was that extensive epidemiological investigation conducted over many years had failed to find any evidence that transmission had occurred. One study in particular, by Brown et al. (1987), had failed to find any evidence that scrapie had transmitted to humans. This epidemiological study investigated if there was a link between scrapie and Creutzfeldt-Jakob disease (CJD), a TSE in humans, over a 15-year period in France. British scientists also had extensive knowledge of scrapie which had been entering the human food chain in contaminated sheepmeat for some 250 years by the time BSE first emerged in cattle (BSE Inquiry Report, Volume 2, 2000). In short, scrapie and its possible transmission to humans had been so thoroughly investigated by 1987 that scientists could confidently claim that if transmission were occurring, then they would know about it. The closed-world assumption was satisfied in this case:

Closed-world assumption: All information that is relevant to a domain D of knowledge is present in a knowledge base B.

The knowledge base in this case was scrapie and what was known about its transmission to other species, most notably humans. But the closed-world assumption on its own cannot ground the conclusion of an argument from ignorance. This assumption must work alongside another epistemic condition known as *exhaustive search*. This condition requires that an exhaustive search be conducted of all the contents of the knowledge base. When this search is perfomed in a comprehensive and systematic way by individuals who have expertise in the domain in question, then the exhaustive search condition is fulfilled. Alongside conducting a 15-year epidemiological study of scrapie and CJD in France, Brown and his colleagues also conducted a review of the world literature. This review was comprehensive and systematic in that all relevant epidemiological studies were scrutinized according to rigorous scientific criteria. The satisfaction of an exhaustive search condition gave scientists further grounds for claiming that scrapie had not transmitted to humans:

Exhaustive search: An exhaustive search is conducted of all information in a knowledge base B. The search is comprehensive in scope and is conducted in a systematic manner.

With both epistemic conditions fulfilled, there was every reason for scientists and others to conclude that scrapie had not transmitted to humans on the ground that there was no evidence of its transmission. A lack of knowledge of transmission was a rationally warranted basis on which to conclude that transmission does not occur. But not every use of the argument from ignorance during the BSE epidemic had the same claim to rational warrant. There were many other uses of the argument that were examples of bad or fallacious reasoning. A prominent instance in which the argument was used fallaciously is shown below:

There is *no evidence* that BSE is transmissible to humans.

Therefore, BSE is *not* transmissible to humans.

Although this argument has the same logical form as the scrapie argument before it, it is not a rationally warranted argument. To understand why this is the case, we need to consider the context in which it was used. Government ministers and public health officials made frequent use of the statement that forms the premise of this argument from the earliest months of the BSE epidemic (see Table 1). In fact, use of this statement was so widespread by those charged with protecting the public's health that it was described by Lord Phillips, the chairman of the public inquiry into BSE, as the 'mantra' of the BSE affair (Cummings, 2011). Officials and government ministers knew that by producing this statement, they could encourage members of the public to draw the conclusion that BSE is *not* transmissible to humans. This conclusion might then reassure the public that BSE would pose no risk to human health. But this 'reassuring' conclusion was also a rationally unwarranted one. In the weeks and months after BSE first appeared in British cattle, there were no grounds for believing that the knowledge base on BSE was closed. In fact, investigations into this new disease were just beginning, with everything from its causal pathogen to host range and routes of transmission still unknown. In the absence of a knowledge base on BSE, the first epistemic condition on the rationally warranted use of the argument from ignorance did not hold. There was no *closed-world assumption* in relation to BSE. Also in the absence of a knowledge base on BSE, the second epistemic condition did not obtain. If there was no knowledge base on BSE, then *a fortiori* there could be no *exhaustive search* of this base. With neither epistemic condition in play, there were no rational grounds to support the above argument from ignorance.

It emerges that the argument from ignorance is not inherently fallacious, as traditional logicians and philosophers would have us believe (Locke, 1959 [1689]; Robinson, 1971). Rather, it can be more or less rationally warranted depending on whether the epistemic conditions described as *closed-world assumption* and *exhaustive search* are fulfilled (Walton, 1995, 1999). That people are aware of these conditions and can make judgements about them is evident in at least two ways. First, a study of 879 members of the public showed that laypeople are adept at evaluating the epistemic conditions associated with use of the argument from ignorance (Cummings, 2014a, 2015a, 2015b). When these conditions were not fulfilled or were fulfilled only partially, participants tended to reject arguments from ignorance that were based on them. They readily accepted these arguments when they believed that a knowledge base was closed and had been exhaustively searched. These evaluative judgements were not only evident in the quantitative performance of participants, but also in the qualitative comments that participants expressed in relation to the test scenarios in the study. Second, people can use, and understand the significance of, a range of linguistic markers that increase the salience of the epistemic conditions examined in this section. For example, expressions such as *at this stage*, *currently* and *to date* remind us that a closed knowledge base is only ever closed at a certain point in time and may very quickly have to be

Table 1 *No Evidence* Statements in the BSE Epidemic

Human health and *no evidence* statements

When BSE first emerged in British cattle in 1986, *no evidence* statements became the mainstay of repeated reassurances by government and health officials that the new disease posed no, or only a remote, risk to human health. Mr. John Suich worked in the Animal Health Division of the Ministry of Agriculture, Fisheries and Food between 1986 and 1989. He was responsible for notifiable and other diseases. On 15 October 1987, Mr. Suich circulated information in Question and Answer form to enable press officers and others to answer questions about BSE (BSE Inquiry Report, Volume 3, 2000: 123). On the central question of the risk that BSE might pose to human health, press officers were advised to respond as follows:

Q. Can it be transmitted to humans?
A. There is no evidence that it is transmissible to humans.

By issuing this *no evidence* response, press officers intended the public to draw the negative inference that BSE is *not* transmissible to humans.

Clearly, many members of the public drew exactly this inference and were reassured by it. But this was a rationally unwarranted use of the argument from ignorance. BSE had only been formally identified 10 months earlier in December 1986 by the Central Veterinary Laboratory in the UK. The closed world assumption could not possibly be satisfied in such a short period of time.

---

reopened if new evidence emerges. The conclusion of an argument from ignorance is defeasible and may have to be overturned if circumstances change (Hinton, 2018). These linguistic markers are an important reminder of this fact. Their logical and epistemic character will be examined in the rest of this section.

One of the ways in which people can be hoodwinked into accepting the conclusions of weak arguments from ignorance is to downplay or suppress the two epistemic conditions that we have examined in this section. If the proponent of a weak argument from ignorance can encourage the recipient of the argument to overlook these conditions, then it is more likely that a weak argument will pass undetected and its conclusion will be accepted. Conversely, if these conditions are made more salient for the recipient through the use of linguistic markers, then we may expect these conditions to hold some logical sway in the recipient's decision to accept or reject the conclusion. When the BSE argument from ignorance was used extensively by government ministers and health officials in the wake of the emergence of BSE, it was asserted categorically with the aim that the public should conclude that BSE is *not* transmissible to humans. A multi-million-pound beef and dairy industry was at serious peril if the public lost confidence in the safety of British beef products. Some form of immediate and definitive reassurance was needed to avoid this adverse outcome. A categorically asserted argument from ignorance appeared to fit the bill perfectly. Let us consider what this same argument might look like if it had been uttered by a different proponent. This proponent might be less concerned to protect commercial interests and might be more interested in encouraging the public to participate in a rational evaluation of the potential risks of BSE to human health. To this end, a *no evidence* statement such as the following may be used:

There is *no evidence* currently that BSE is transmissible to humans.

The addition of the adverb *currently* in this statement is significant in the following respect. The inclusion of this linguistic marker has the effect of blocking the inference to the conclusion that BSE is *not* transmissible to humans. When presented with this statement, the public would rightly conclude that it was not possible to state if BSE is or is not transmissible to humans on the basis of the limited knowledge base on this new bovine disease that existed in the late 1980s. The closed-world assumption that this marker made salient would be assessed by the public and would be found to be wanting. No conclusion about BSE's transmissibility to humans was possible given the incomplete state of knowledge of BSE that existed at this time. Clearly, this conclusion was neither politically expedient for government ministers or commercially desirable for the beef industry. However, it was a conclusion that would have reflected the public's engagement in a process of rational evaluation of the risks that BSE might pose to human health.

It emerges that linguistic markers can alter the salience of the epistemic conditions that are central to a rational evaluation of the argument from ignorance. Markers like *currently*, *at this stage* and *to date* alert the recipient of the argument to the fact that a knowledge base may only be partially developed, or may be complete at a certain point in time but may have to be reopened as new findings and evidence emerge. In neither of these scenarios would a rational public be inclined to accept a claim about disease transmission or any other serious health issue on anything but a tentative basis. Still other markers can increase our confidence that a knowledge base is truly complete. If we learn that there has been *no evidence* that disease *X* in cattle has transmitted to humans *since 1970* when it first emerged, then we can be reasonably certain that the closed-world assumption is satisfied in this case and that a claim based on this assumption is rationally warranted. The lapse of 50 years is sufficient time in which to establish transmission to humans. So if transmission were occurring through either direct contact with cattle or consumption of beef and other bovine products, then we would presumably know it. The knowledge base on *X* can be considered complete to all intents and purposes, so that any claim that is not part of this base may be judged to be false. The extensive time period represented by the linguistic marker *since 1970* is the warrant we need to treat the knowledge base as complete. In the next section, we will examine how linguistic markers are used in the *no evidence* claims of public health agencies in Hong Kong and the UK. It will be argued that significant differences in the use of these markers reflect two different conceptions of how public health communication should be conducted.

3   Arguments from Ignorance in Public Health

The *no evidence* statements that form the premise of an argument from ignorance are used extensively in public health. It is not difficult to see why this is the case. When they assess health risks and recommend protective actions, public health agencies are guided by the best available evidence. Quite often, the best available evidence indicates that a statement or claim is either true or false. So it is true that HIV is a viral infection that can be transmitted through sexual intercourse. But let us imagine it is June 1981 and we are reading the first report of what were later known to be cases of AIDS in the *Morbidity and Mortality Weekly Report* (Centers for Disease Control, 1981). The new disease that is described in this report has no identifiable causal pathogen. Under these circumstances, only an imprudent scientist with disregard for evidence would state that the new disease is a viral infection. A more cautious approach would be to state that there is currently *no evidence* that the new disease is a viral infection. Appeals to *no evidence* are a scientifically responsible way of framing claims when there is insufficient evidence to settle a matter one way or the other. But there is another context in which *no evidence* statements are used in public health. This context arises when an investigation or an inquiry has been conducted, and a statement is produced that summarizes its findings. In this scenario, a large amount of evidence is available and is systematically examined. A statement of *no evidence* then leads us to conclude that a particular claim is false. It is this second use of *no evidence* statements that is most closely associated with the argument from ignorance. Examples of this second type of *no evidence* statement are shown below. They are taken from the press releases of the Department of Health in Hong Kong and Public Health England in the UK:

(A)

Title	Investigation into unsatisfactory water samples from aircraft completed
Source	Press release, Department of Health, Hong Kong, 6 July 2015

"The investigation of this incident has been completed. There is **no evidence** to suggest a contaminated water source at the water filling points of the airport. However, the trace amount of coliform bacteria detected earlier in the two water samples from water tankers of Hong Kong Aircraft Engineering Company Limited and Pan Asia Pacific Aviation Services Limited suggested a suboptimal standard of water quality, which may likely be related to the hygienic conditions of the water tankers. No pathogen or coliform bacteria were detected in the post-disinfection water samples from these two tankers", the spokesman said.

(B)

Title	Bacillus cereus infections: 1 July 2014
Source	Press release, Public Health England, UK, 1 July 2014

"Gerald Heddell, the Medicines and Healthcare products Regulatory Agency's Director of Inspection, Enforcement and Standards, said: "There is **no evidence** to suggest that individual ingredients, components or materials used for the manufacture of Total Parenteral Nutrition (TPN) on 27 May 2014 were the cause of the contamination. However, what we do know from our investigation is that the strain of Bacillus cereus which infected the babies has also been identified at ITH Pharma's manufacturing facility and within some of the unopened TPN supplies manufactured on the 27 May 2014.""

The *no evidence* statements in these press releases constitute the conclusions of two public health investigations, one (A) into water quality in aircraft at Hong Kong International Airport, and the other (B) into the source of contamination of Total Parenteral Nutrition (TPN) for babies. These investigations were comprehensive and systematic in that they reviewed all available evidence relating to water quality and the source of TPN contamination. The two epistemic conditions that must obtain for an argument from ignorance to be rationally warranted—closed-world assumption and exhaustive search—are both satisfied by the investigations conducted by these public health agencies. The conclusions of the following arguments from ignorance are therefore rationally warranted:

(A1)

There is *no evidence* that the water filling points at the airport were contaminated. Therefore, the water filling points at the airport were *not* contaminated.

(B1)

There is *no evidence* that individual TPN ingredients, components or materials were contaminated.
Therefore, individual TPN ingredients, components or materials were *not* contaminated.

In the absence of linguistic markers, the inference to a negative conclusion from the *no evidence* premise in each of these arguments is effectively automatic. There is a default inference in operation in the absence of these markers—if the closed-world assumption and exhaustive search conditions are satisfied, then it can be automatically inferred that X is *not* the case. In order to override this default inference, one or more linguistic markers must be used. The effect of these markers is to make the closed-world assumption and exhaustive search conditions highly salient so that they become the focus of greater critical scrutiny than might otherwise be the case. Under these circumstances, an incomplete knowledge base or a knowledge base that has only been partially searched is more likely to be discovered and exposed. When this occurs, the inference to a negative conclusion is blocked. To illustrate, consider the following extract from a press release from Hong Kong's Department of Health:

(C)

Title	Control of infectious diseases in prisons satisfactory
Source	Press release, Department of Health, Hong Kong, 21 April 2008

> "In response to media enquiries, the Department of Health reiterates it, together with the Correctional Services Department, achieve satisfactory control of tuberculosis (TB), human immunodeficiency virus (HIV), and other infectious diseases in prisons […] The apparently excess prevalence of TB and HIV among prisoners as compared with the general population in Hong Kong is attributable to major high-risk groups that contribute the prison population, e.g., illegal immigrants and drug addicts. It is not due to transmission of these infections in the prison. There is **no evidence** from available records to indicate there has been any outbreak of TB and HIV in the prison affecting multiple persons."

The linguistic marker *from available records* in the *no evidence* statement in this extract has the effect of making the closed-world assumption particularly salient. We are forced to consider if the knowledge base on outbreaks of TB and HIV in Hong Kong's prisons is complete. We may decide that record-keeping and infectious disease monitoring are conducted in a robust fashion in the prison system in Hong Kong and that the available records are likely to be complete. In this case, we may reason in accordance with (C_1) below. But we may also judge that this linguistic marker introduces sufficient uncertainty about the completeness of this knowledge base that we are inclined to reject the conclusion of (C_1)—the inference to this negative conclusion is blocked:

(C_1)

There is *no evidence* from available records that there have been outbreaks of TB and HIV in Hong Kong's prisons.

Therefore, there have *not* been outbreaks of TB and HIV in Hong Kong's prisons.

It is noteworthy that the Department of Health in Hong Kong makes extensive use in its press releases of arguments from ignorance in which default inferences to a negative conclusion are blocked by linguistic markers. These arguments occur only rarely in the press releases of public health agencies in the UK. Consider the *no evidence* statements in the press releases in (D) to (J) below:

(D)

Title	Update of influenza situation
Source	Press release, Department of Health, Hong Kong, 23 April 2008

"The Centre for Health Protection (CHP) of the Department of Health received two reports of outbreaks of influenza-like illness today involving a primary school and a residential home for the disabled, affecting a total of 10 people […] An eleven-year-old boy passed away in Prince of Wales Hospital this morning. A spokesman for the CHP said the boy was admitted to the hospital on April 17 because of convulsion and fever. Preliminary examination of the boy's respiratory sample yielded negative results for Influenza A and B, parainfluenza, adenovirus and respiratory syncytial virus. "There is **no evidence** at the present stage suggesting the boy has contracted influenza. He had no history of recent travel. Further investigation is ongoing and the case has been submitted to Coroner's Court for investigation", the spokesman said."

(E)

Title	Interdepartmental task force closely monitors development of Streptococcus suis infection
Source	Press release, Department of Health, Hong Kong, 31 July 2005

"The interdepartmental task force of the Health, Welfare and Food Bureau today continues to closely monitor the latest development with respect to the Streptococcus suis infection in Sichuan. A spokesman for the task force said at this moment, there was **no evidence** to suggest that Hong Kong had a risk of outbreak."

(F)

Title	Serious influenza response stands down
Source	Press release, Department of Health, Hong Kong, 8 April 2015

"A spokesman for the Centre for Health Protection of the Department of Health said that the "Alert" response level was activated in view of the ongoing activity of highly pathogenic avian influenza among poultry outside Hong Kong. "We will continue to closely monitor the global situation of avian influenza. So far, there is **no evidence** of efficient human-to-human transmission", the spokesman added."

(G)

Title	Briefing for financial sector on flu pandemic
Source	Press release, Department of Health, Hong Kong, 7 November 2005

"Medical professionals from the Centre for Health Protection (CHP) of the Department of Health today briefed about 250 representatives from the financial sector on the latest situation of avian influenza and advised them in formulating their own preparedness plans for influenza pandemic.

Acting Controller of the CHP, Dr Regina Ching said at the briefing that the Government had been working closely with the World Health Organization (WHO) as well as the Mainland and overseas counterparts in monitoring the situation.

"Hong Kong is now at the Alert Response Level, in accordance with the Framework of Government's Preparedness Plan for Influenza Pandemic. We acknowledged that the threat of avian flu has raised international concern but there is no cause for panic as **no evidence** to date suggests that the virus had mutated to human-to-human transmission", she said."

(H)

Title	Avian flu in China: Guidance for health professionals
Source	Press release, Public Health England, UK, 18 April 2013
"Over 1,000 close contacts of confirmed cases of A/(H7N9) bird flu have been followed up and there is **no evidence** of person-to-person spread."	

(I)

Title	Low risk of infection with Mycobacterium bovis in the UK – 1 July 2013
Source	Press release, Public Health England, UK, 1 July 2013
"Dr John Watson, head of respiratory diseases at Public Health England, said: "On the basis of the recent epidemiology of Mycobacterium bovis infections in the human population in the UK, there is **no evidence** of a significant public health problem associated with the consumption of meat. The risk to humans remains very low.""	

(J)

Title	Middle East respiratory syndrome coronavirus (MERS-CoV): Update
Source	Press release, Public Health England, UK, 30 May 2013
"Public Health England remains vigilant to the developments in the Middle East and in the rest of the world where new cases have emerged and continue to liaise closely with our international colleagues to assess whether our recommendations need to change. Although some person-to person transmission has been reported, there remains **no evidence** of sustained person-to-person transmission."	

The press releases in (D) and (E) concern, respectively, an unexplained illness and subsequent death of an 11-year-old boy, and an outbreak of a potentially fatal bacterial infection, *Streptococcus suis*, in people with occupational exposure to infected pigs in Sichuan Province in Mainland China. In both press releases, *no evidence* statements would ordinarily lead to the negative conclusions that the 11-year-old boy did *not* contract influenza, and that Hong Kong was *not* at risk of an outbreak of *S. suis* infection. But the default inferences to these negative conclusions are effectively blocked by two linguistic markers. These markers—*at the present stage* and *at this moment*—force further consideration of the knowledge bases upon which these negative conclusions are based. To the extent that these bases appear to be complete only to a certain point in time, we may consider the closed-world assumption in these cases to be weakly warranted at best. *A fortiori*, the negative conclusions that are based on this assumption are also weakly warranted. No-one would be surprised to discover that the *no evidence* statements in these press releases lead nowhere in logical terms—most rational observers would not be inclined to base negative conclusions on these statements.

The extracts in (F) and (G) are taken from press releases that are spaced 10 years apart. Yet, they both express very similar concerns about the human health risks associated with avian influenza. The extracts address the possibility that the viral pathogen in avian influenza may mutate, permitting human-to-human transmission to occur. The linguistic markers *so far* in (F) and *to date* in (G) raise the salience of the closed-world assumption. These markers serve to remind us that the current knowledge base on this pathogen may be incomplete in an essential respect. Although evidence *so far* and *to date* strongly suggests that human-to-human transmission does *not* occur, we may quickly need to revisit this claim and the knowledge base on which it is based should the virus mutate. Once again, linguistic markers function by blocking a negative conclusion—human-to-human transmission does *not* occur—that we might otherwise be inclined to accept.

The effect of these markers can be clearly illustrated by comparing these cases to the extracts from press releases issued by Public Health England in (H) to (J). The extract in (H) also addresses avian flu and the risk that human-to-human transmission may occur. The *no evidence* statement in this extract is much more likely to generate an inference to a negative conclusion—person-to-person spread of A/(H7N9) bird flu does *not* occur—in the absence of qualification from linguistic markers. That readers are encouraged to draw such a conclusion is confirmed by the fact that the press release also states that over 1,000 close contacts of confirmed cases of bird flu have been investigated with no evidence of human-to-human transmission. Public Health England is strongly implying that the knowledge base is complete in this case and that human-to-human transmission of avian flu does *not* occur. Mycobacterium bovis is the causative agent of bovine tuberculosis. It is also responsible for some cases of tuberculosis in human beings. Although it has been recognized for over a century, this form of human tuberculosis is still poorly understood, including transmission between people, and between infected cattle and humans (Grange, 2001). The extract in (I) addresses the human health risks associated with the consumption of meat. Once again, an unqualified *no evidence* statement leads readers to draw the inference that there is *not* a significant public health problem associated with the consumption of meat. Finally, in the absence of linguistic markers, the *no evidence* statement in the extract in (J) triggers a default inference to the negative conclusion that sustained person-to-person transmission of Middle East Respiratory Syndrome (MERS) does *not* occur. This difference in the use of *no evidence* statements by public health agencies in Hong Kong and the UK is significant for what it can tell us about the approaches of these agencies to public health communication. This point is developed in the following sections.

4   No Evidence and Systematic Versus Heuristic Reasoning

It was argued in the previous section that public health agencies can promote two different modes of reasoning based on *no evidence* statements by means of their use or omission of linguistic markers in press releases to the public. In one mode of reasoning, *no evidence* statements are used in the absence of linguistic markers. In the absence of these markers, a default inference is generated from the claim of *no evidence* to a negative conclusion that X is *not* the case. This inference is triggered by the apparent satisfaction of the epistemic conditions referred to in this chapter as *closed-world assumption* and *exhaustive search*. These conditions may ultimately be found not to be adequately satisfied, and the negative conclusion may have to be rejected. But the inference has still enabled a public health agency to communicate a negative claim by merely issuing a *no evidence* statement. There are many circumstances where this mode of reasoning may be rationally warranted. Scientists who believe and who want the public to believe that the MMR vaccine does *not* cause autism are nonetheless compelled to produce cautiously worded statements to the effect that there is *no evidence* that MMR vaccine causes autism. These statements afford protection to scientists should they later be found to be incorrect—scientists can deflect the charge of error by claiming that they only stated that there was *no evidence* that X is the case. At the same time, these statements enable a negative conclusion (e.g. MMR vaccine does *not* cause autism) to take root in the public's consciousness. Unqualified *no evidence* statements encourage little interrogation of the closed-world assumption and exhaustive search conditions—if these conditions *appear* to be satisfied, the inference proceeds automatically (Fig. 1).

In their press releases to the public, public health agencies also make use of the second mode of reasoning based on *no evidence* statements. This occurs when *no evidence* statements are used alongside linguistic markers such as *at the present stage* and *from the available evidence*. The effect of these markers is to increase the salience of the closed-world assumption and exhaustive search conditions. The purpose of these markers is to encourage the public to undertake a systematic examination of these epistemic conditions with a view to determining the extent to which they are satisfied. If the public suspects that a knowledge base is incomplete in some respect, then it is unlikely to draw a negative conclusion from the fact that a proposition or claim is absent from the base. The inference from the *no evidence*

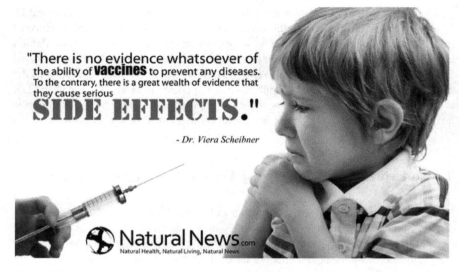

Fig. 1 Both sides in the vaccine safety controversy can use *no evidence* statements to imply or suggest claims (reproduced courtesy of Naturalnews.com, 2013)

statement to the conclusion that *X* is *not* the case is effectively blocked. Where the first mode of reasoning based on a *no evidence* statement involves an automatic inference to a negative conclusion, this second mode of reasoning encourages an extended process of deliberation that can overturn a negative conclusion. The distinction between these two modes of reasoning reflects another, well-known distinction in the psychology and philosophy of reasoning, namely, that between heuristic and systematic reasoning. Heuristic reasoning embodies speed and automaticity. It involves default inferences to conclusions. These inferences are rapid, take shortcuts through complex domains and make limited use of cognitive resources (Gigerenzer, 2008; Gigerenzer and Brighton, 2009). They are in stark contrast to the inferences in systematic reasoning which is a slow, deliberative process that is resource intensive. This is how one informal logician, Douglas Walton, characterizes these different approaches to reasoning:

> In recent years there has been great interest in so-called dual-process theories of reasoning and cognition. According to dual-process theories in cognitive science, there are two distinct cognitive systems underlying human reasoning. One is an evolutionarily old system that is associative, automatic, unconscious, parallel, and fast. It instinctively jumps to a conclusion. In this system, innate thinking processes have evolved to solve specific adaptive problems. The other is a system that is rule-based, controlled, conscious, serial, and slow. In this cognitive system, processes are learned slowly and consciously, but at the same time need to be flexible and responsive. (2010:" 161)

It is the contention of this chapter that public health agencies can directly influence how the public processes *no evidence* statements in its press releases through the inclusion or omission of linguistic markers. By omitting these markers, these agencies can encourage the public to engage in heuristic processing of *no evidence* statements. A default inference from a *no evidence* statement to a negative conclusion is automatically generated. This achieves speed of processing by circumventing an extended examination of the two epistemic conditions on the rationally warranted use of the argument from ignorance, namely, the closed-world assumption and exhaustive search condition. By introducing one or more linguistic markers into *no evidence* statements, public health agencies can encourage the public to engage in systematic processing of these statements. This slower, deliberative process of reasoning exposes the closed-world assumption and the exhaustive search condition to extensive critical scrutiny. The outcome of this scrutiny may be that it is decided that these conditions are not fulfilled in a certain case. The default inference that takes us from a *no evidence* statement to a negative conclusion is then overridden. The view that health messages can be manipulated to encourage heuristic versus systematic reasoning is not without precedent. There is clear evidence that message framing can influence the processing of health and other messages (Meyers-Levy and Maheswaran, 2004; Smith and Petty, 1996; Yan, 2015). But where the argument of this chapter is novel is in its claim that an informal fallacy can be an effective rational resource under conditions of both heuristic and systematic processing.

Thus far, it has been argued that *no evidence* statements in the press releases of public health agencies undertake considerable logical work. Under certain epistemic conditions, these statements permit the public to infer that claim X is false (true) because there is *no evidence* that X is true (false). It has also been argued that public health agencies can exercise control over the type of processing—heuristic versus systematic processing—that the public undertakes when it uses *no evidence* statements in its reasoning. This latter point raises the issue of when it might be beneficial for these agencies to encourage the public to undertake heuristic versus systematic processing of *no evidence* statements. With its emphasis on quick, automatic inferences and bypassing of information, heuristic processing encourages the public to come to a rapid judgement about a claim. This can be advantageous when a public health problem (e.g. an infectious disease outbreak) requires urgent action by the public. Under these circumstances, a protracted examination of the closed-world assumption and exhaustive search conditions is discouraged. The public is encouraged to place its trust in the public health agency that produces the *no evidence* statement and defer to the greater expertise of the agency. Trust is ultimately founded on the assumption that the agency has undertaken the more extensive deliberations that it is urging the public to suspend. To the extent that this assumption is correct, a strong steer to the public to accept a certain claim is warranted. The stance of the public health agency can be captured as follows: *When we state that there is 'no evidence' that X is true, you can confidently conclude that X is false.* On this view, the public is led in judgement-making by the public health agency and is encouraged to accept its pronouncements with little in the way of rational reflection.

Public health agencies can also steer the public towards systematic reasoning using *no evidence* statements. Through the inclusion of linguistic markers such as *from the available evidence* and *at the present stage*, public health agencies can increase the salience of the closed-world assumption and exhaustive search conditions. These conditions are emphasized as worthy of the public's rational scrutiny and examination. Where we might overlook these conditions, or simply give them a cursory glance in heuristic reasoning, our sustained attention is directed towards them in systematic reasoning. The public is encouraged to interrogate these conditions and consider what, if any, rational warrant they provide for the claims that are based on them. Public health agencies may consider it beneficial to steer the public towards systematic reasoning when deliberation can proceed in the absence of time constraints and when the public is viewed as competent to assess an issue. The relationship between the public and the public health agency that promotes systematic reasoning is one of the equal participation in a shared rational enterprise. The agency does not presume to possess all the expertise in the relationship which is then bestowed on an inexpert public. The agency is also not alone in possessing a rational competence which only it can exercise. Instead, the public is viewed as a rational agent that can be trusted to undertake an independent, rational assessment of public health issues. The stance of the public health agency that promotes systematic reasoning can be captured as follows: *When we state that there is no evidence that X is true, you should determine if that means X is false.* On this view, the public is urged to be a proactive, rational actor alongside the public health agency.

It emerges that public health agencies that promote heuristic processing versus systematic processing of *no evidence* statements possess two different conceptions of the public as a rational actor. The public health agency that promotes heuristic processing of these statements does not prioritize rational engagement with the public. Instead, the agency aims to secure the public's acceptance of a conclusion based on trust and its presumed expertise. There is relatively little attempt to foster independent rational competence on the part of the public. Instead, the public is expected to follow the strong logical steer of the public health agency. A very different rational stance towards the public is taken by the public health agency that promotes systematic processing of *no evidence* statements. The public is entrusted by the agency to arrive at rational judgements of the logical significance of these statements based on an evaluation of the closed-world assumption and exhaustive search conditions. Indeed, such an evaluation is encouraged through the agency's use of linguistic markers that make these conditions salient for the public. The agency fosters the development of an independent rational competence on the part of the public. The rational attitudes associated with these two approaches to the processing of *no evidence* statements are displayed in Table 2. In the final section, we discuss these approaches further in the context of public health agencies in Hong Kong and the UK. These agencies do not promote heuristic and systematic processing of *no evidence* statements to equal extents. The differences, it is argued, reflect a more fundamental divergence in the conduct of public health communication.

Table 2 Rational Attitudes Associated with Heuristic and Systematic Reasoning

No evidence statements	
Heuristic reasoning	**Systematic reasoning**
• *No evidence* statements used without linguistic markers	• *No evidence* statements used with linguistic markers
• Public health agency provides strong logical steer to the public to accept a claim	• Public health agency encourages the public to assess a claim independently
• Public is perceived to be reliant on the expertise of the public health agency in forming rational judgements	• Public is perceived to be competent in exercising its own rational judgements apart from the public health agency
• The public places trust in the public health agency	• The public health agency places trust in the public
• The public and public health agency are unequal rational partners in public health	• The public and public health agency are equal rational partners in public health

5 The 'Public' in Public Health Communication

The ten *no evidence* statements that were examined in Sect. 3 were taken from the press releases of just two public health agencies, namely, the Department of Health in Hong Kong and Public Health England in the UK. Clearly, claims based on only ten *no evidence* statements across two public health agencies must be treated with caution. But they do suggest a tendency or pattern that is consistent with other research findings (Cummings, 2010, 2015a, 2020). The pattern is one in which public health authorities in the UK use *no evidence* statements in press releases with the intention of strongly encouraging the public to accept a certain claim. On this view, the public is not an autonomous rational agent and must be logically led to the conclusion that it is in its best interests to accept. This type of public health communication is strongly paternalistic in nature (Bernhardt, 2004; Guttman, 2000; Grill, 2013). One of its most striking manifestations in the UK was the public health response to the emergence of BSE in British cattle. The official communication strategy—to the extent that there was a strategy—involved repeated reassurances by public health officials, including the Chief Medical Officer, that beef was safe to eat. These reassurances were based on the claim that there was *no evidence* that BSE had transmitted to humans. That these reassurances lulled the British public into a false sense of security that BSE would pose no risk to human health was amply demonstrated by the sense of betrayal the public felt when the Government announced to British Parliament on 20 March 1996 that BSE had transmitted to humans (BSE Inquiry Report, Volume 1, 2000: xviii). The public had diligently followed the strong logical steer of public health officials, only for that steer to be shown to be catastrophically flawed.

Public health authorities in Hong Kong also make extensive use of *no evidence* statements in their press releases to the public. But these authorities have a different type of rational engagement with the public they serve. Specifically, public health agencies in Hong Kong avoid strongly steering the public towards acceptance of a certain claim. Instead, the public is encouraged by these agencies to reflect on the epistemic conditions that a rational actor should prioritize in public health reasoning. As far as *no evidence* statements are concerned, these conditions are the closed-world assumption and exhaustive search conditions that have been examined throughout this chapter. The salience of these conditions is increased through the inclusion of linguistic markers in the press releases issued by these public health agencies. Unlike their counterparts in the UK, public health agencies in Hong Kong view the public as an autonomous actor that *can* exercise rational choices in relation to its health even if there are circumstances in which this does not occur. The decision to accept or reject a claim based on a *no evidence* statement is one such choice. On this view, the public should not be compelled to make decisions or take courses of action as strong paternalism would have it. Rather, the public can be 'nudged' in the direction of more rational choices in relation to its health. It is the function of linguistic markers in *no evidence* statements to nudge the public towards these choices. The term 'nudge' is borrowed from Thaler and Sunstein (2008). These theorists propose a much gentler paternalism than that which forcefully directs us to accept certain conclusions or claims. So-called libertarian paternalism recognizes that people want to exercise freedom in the choices that they make but that they should be gently nudged in directions that will improve their lives:

> Libertarian paternalism is a relatively weak, soft, and nonintrusive type of paternalism because choices are not blocked, fenced off, or significantly burdened. If people want to smoke cigarettes, to eat a lot of candy, to choose an unsuitable health care plan, or fail to save for retirement – libertarian paternalists will not force them to do otherwise – or even make things hard for them. Still, the approach we recommend does count as paternalistic, because private and public choice architects are not merely trying to track or to implement people's anticipated choices. Rather, they are self-consciously attempting to move people in directions that will make their lives better. They nudge. (Thaler and Sunstein, 2008: 5-6)

Public health agencies in Hong Kong are a type of 'public choice architect'. A choice architect has the responsibility for organizing the context in which people make decisions. In its press releases to the public, the Department of Health in Hong Kong elected to include linguistic markers in its *no evidence* statements that public health agencies in the UK opted to omit. These markers do not constrain the decisions that the Hong Kong public makes in relation to its health—the public is at liberty to disregard these markers and to draw whatever implications it wants from *no evidence* statements, or equally to draw no implications at all. Instead, these markers gently nudge the public in a direction that will improve its decision-making ability in relation to health. By raising the salience of the epistemic conditions under which *no evidence* statements are a rationally warranted basis on which to accept claims about health, the Department of Health in Hong Kong is organizing the context in which health decisions are made. It is an effective choice architect. An analogy with Thaler and Sunstein's example of encouraging healthy food choices in students seems pertinent at this point. Thaler and Sunstein argue that students can be encouraged to select a healthy food option over junk food by placing fruit at eye level in the cafeteria. Food layout, in which healthy options are displayed prominently and are easily accessible, serves to organize the context in such a way that students are nudged in the direction of making healthy choices. In much the same way, public health agencies such as the Department of Health in Hong Kong can place conditions for rational decision-making about health at 'eye level' through its use of linguistic markers. The public's freedom of choice is not constrained by these markers. But they do serve to nudge us in the direction of better health decision-making.

It emerges that public health authorities in the UK exercise a strong paternalism in which the public is compelled to accept a claim that is judged to be in its best interests. The public is discouraged from exercising its own rational judgements about health risks. Instead, it is forcefully steered towards acceptance of a claim that a more expert authority has deemed is the most rationally warranted position for the public to hold. Public health authorities in Hong Kong exercise a quite different form of paternalism during public health communication. The public is gently nudged in the direction of making better choices in relation to its health. The libertarian paternalism that is practiced by these authorities does not seek to constrain the public's choices—the public can choose to reject a health risk and continue to practice risk-taking behaviours. That these two forms of paternalism should be played out in public health communication is unremarkable. Paternalism has, after all, a long history in the public health arena (Schramme, 2015). But what is remarkable is that it should shape the logical structures and rational processes by means of which public health communication is conducted. The paternalistic stance of a public health agency was enacted through the agency's promotion of either heuristic reasoning or systematic reasoning on the part of the public. When a public health agency exercised strong paternalism, the public was encouraged to suspend its own assessment of a health risk, and draw a quick, automatic inference to a conclusion. When a public health agency practiced libertarian paternalism, the public was nudged in the direction of making rational choices about its health and undertaking a systematic evaluation of risk. Paternalism profoundly shaped the type of reasoning promoted by a public health agency.

In summary, it has been argued in this chapter that the argument from ignorance is a powerful rational resource in public health reasoning. This resource has been overlooked amidst the largely negative logical characterizations of this argument as a fallacy. In some contexts, the title of 'fallacy' is warranted—examples of the abuse and misuse of this argument are not difficult to find in public health and elsewhere. But even in public health we must acknowledge the many rationally warranted uses of this argument. Instances of the fallacious and rationally warranted use of the argument from ignorance are commonly found in public health communication. The single premise of this argument is a *no evidence* statement. These statements were examined in the press releases of two public health agencies, namely, Public Health England in the UK and the Department of Health in Hong Kong. These agencies both made extensive use of *no evidence* statements to characterize potential risks to human health. However, they differed in whether these statements were qualified by linguistic markers. These markers, it was argued, served the purpose of raising the salience of two epistemic conditions—the closed-world assumption and exhaustive search condition—that must be satisfied for an argument from ignorance to be rationally warranted. The omission and inclusion of these markers by public health authorities in the UK and Hong Kong, respectively, revealed two different modes of reasoning using *no evidence* statements. Where UK public health authorities promoted heuristic reasoning based on these statements, public health authorities in Hong Kong promoted the public's use of systematic reasoning. These modes of reasoning, it was argued, reflected different paternalistic stances on the part of these public health agencies.

6   A Final Note for Public Health Professionals

The discussion in this chapter is particularly relevant to the professionals who are charged with protecting the health of populations. Central to this effort is effective public health communication. It has been argued in this chapter that the way in which this communication is conducted can directly affect the public's compliance with health recommendations. When the public is strongly steered by public health agencies to suspend judgement and follow the recommendations of authorities 'who know best', the type of quick, reflexive thinking that ensues is not always conducive to rational decision-making. In fact, it may even be strongly counter-productive to achieving the aims of a public health agency if the public feels coerced by the type of health communication employed and develops a stance of resistance as a result. It is much better to view the public in health communication as a cooperative partner which is striving to make most effective use of its rational resources in decision-making related to health. These decisions can be helpfully guided by a public health agency through the provision of key supports (e.g. accessible health literature). Through gentle nudges, the public can be directed towards courses of action that protect health without instilling a strong stance of resistance and mistrust. This chapter illustrated the way in which these nudges may be achieved in the type of linguistic communication that is employed. It is hoped that these simple linguistic strategies may be more directly integrated into future efforts at public health communication.

References

Arroyo-Johnson, C., & Mincey, K. D. (2016). Obesity epidemiology trends by race/ethnicity, gender, and education: National Health Interview Survey, 1997-2012. *Gastroenterology Clinics of North America, 45*(4), 571–579.

Bernhardt, J. M. (2004). Communication at the core of effective public health. *American Journal of Public Health, 94*(12), 2051–2053.

Brown, P., Cathala, F., Raubertas, R. F., Gajdusek, D. C., & Castaigne, P. (1987). The epidemiology of Creutzfeldt-Jakob disease: Conclusion of a 15-year investigation in France and review of the world literature. *Neurology, 37*(6), 895–904.

BSE Inquiry Report. (2000a). *Volume 1: Findings and conclusions.* London: The Stationery Office.

BSE Inquiry Report. (2000b). *Volume 2: Science.* London: The Stationery Office.

BSE Inquiry Report. (2000c). *Volume 3: The early years, 1986-88.* London: The Stationery Office.

Centers for Disease Control. (1981). *Pneumocystis* pneumonia – Los Angeles. *Morbidity and Mortality Weekly Report, 30*(21), 1–3.

Christakos, G., Olea, R. A., Serre, M. L., Yu, H.-L., & Wang, L.-L. (2005). *Interdisciplinary public health reasoning and epidemic modelling: The case of black death.* The Netherlands: Springer.

Cummings, L. (2005). Giving science a bad name: Politically and commercially motivated fallacies in BSE inquiry. *Argumentation, 19*(2), 123–143.

Cummings, L. (2010). *Rethinking the BSE crisis: A study of scientific reasoning under uncertainty.* Dordrecht: Springer.

Cummings, L. (2011). Considering risk assessment up close: The case of bovine spongiform encephalopathy. *Health, Risk & Society, 13*(3), 255–275.

Cummings, L. (2014a). Informal fallacies as cognitive heuristics in public health reasoning. *Informal Logic, 34*(1), 1–37.

Cummings, L. (2014b). The 'trust' heuristic: Arguments from authority in public health. *Health Communication, 29*(10), 1043–1056.

Cummings, L. (2015a). *Reasoning and public health: New ways of coping with uncertainty.* Cham, Switzerland: Springer.

Cummings, L. (2015b). The use of 'no evidence' statements in public health. *Informal Logic, 35* (1), 32–65.

Cummings, L. (2020). *Fallacies in medicine and health: Critical thinking, argumentation and communication.* Houndmills, Basingstoke: Palgrave Macmillan.

De Cornulier, B. (1988). Knowing whether, knowing who, and epistemic closure. In M. Meyer (Ed.), *Questions and questioning* (pp. 182–192). Berlin: Walter de Gruyter.

Gigerenzer, G. (2008). Why heuristics work. *Perspectives on Psychological Science, 3*(1), 20–29.

Gigerenzer, G., & Brighton, H. (2009). Homo heuristicus: Why biased minds make better inferences. *Topics in Cognitive Science, 1*(1), 107–143.

Grange, J. M. (2001). Mycobacterium bovis infection in human beings. *Tuberculosis, 81*(1–2), 71–77.

Grill, K. (2013). Normative and non-normative concepts: Paternalism and libertarian paternalism. In D. Strech, I. Hirschberg, & G. Marckmann (Eds.), *Ethics in public health and health policy: Concepts, methods, case studies.* Public Health Ethics Analysis 1 (pp. 27–46). Dordrecht: Springer Science + Business Media.

Guttman, N. (2000). *Public health communication interventions: Values and ethical dilemmas.* Thousand Oaks, California: Sage Publications.

Hinton, M. (2018). *On arguments from ignorance. Informal Logic, 38*(2), 184–212.

Lenzer, J. (2016). Conflicts of interest compromise US public health agency's mission, say scientists. *BMJ, 355*, i5723.

Locke, J. (1959/1689). *An essay concerning human understanding*. Ed. by A. C. Fraser, New York: Dover.

Meyers-Levy, J., & Maheswaran, D. (2004). Exploring message framing outcomes when systematic, heuristic, or both types of processing occur. *Journal of Consumer Psychology, 14* (1–2), 159–167.

Mosley-Jensen, W., & Panetta, E. (2017). Patterns of reasoning. *Oxford Research Encyclopedia of Communication*. https://doi.org/10.1093/acrefore/9780190228613.013.301.

Newman, L., Rowley, J., Hoorn, S. V., Wijesooriya, N. S., Unemo, M., Low, N., et al. (2015). Global estimates of the prevalence and incidence of four curable sexually transmitted infections in 2012 based on systematic review and global reporting. *PLoS ONE, 10*(12), e0143304.

Ng, M., Freeman, M. K., Fleming, T. D., Robinson, M., Dwyer-Lindgren, L., Thomson, B., et al. (2014). Smoking prevalence and cigarette consumption in 187 countries, 1980–2012. *JAMA, 311*(2), 183–192.

Robinson, R. (1971). Arguing from ignorance. *The Philosophical Quarterly, 21*(83), 97–108.

Schramme, T. (Ed.). (2015). *New perspectives on paternalism and healthcare. Library of Ethics and Applied Philosophy 35*. Cham, Switzerland: Springer International Publishing.

Smith, S. M., & Petty, R. E. (1996). Message framing and persuasion: A message processing analysis. *Personality and Social Psychology Bulletin, 22*(3), 257–268.

Thaler, R. H., & Sunstein, C. R. (2008). *Nudge: Improving decisions about health, wealth, and happiness*. New Haven and London: Yale University Press.

Walton, D. (1995). *Arguments from ignorance*. University Park, PA: The Pennsylvania State University Press.

Walton, D. (1999). Profiles of dialogue for evaluating arguments from ignorance. *Argumentation, 13*(1), 53–71.

Walton, D. (2008). *Informal logic: A pragmatic approach* (2nd ed.). New York: Cambridge University Press.

Walton, D. (2010). Why fallacies appear to be better arguments than they are. *Informal Logic, 30* (2), 159–184.

Ward, P. R. (2017). Improving access to, use of, and outcomes from public health programs: The importance of building and maintaining trust with patients/clients. *Frontiers in Public Health*. https://doi.org/10.3389/fpubh.2017.00022.

World Health Organization. (2014). *Global status report on alcohol and health 2014*. Geneva: Switzerland.

Yan, C. (2015). Persuading people to eat less junk food: A cognitive resource match between attitudinal ambivalence and health message framing. *Health Communication, 30*(3), 251–260.

Louise Cummings is Professor in the Department of English at The Hong Kong Polytechnic University. She teaches and conducts research in pragmatics, clinical linguistics, and public health reasoning and argumentation. She is particularly interested in the application of logical fallacies to the study of public health reasoning by both experts and laypeople. Her publications in public health include the books Rethinking the BSE Crisis (Springer, 2010), Reasoning and Public Health (Springer, 2015) and Fallacies in Medicine and Health (Palgrave Macmillan, 2020). She has also published her work on public health reasoning in international journals including Health, Risk & Society and Health Communication. She is a member of the International Research Centre for the Advancement of Health Communication (IRCAHC) at The Hong Kong Polytechnic University, the Royal College of Speech and Language Therapists in the UK, and the Health & Care Professions Council in the UK.

Visualizing Conversations in Health Care: Using Discursis to Compare Cantonese and English Data Sets

Alice Yau, Margo Turnbull, Daniel Angus, and Bernadette Watson

Abstract Health care is shaped by often complex communication between multiple people such as doctors, nurses, patients and carers. Research has repeatedly shown that effective communication is key to safe and high-quality care yet improving communication remains a challenge across health systems. In recent years, the field of natural language processing has developed analytic tools to supplement the study of verbal communication through visual representation of analysis. To date, these tools have primarily been used on English data. This study used the software tool Discursis to compare visual representations of Cantonese conversational data that were analysed before and after English translation. Results indicate that some linguistic features of Cantonese that carry meaning may be lost in translation into English. Specific concerns relate to the multidimensional issues of equivalence, ranging from cultural and social associations to semantic, lexical and conceptual differences. These results highlight the importance of developing visual analytic tools that can be used on Cantonese data. Generating visual representations of such data contributes to local and international understandings about communication in health care.

Keywords Discursis · Cantonese · Natural language processing

A. Yau (✉)
Centre for the Applied English Studies, The University of Hong Kong,
Hong Kong SAR, China
e-mail: aliceyau.alice@gmail.com

M. Turnbull
International Research Centre for the Advancement of Health Communication, Department
of English, The Hong Kong Polytechnic University, Hung Hom, Hong Kong SAR, China

D. Angus
Digital Media Research Centre School of Communication, Queensland University
of Technology, Brisbane, Australia

B. Watson
International Research Centre for the Advancement of Health Communication Department
of English, The Hong Kong Polytechnic University, Hung Hom, Hong Kong SAR, China

© Springer Nature Singapore Pte Ltd. 2020
B. Watson and J. Krieger (eds.), *Expanding Horizons in Health Communication*,
The Humanities in Asia 6, https://doi.org/10.1007/978-981-15-4389-0_13

1 Introduction

Communication in health care is complex and involves ongoing and dynamic interactions between people. Communication incorporates multiple modes of interaction (such as spoken and written formats), speakers, contexts and communicative events (such as meetings, conversations, emails, etc.: Bondi, 2017). Effective and meaningful communication involves both the transfer of information *and* the generation of shared meaning between doctors, nurses, patients and carers. Meaningful communication in health care is vital in terms of safety and quality of care, as well as empowering people to improve their own health by taking up preventative and curative advice (Goldstein, MacDonald, & Guirguis, 2015; Street, Makoul, Arora, & Epstein, 2009).

Although health-related information can be shared across a range of modalities, such as electronically or in print, *conversations* between people remain a key element of health communication. Conversation involves multiple interactants and is dynamic, purpose-driven and reflective (Bondi, 2017). As conversation unfolds meaning is generated and shared, as the interactants come to discuss a shared topic. This can be described as semantic alignment (Tolston, Riley, Mancuso, Finomore, & Funke, 2018). Semantic alignment can be achieved within a conversation even if participants do not agree or reach consensus.

Human conversation and dialogue has been studied extensively using a range of well-established theoretical and methodological approaches (see Weigand, 2017). Recent developments in Natural Language Processing (NLP), a sub-field of computer science concerned with analysing and understanding human language (Hirschberg & Manning, 2015), have seen the increasing use of computer programs to process conversational data and supplement other methods of qualitative and quantitative analysis. Discursis, one such NLP tool, has been used successfully in recent studies of health care in both clinical and managerial contexts (Atay et al., 2015; Chevalier, Watson, Barras, Cottrell, & Angus, 2018; Watson, Angus, Gore, & Farmer, 2015). Although Discursis and other NLP tools may be theoretically able to process non-alphabetic input, most published work to date has reported on the analysis of data sourced in or translated to alphabetic languages (in the case of the related software Leximancer: English, Italian and Danish: Evers, Marroun & Young, 2017; Franzoni & Bonera, 2019).

This chapter reports on a novel study that compared the analytic outputs produced by Discursis following the analysis of conversational data uploaded to the program written both in Cantonese Chinese characters and English. Analytic outputs were compared in terms of the representation of inter-speaker engagement, conceptual alignment and levels of interaction. The comparison of data outputs based on Cantonese and translated data highlighted important conversational markers that are at risk of being lost through either translation or inadequate customization of software for use with a logographic language.

This chapter begins by briefly examining the importance of conversation in health care, as both a tool for information exchange and as a process through which meaning is generated. We then introduce Discursis as an analytic tool that can supplement other qualitative and quantitative approaches to conversational analysis. We pay particular attention to Discursis's visualization plots which represent data-grounded, time-ordered exchanges between conversational participants (Chevalier et al., 2018, p. 3). These plots show map patterns of conversational features such as turn taking, concept sharing and topic maintenance, which contribute to the generation of meaning through ongoing exchanges. We draw on the analytic outputs from Discursis to discuss three key features of Cantonese that influence analysis in Discursis. These features include the logographic nature of written Cantonese, the significance of the 'word' units used in the software analysis and the need for software adaptation to accommodate the lexical and semantic role of tone in Cantonese. We conclude this chapter by examining how the results of this research underscore the need for continued investment in the development of analytic tools like Discursis that can be used for the analysis of alphabetic and logographic data in health communication research.

1.1 Conversations in Health Care

Health care is shaped by a diverse range of interactions between people. Recent research has noted the impact of spoken communication and conversation on knowledge, motivation, diagnosis, treatment and management of health conditions (Nouri & Rudd, 2015). It has also been argued that as doctors spend *decreasing* amounts of time with patients yet need to exchange *increasingly* large and detailed amounts of information associated with treatment and diagnosis, the need for effective and efficient communication has grown (Nouri & Rudd, 2015). Communication about health in a broader sense involves a discussion about a wide range of information including physical conditions, lifestyle factors and the broader context in which people live.

Despite technological advances reflected in the growth of tools associated with e-health and telehealth, conversation remains a core element of health care. Conversations are made up of linguistic interactions and exchanges between people which results in the transmission of information and generation of shared meaning even when speakers do not agree about the subject being discussed. These exchanges are shaped by the use of semantic and lexical features including vocabulary and grammar as well as contextual and relational markers that connect words, phrases and spoken sentences in meaningful ways. Importantly, the language used in the conversation also reflects the relationships that connect people in terms of familiarity, authority and professional expertise.

As the conversation unfolds between participants, meaning is shared and generated through various linguistic devices such as turning taking, asking questions, making statements or repeating what another speaker has said. Through this process, interpersonal and semantic alignment (Tolston et al., 2018) is achieved. Semantic alignment is not predetermined but is generated as a conversation progresses and meaning is negotiated and debated. Spevack et al. (2018) described conversation as marked with ambiguities that are progressively addressed and resolved through dynamic and unpredictable interaction. This dynamic nature of conversation can be contrasted with comparatively static types of interactions such as letters or emails and other verbal interactions such as giving instructions which feature a predominantly one-way flow of information.

Tolston et al. (2018) argued that semantic and interpersonal alignment are important features of conversation that can be quantitatively and qualitatively measured. Markers such as turn taking, cross-referencing of ideas and links across time periods are features that can be identified, measured and described. Similarly, Chevalier et al. (2018) noted that effective communication between participants can be reflected in the mapping of the extent of engagement between speakers, the relative contributions each speaker makes and how consistently topics are maintained within a conversation.

1.2 Natural Language Processing and Using Discursis to Produce Visual Analysis

Various methodologies have been developed to study and describe how people interact through conversation including Communication Accommodation Theory (CAT), Conversational Analysis (CA) and Discourse Analysis (DA) (see chapters by Harrison & Lam; Yip & Zhang; Schoeb & Yip in this edition). These approaches focus in different ways on the analysis of the content and process of linguistic communication—that is, the study of what is said or understood by participants in a conversation and how these messages are conveyed, modified, accepted or rejected. These approaches can be described as *process analysis* which focuses on in-depth coding of data and the *microanalysis* of conversational features (Heritage & Maynard, 2006). Various elements of conversation are described in terms such as syntax, semantics and phonetics (Spevack et al., 2018).

In recent years, the field of NLP has developed a range of computer-based tools which can be used to provide additional and supplementary data to the study of conversational content and process by focusing on multiple dimensions of conversation. Analysis of these multiple dimensions aims to identify patterns, structures and orderliness of exchanges and interactions and to present these findings visually (Angus, Smith, & Wiles, 2012). Examples of such machine-based or automatic analytic methods include latent semantic analysis and word2vec (Tolston et al., 2018). These tools map semantic alignment through the analysis of large amounts of data and by quantifying 'linguistic and communicative co-ordination… the alignment of the meaning of the content of the utterances rather than the syntactical, morphological, or lexical alignment' (Tolston et al., 2018, p. 3).

In contrast to these tools which draw on large quantities of data, the Discursis software described in this chapter can analyse relatively small data sets. The software is straightforward to use as the analyst simply uploads a transcript or text as a comma-separated value (.csv) file, makes a few parameter selections, then analyses the resulting visual and metric outputs. A transcript of as few as 10 conversational turns can be used as the basis for Discursis' language corpus, thereby enabling analysis of very brief conversational exchanges (Tolston et al., 2018).

Once a transcript is selected, Discursis automatically builds a data-grounded natural language model from this same input text (and only this input text) by using Leximancer's conceptual modelling algorithm (Smith & Humphreys, 2006). The Leximancer concept model uses Bayesian statistics to identify groups of words that co-occur within an input text. This bottom-up approach is based on a bag-of-words assumption that draws on the idea that words which collocate often have an associated meaning, or in the words of John Firth: 'You shall know a word by the company it keeps!' (Firth, 1962, p.11). Leximancer and Discursis refer to these bags-of-words as concepts. By identifying and grouping words in this way, input text can be reduced in length from thousands of unique words, to a smaller number of concepts. This process is preceded by the removal of words included in a stop word list. This stop word list consists of words that occur frequently but carry little or no semantic meaning. Examples of such words in English include *a, an, and, the*. A default stop word list is used by Discursis and this can also be manually generated or customized by the analyst depending on the text and communicative interaction being analysed.

After building a language model from the entire input transcript, Discursis then codes the transcript to indicate which concepts are present per turn. This coding process involves the automatic identification and labelling of concepts within each conversational turn. Discursis performs this coding by looking for words within a single turn that can be considered evidence of the presence of specific concepts, and if found, uses these words as markers that this concept is present in this turn.

Once a transcript is coded, Discursis uses a graphical interface to present this coding visually as a recurrence plot. A Discursis recurrence plot features vertically and horizontally adjacent coloured squares (recurrence elements) that highlight instances of conceptual repetition between pairs of conversation turns (see Fig. 1 for an example). These plots are a useful tool for the analyst who can then click on squares to see detail about the concepts identified as well as their actual location within a text. Discursis can also produce other statistical and visual data to support quantitative and qualitative analysis (Angus, Rintel, & Wiles, 2013; Angus et al., 2012).

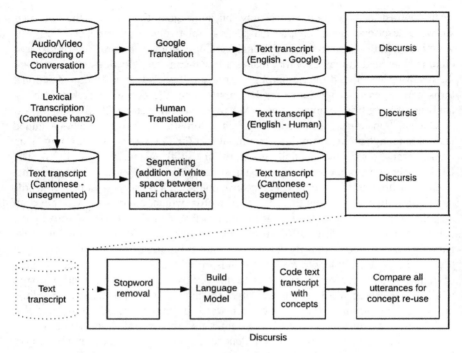

Fig. 1 Workflows used in the analysis of cantonese and translated data: workflow begins with the transcription of the Conversation

1.3 Studying a Logographic Language: Contrasting Features of Cantonese and English Data

As previously discussed, Discursis has been used to analyse a range of health-related data. However, at the time of writing, this growing body of published work described the analysis of alphabetic data (i.e. data sourced or translated into English or other alphabetic languages). Cantonese, the version of Chinese spoken in Hong Kong and the broader Guangdong province including Macau, is a logographic language and is written in Chinese (hanzi) characters (Ho & Bryant, 1997). From a historical perspective, Cantonese developed as a predominantly spoken, rather than written, language. This is reflected in Cantonese's linguistic subtlety and complexity (Snow, 2004). Cantonese has been the focus of significant linguistic analysis but discussion of this is beyond the scope of this chapter (see Matthews & Yip, 2011; Snow, 2004). There are, however, three key features of Cantonese that can be contrasted with English and are relevant to this discussion of Discursis and the ongoing development of NLP models.

Firstly, written Chinese characters and symbols used in other logographic systems do not correspond directly to spoken components (phonemes or morphemes) as they do in alphabetic languages like English. In contrast, Chinese characters map onto spoken syllables and carry semantic and lexical significance (Liu & Hsiao, 2014; Wong, Juang, & Chen, 2012). The semantic and lexical information that is encoded within the characters is often carried within English sentences. For example, the Cantonese 多謝 (do1ze6) and 唔該 (m4goi1) can both be translated into the English form 'thank you.' However, 多謝 (do1ze6) is used when someone offers you a gift while 唔該 (m4goi1) is used when someone offers you a service or help. In English, these differences and the additional information would be set out in the context of the phrase or sentence in which 'thank you' is embedded. For example, 'thank you for the gift' or 'thank you for helping me.'

Secondly, Cantonese is a *tone* language and each spoken unit, 'has a lexical tonal pattern' (Fok 1972, p. 1 in Chan & Li, 2000, p. 76). The significance of tone in Cantonese is not the same as intonation in English. A change in intonation in English usually suggests a difference in attitude or significance rather than a change in meaning (Chan & Li, 2000). For example, changing emphasis on the italicised words below does not change the underlying meaning of the sentence [i.e. the doctor (subject) walked (verb) to the hospital (object)]:-

The doctor *walked* to the hospital.

The doctor walked to the *hospital*.

In contrast, tone in Cantonese carries fundamental lexical and semantic significance. Changing the tone in a Cantonese word changes the meaning of the word. There are six distinctive tones in Cantonese (Bauer & Benedict, 1997; Matthews & Yip, 2011), which are indicated by numbers when transcribed in the Romanized form of Jyutping[1] (as shown in the example below). The tone used with the morpheme or word partly determines lexical and semantic meaning and additional meaning is determined by the broader context of the utterance. This can be seen in the examples given below:

- First tone (high level): *maa1* 媽 (mother), 孖 (twin)
- Second tone: not possible
- Third tone (mid level): *maa3* 嗎 (question particle)
- Fourth tone (low falling): *maa4* 麻 (hemp)
- Fifth tone (low rising): *maa5* 馬 (horse)
- Sixth tone (low level): *maa6* 罵 (scold, abuse)

However, this tonal system restricts a speaker's ability to manipulate pitch which usually conveys a range of communicative information about speaker's interactions including attitudes (surprise, doubt, hesitation, reluctance, etc.) as well as speech-acts such as asking, requesting, refusing or persuading (Bauer & Benedict, 1997). While

---

[1]Jyutping is a Romanised written version of Cantonese, introduced by the Linguistic Society of Hong Kong in 1993 and is the most widely used system of Romanization (https://www.lshk.org/). The numbers used in the in the Romanized examples indicate the relevant tone for that word/ utterance. When written Chinese characters are used tone is embedded within the character itself and is not indicated separately.

English largely expresses this information through intonation, Cantonese relies on a rich variety of sentence-final particles (SFPs) (also referred to as utterance particles (Gibbons, 1980; Luke, 1990)) to compensate for this limitation (see Matthews and Yip (2011) and Luke (1990) for discourse-related functions and meanings of these particles). For instance, 咩 (me1) can change a statement into a question while 啩 (gwaa3) conveys the speaker's uncertainty about the truth of the statement.

The third contrasting feature relevant to this discussion relates to the identification of semantic 'word' units and how these are embedded within larger 'sentences'. The majority of alphabetic writing systems segment words by using spaces and punctuation as word delimiters. Logographic Asian languages, such as Cantonese, Japanese and Korean, do not delimit words by whitespace (Bai, Yan, Zang, Liversedge, & Rayner, 2008) (see Taylor & Taylor (2014) for an overview of literacy and writing in these languages). This is illustrated in the following example:

你老人著得少衫呢

You old people are wearing so few

This Cantonese sentence contains eight characters but these are not separated by spaces. Each character in this sentence can be considered to be the semantic equivalent of a 'word' unit. However, this is not always the case. Cantonese words can be made up of multiple characters. Segmentation, the process of the separation of characters into semantic word units, is subjective and open to interpretation by the analyst rather than being governed by rules (Fung & Bigi, 2015; Luke & Wong, 2015).

There are also significant differences in the way in which Cantonese sentences are structured. For example, in English verb tenses are used to indicate temporal features such as time. In Chinese, adverbs and contextual information are used. When translating written Chinese into English, the translator has to make word choices based on contextual understanding rather than relying on word for word translation.

These contrasting features between languages raise issues in terms of translation and the potential loss of important semantic, social and cultural meaning all of which are relevant in the study of health communication. For example, it is quite common in Cantonese to address a person using his or her family role especially in a medical consultation, for example, 媽咪 (maa1 mi5), 哥哥 (go1 go1), 爹哋 (de1 dei2) and 阿仔 (aa3 zai2). These terms could be accurately translated into 'you', the common form of address in English, or their literal translation of 'mummy', 'elder brother', 'daddy' and 'son'. Although these translations correspond to the original meaning, the *relational* aspects of the speakers involved in that conversation are difficult to translate into another language. The loss of this relational information could have implications for researchers in interpreting and analysing data.

As will be discussed further, these issues of equivalence of language as well as cultural and social associations and semantic, lexical and conceptual differences (Al-Amer, Ramjan, Glew, Darwish, & Salamonson, 2015; Hilton & Skrutkowsky, 2002; Twin, 1997) raise important questions about how NLP tools such as

Discursis can be customized for use on first or native languages. These questions will be addressed through a comparative analysis of the same texts in Cantonese characters and in English translation.

2 Methods

Conversational data used in the research[2] discussed in this chapter were collected in 2008 and 2009 in a number of government-run health settings in Hong Kong S.A. R. Data collection was approved by The Hong Kong Polytechnic University Human Research Ethics Committee (HREC), and relevant hospital bodies in accordance with local requirements. Research participants provided written and informed consent prior to the audio recording of conversations between them and a research assistant. Research participants were native speakers of Cantonese and Hong Kong residents. Conversations were audio recorded, de-identified and transcribed verbatim into Cantonese (written in Chinese Hanzi characters) following the standard of the Hong Kong Supplementary Character Set (HKSCS) (https://www. ogcio.gov.hk/en/). Three extracts from the de-identified Cantonese transcripts were shared with the authors of this chapter in May 2018.[3] A total of 155 conversational turns were analysed in the research described in this chapter.

Data were entered into Discursis in three formats—Cantonese, English translated from Cantonese by the first author and English translated from Cantonese using Google Translate. Each set of data was entered into Discursis twice and analysed using (i) a default stop word list; and (ii) a customized stop word list generated by the first and second authors. These workflows are shown in Fig. 1. On this basis, six Discursis visualization plots were produced per transcript and there were 18 plots in total. Although Google Translate draws on a corpus of simplified Mandarin Chinese characters rather than Cantonese, as this is the most widely used and freely available tool for translation, it was included in the initial analysis. The low quality of the translation produced by Google Translate, however, limited its usefulness for analysis in Discursis. Therefore, the two data sets (12 plots) discussed in this chapter are based on the Cantonese (written in traditional Chinese characters) transcript and the transcript translated into English by the first author.

Comparison of the plots was based on a combination of visual qualitative examination and quantitative assessment of differences in outputs. For the quantitative comparison, each plot was directly compared via the number of recurrence elements (and shared absence of recurrence) each plot has in common. In Discursis, there is a unique recurrence element for each pair of utterances. For example, if

[2]This research was funded by a grant from the Faculty of Humanities, Dean's Reserve, The Hong Kong Polytechnic University.

[3]The authors would like to acknowledge and thank the original research team at The Hong Kong Polytechnic University and its' representatives who allowed the data to be used in this research. Details of that research are recorded under approval code HSEARS20131104001.

turns 2 and 34 of a transcript share concepts, then there will be a recurrence element visible at position (2, 34) that contains a value more than zero and less than or equal to one that indicates the strength of this conceptual overlap. These recurrence elements combine to create the recurrence plot and can also be compared directly. This is the case here where we have two versions of a transcript in different languages, but whose utterances should be equivalent. Differences between corresponding recurrence elements in the case of this study are an indicator of disparity between how transcripts are coded and processed by Discursis' language model. To measure the overall similarity of any two Discursis plots we simply sum the similarity (measured as 1—difference between two corresponding recurrence elements) of all paired recurrence elements across two plots, and divide this sum by the total number of recurrence elements.

3 Findings and Analysis

The results of the analysis of these three transcripts using the customized stop word lists are shown in Figs. 2, 3, 4. The letter 'a' refers to Cantonese transcripts and letter 'b' refers to transcripts translated into English prior to analysis in Discursis. Analysis of the comparison of the (a) and (b) figures will be discussed in turn in order to highlight changes in the visual representation of speaker engagement, interaction and the sharing of meaning and concepts through the conversation. Quantitative results (shown in Table 1 at the end of this chapter) suggest that, at least in the case of the customized stop word list, the workflows were mostly comparable (with an average 92% similarity according to a direct comparison of recurrence elements between plots), however the differences that do exist are enough to affect and potentially alter qualitative interpretations as discussed below. Note also that for the quantitative comparison, the presence of corresponding white space on two plots (recurrence elements with a value of zero) will count towards overall similarity, making it easy to qualitatively assess two plots as being more dissimilar than they are.

Visual comparison of Fig. 2a and 2b highlights differences in colours and sizes of the recurrence elements (shown in the plots as coloured squares). Figure 2b shows a large white space in the first half of the plot. The white space indicates no engagement between the speakers. This suggests that the speakers were neither repeating each other's nor their own concepts. However, Fig. 2a shows a higher level of speaker engagement reflected by the two-colour off-diagonal blocks in the same area of Fig. 2b. By clicking on the coloured block within the plot the analyst can take a closer look and identify recurring concepts. In this case, the recurring concept is '住' (zyu6) (live) which occurred in five turns. The moderate–high level speaker engagement was also attributed to the association between this concept and three other words '大廈' (daai6haa6) (building), '雜' (zaap6) (dodgy) and '長大' (zoeng2daai6) (grew up). That means when the utterance includes either of these words, they will be categorized into the concept of '住'. However, in Fig. 2b, all

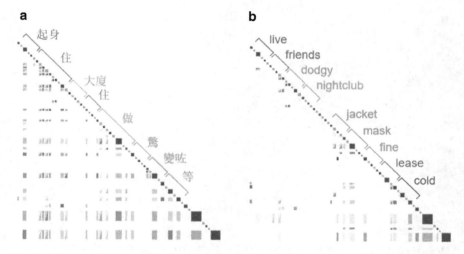

Fig. 2 Discursis plots showing analysis of **a** the Cantonese and **b** the English transcripts of Extract 1

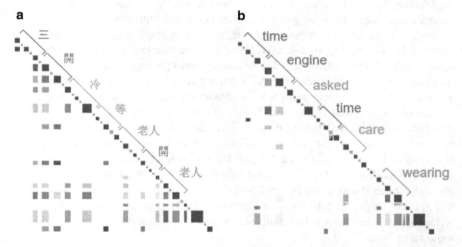

Fig. 3 Discursis plots showing analysis of **a** the Cantonese and **b** the English transcripts of Extract 2

these words were identified as separate concepts, showing no connection between each other. One possible explanation of this difference is that '住' (zyu6) was not always translated as live/living in English. For example, '哦!住 邊 頭 呀?' was translated as 'Oh, where?' as a question raised following the response 'I have some friends who used to live there'. In another instance, 住宅 was translated as residential building, instead of living home. Although the translation into English

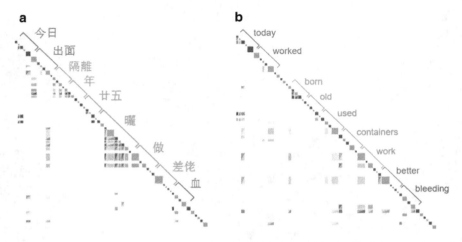

Fig. 4 Discursis plots showing analysis of **a** the Cantonese and **b** the English transcripts of Extract 3

maintained the semantic and syntactic relations within the utterance, some of the nuances and implied meaning of the original communication was lost.

Both Fig. 3a and 3b shared similar recurrence in the initial opening and final sections, but there was a significant difference in the intersection of the first half and second half of these conversations. Recurring concepts in Fig. 3a are '開' (hoi1) (start/turn on) and '冷' (laang5) (cold) yet these are absent in Fig. 3b. Other words associated with these two concepts were also identified. For example, 開 (start/turn on)–車 (ce1) (car) and 冷氣 (laang5hei3) (air-conditioner); 冷 (cold)–衫 (saam1) (clothes) and 脾氣 (pei4hei3) (temper). The Cantonese word '開' (open/start/turn on) can collocate with car and air-conditioner while different verbs were needed to collocate with those nouns in the English transcript, for example, *start* the car, *turn on* the air-conditioner. This contextual information was not added into the English transcript when it was translated and thus the relationship between these words was lost and not shown in Fig. 3b. This suggests that the process of translation, while technically correct from a linguistic perspective, has altered the representation of topic recurrence.

The visual differences between Fig. 4a and 4b in the first and middle sections of the plots indicate different levels of speaker engagement. Figure 4a shows a higher engagement level with more blocks of darker colours, indicating a higher concept similarity compared with Fig. 4b. It is a more accurate representation of the original conversation as the recurring concepts '做' (zou6) (do) and '曬' (saai3) (expose in the sun) appeared consecutively in conversational turns. The differences between these two figures can be attributed to some translation issues similar to those discussed in relation to Figs. 2 and 3. For example, '年' (nin4) (year) occurred five times in the initial opening of the conversation which was accurately represented by the moderate-high level of speaker engagement in Fig. 4a. The reason why this

Table 1 Results of pairwise quantitative comparison between recurrence plots generated using the original Cantonese (**a**), and hand-translate English (**b**) transcripts, using both the default (i) and modified custom (ii) stop word lists (similarity between plots: 1.0 = identical, 0.0 = opposite)

	Dataset1ai	Dataset1aii	Dataset1bi
Dataset1aii	0.77		
Dataset1bi	0.75	0.87	
Dataset1bii	0.76	0.92	0.92

	Dataset2ai	Dataset2aii	Dataset2bi
Dataset2aii	0.95		
Dataset2bi	0.90	0.95	
Dataset2bii	0.90	0.9	0.99

	Dataset3ai	Dataset3aii	Dataset3bi
Dataset3aii	0.76		
Dataset3bi	0.75	0.92	
Dataset3bii	0.73	0.94	0.97

level of speaker engagement was not shown in Fig. 4b is because '年' was not always translated as 'year', for example, in the case of '七九年' (79 years) which should be 1979 in the translation. Another translation issue is related to verb inflection. Tense in English is often reflected by verb inflection such as-*ed*. In Cantonese, however, this is expressed lexically with the help of, for example, temporal phrases such as ('而家' (ji4gaa1) (now) and '之前' (zi1cin4) (before)) (Lin, 2006). In this case, '做' was translated into three different words (*worked*, *working* and *work*) and then three separate concepts in the English plot. This affected the level of speaker engagement that was shown in the plots. As was discussed earlier, the inherent differences between Chinese and English make transcription and translation challenging and even high-quality translations may have discrepancies or inconsistencies in meaning.

4 Discussion

The process of translating the Cantonese data into English and preparing it for analysis in Discursis involved modification of syntactic and lexical markers. This included the initial translation from Cantonese to English as well as segmentation of the written Chinese characters and development of stop word lists for both languages. Within the context of studies of health communication, the complexity of these processes and the risk of losing important relational data supports the argument for the ongoing development of software that can facilitate bottom-up, first-language analysis. Each of these stages of data preparation is discussed below.

4.1 Transcription and Translation of Conversation into Chinese Characters

Many Cantonese words can have identical sounds and tones and share similar meaning yet can be written differently. For example:

Cantonese words	Jyutping (Cantonese Romanization)	Translation
嗽/咁	(gam2)	Like this/that; in this way
喺/係	(hai6)	To be; yes; right
哋/地	(dei6)	To indicate plurality after a personal pronoun
返/番	(fann1)	Return; come/go back
冇/無	(mo5)	Do not; not
畀/俾	(bei2)	Give
晒/嗮	(saai3)	Completely; show off; bask in the sun

When preparing a transcript for analysis, consistent and accurate use of Chinese characters becomes crucial as it can affect the level of speaker engagement shown in the analysis. This characteristic of Cantonese is also the reason why the Cantonese transcripts were transcribed using Chinese characters, rather than Jyutping. Jyutping can show six lexical tones; however, many Cantonese words can have identical sounds and tones yet be written differently and carry different meaning, e.g. soeng2— 想 (want, hope), 相 (photo); coi3—菜 (vegetables), 蔡 (surname), 賽 (race, competition). This complicates the transcription and process of segmentation and requires verification of the accuracy of the representation of tone. Additionally, Discursis can only identify different characters or words for data coding. Showing identical sounds and tones will affect how Discursis identifies concepts and depicts relationships as well as the level of speaker engagement in the plot. This consideration also impacts upon the creation of the stop word list for a transcript, for example, in the case of 喎 (wo5) (a model particle included in the stop word list) which shares the same sound and tone as 禍 (calamity) (a content word which should be excluded from the stop word list). As demonstrated in this research, Discursis can analyse *logographic* characters. This suggests that transcribing Cantonese health-related conversations in Chinese characters and then segmenting the utterances prior to analysis in Discursis is preferable to using the Romanized Jyutping format. As written Chinese characters convey significant semantic and relational information and more accurate Discursis plots can be produced, the additional preparation time is warranted.

4.2 Segmentation of Chinese Characters

As noted earlier in this chapter, one of the most important differences between alphabetic writing systems such as English and the Chinese logographic system from the perspective of text analytics is that the latter is written without spaces between characters (Bai et al., 2008). However, NLP tools such as Discursis which aim to work with logographic and alphabetic languages, need to draw on semantic word units as essential parts of their analysis. The segmentation of a Cantonese transcript is, therefore, a fundamental but complicated step in the preparation of data for analysis. Segmentation not only delimits the words into meaningful semantic units, but also provides a unit (i.e. the word) which can be analysed. The analyst can then identify parts of speech or grammatical functions of words or units in order to generate the stop word list.

4.3 Generation and Modification of Stop Word Lists

As has been discussed, stop word lists generated for the analysis of English transcripts usually include words which do not have a specific meaning but rather fulfil a predominantly grammatical function such as particles, auxiliaries, connectives (also referred to as conjunctions, prepositions, adverbs). Common examples of these words include *the, and, of, a, be*. Cantonese stop word lists also include words that have similar functions as the English ones. However, there are two main issues in relation to translating stop word lists across languages which have also been well-documented in previous studies in English–Cantonese translation (e.g. Lin, 2006; Yip & Matthews, 2017).

Firstly, no single English words can be translated as equivalent to a Cantonese sentence-final particle. Sentence-final particles do not have any semantic content and their meaning comes from the sentence, clause, phrase or word they are attached to in a specific discourse context (Luke, 1990). For example, the accompanying response 金國大廈 'Kam Kwok Building' with the sentence-final particles 吖嘛 (aa1maa3) attached can be translated as 'Kam Kwok Building of course. Don't you know?' The additional words 'of course. Don't you know?' in the translation express the intonation and speaker's intention as naturally and closely as in that context where the speaker might have assumed the listener should have known this building prior to this discourse. Also, these particles are used primarily in relatively informal colloquial speech and are rarely found in written Chinese (Luke & Nancarrow, 1997). In contrast, many of the words in the English stop word lists can appear in both informal and formal English writing. This suggests that these sentence-final particles might only be understood through additional words or punctuation at the sentence level rather than at the word level as may be possible in English. This distinctive difference between Cantonese and English makes the application and translation of the English stop word list to Cantonese almost impossible.

Secondly, in English, verbs are conjugated to express tense, e.g.-*ed* for past events. However, this kind of inflection is absent in Cantonese as tense is realized through aspect and verbal particles. For example, the possible Cantonese equivalents of 'went' (which is a verb in the default English stop word list) could be 有去, 去咗, 去過, 去完. If a conjugated verb is translated, all the possibilities may also have to be included in the Cantonese stop word list. However, in some cases, these particles may not be necessary as tense can also be indicated through temporal phrases as discussed in the analysis of Fig. 4. The tense of 去 (go/went) can already be clearly understood if the contextual information is sufficient.

In view of these two major issues, the translation and application of English stop word lists to Cantonese transcripts is not a feasible option for generating a meaningful analysis of a Cantonese plot in Discursis. Results of the analysis in this chapter, therefore, suggest that as Discursis provides a dynamic analysis of language, the generation of a customized stop word list for different languages is fundamental. This is a time-consuming step in the process but is important for the validity of the analysis.

5   Conclusion

This chapter has detailed the findings of a unique research study that compared the visual analysis of Cantonese and English data using Discursis. As was discussed earlier in this chapter, the analytic value of using Discursis has been demonstrated in other research. Although the program can be theoretically used on non-alphabetic data, at the time of writing this is the first published study using logographic transcripts. The results described in this chapter have highlighted the relational information, which can be lost through the translation of Cantonese into English. This emphasizes the importance of developing visual analytic tools that can be used on Cantonese data sets particularly in health-related research in which relational information embedded within the semantic and lexical features of a language is important. Generating visual representations of such data has benefits in terms of contributing to local and international understandings about how health and health care are discussed in different communities and cultures.

Research has consistently shown that communication about health and care is more effective when conversational features such as turn taking and semantic alignment are balanced between participants rather than dominated by experts such as doctors. Complex yet critical interpersonal components of health care such as building trust and rapport, decision-making, managing medication and explaining risk and uncertainty unfold through dynamic processes of interaction and communication and often involve talking about broad lifestyle-related information that goes beyond the description of symptoms or treatments. Language is a fundamental data source in research into this area yet relational data can be lost through the process of translation from one language to another (Squires, 2009).

Conversational transcripts recorded in first or native languages, therefore, provide unique insights into cultural and social perceptions of health. Throughout this chapter, we have argued that the complex processes of both the transcription of spoken language and translation between languages present unique challenges to language and communication researchers. Developing analytic tools that can be used with logographic *and* alphabetic languages without requiring translation will help to preserve the subtle and relational aspects of language that shape communication about health and health care. Expanding the field of health communication in Asia will be supported through the continued development of analytic tools that can be used with first-language, logographic data. Discursis outputs have been used to inform the development of training programs for a variety of professions that aim to increase awareness of communication between people. Such insights could be of benefit across multiple language groups if the software can be appropriately customized. Expanding this work with Asian languages will also make significant contributions to the fields of NLP and machine translation.

Funding The research reported in this chapter was funded by the Faculty of Humanities, Dean's Reserve, The Hong Kong Polytechnic University.

References

Al-Amer, R., Ramjan, L., Glew, P., Darwish, M., & Salamonson, Y. (2015). Translation of interviews from a source language to a target language: examining issues in cross-cultural health care research. *Journal of Clinical Nursing, 24*(9–10), 1151–1162.

Angus, D., Rintel, S., & Wiles, J. (2013). Making sense of big text: a visual-first approach for analysing text data using Leximancer and Discursis. *International Journal of Social Research Methodology, 16*(3), 261–267.

Angus, D., Smith, A., & Wiles, J. (2012). Conceptual recurrence plots: revealing patterns in human discourse. *IEEE Transactions on Visualizations and Computer Graphics, 18*(6), 988–997.

Atay, C., Conway, E., Angus, D., Wiles, J., Baker, R., & Chenery, H. (2015). An automated approach to examining conversational dynamics between people with dementia and their carers. *PLoS ONE, 10*(12), e0144327.

Bai, X., Yan, G., Zang, C., Liversedge, S. P., & Rayner, K. (2008). Reading spaced and unspaced Chinese text: Evidence from eye movements. *Journal of Experimental Psychology: Human Perception and Performance, 34*(5), 1277–1287.

Bauer, R., & Benedict, P. (Eds.). (1997). *Modern Cantonese phonology*. Berlin and New York: Mouton de Gruyter.

Bondi, M. (2017). Corpus linguistics. *The Routledge handbook of language and dialogue* (pp. 46–61). New York: Routledge.

Chan, A., & Li, D. (2000). English and Cantonese phonology in contrast: explaining Cantonese ESL learners' English pronunciation problems. *Language, Culture and Curriculum, 13*(1), 67–85.

Chevalier, B., Watson, B., Barras, M., Cottrell, W., & Angus, D. (2018). Using Discursis to enhance the qualitative analysis of hospital pharmacist-patient interactions. *PLOSone* (May).

Evers, W., Marroum, S., & Young, L. (2017). A pluralistic, longitudinal method: Using participatory workshops, interviews and lexicographic analysis to investigate relational evolution. *Industrial Marketing Management, 61*(February), 182–193.

Firth, J. (1962). A synopsis of linguistic theory 1930–1955. *Studies in Linguistic Analysis*.

Franzoni, S., & Bonera, M. (2019). How DMO can measure the experiences of a large territory. *Sustainability, 11*(2), 492.

Fung, R., & Bigi, B. (2015). Automatic word segmentation for spoken Cantonese. In: *Paper presented at the international conference oriental and conference on asian spoken language research and evaluation*. China: Shanghai.

Gibbons, J. (1980). A tentative framework for speech act description of the utterance particles in conversational Cantonese. *Linguistics, 18*, 763–775.

Goldstein, S., MacDonald, N. E., & Guirguis, S. (2015). Health communication and vaccine hesitancy. *Vaccine, 33*(34), 4212–4214.

Heritage, J., & Maynard, D. (Eds.). (2006). *Communication in Medical Care*. Cambridge: Cambridge University Press.

Hirschberg, J., & Manning, C. (2015). Advances in natural language processing. *Science, 349* (6245), 261–266.

Hilton, A., & Skrutkowsky, M. (2002). Translating instruments into other languages: development and testing process. *Cancer Nursing, 25*(1), 1–7.

Ho, C. S.-H., & Bryant, P. (1997). Development of phonological awareness of Chinese children in Hong Kong. *Journal of Psycholinguistic Research, 26*(1), 109–126.

Lin, J.-W. (2006). Time in a language without tense: The case of Chinese. *Journal of Semantics, 23*(1), 1–53.

Liu, T., & Hsiao, J., H-W. (2014). Holistic processing in speech perception: experts' and novices' processing of isolated Cantonese syllables. In *Proceedings of the annual meeting of the cognitive science society* (vol. 36, pp. 869–874).

Luke, K., & Nancarrow, O. (1997). *Sentence particles in Cantonese: A corpus-based study*. Presented at The Yuen Ren Society Meeting, University of Washington.

Luke, K., & Wong, M. (2015). The Hong Kong Cantonese corpus: Design and uses. *Journal of Chinese Linguistics, 25*, 309–330.

Luke, K. K. (1990). *Utterance particles in Cantonese conversation*. John Benjamins Publishing.

Matthews, S., & Yip, V. (2011). *Cantonese: A comprehensive grammar* (2nd ed.). London and New York: Routledge.

Nouri, S., & Rudd, R. (2015). Health literacy in the "oral exchange": An important element of patient–provider communication—ScienceDirect. *Patient Education and Counseling, 98*(5), 565–571.

Smith, A., & Humphreys, M. (2006). Evaluation of unsupervised semantic mapping of natural language with Leximancer concept mapping. *Behaviour Research Methods, 38*(2), 262–279.

Snow, D. (2004). *Cantonese as Written Language: The growth of a written Chinese Vernacular*. Hong Kong S.A.R.: Hong Kong University Press.

Spevack, S., Falandays, J., Batzloff, B., & Spivey, M. (2018). Interactivity of language. *Language and Linguistics Compass, 12*(e12282), 1–18.

Street, R., Makoul, G., Arora, N. K., & Epstein, R. (2009). How does communication heal? Pathways linking clinician-patient communication to health outcomes. *Patient Education and Counseling, 74*(3), 295–301.

Squires, A. (2009). Methodological challenges in cross-language qualitative research: A research review. *International Journal of Nursing Studies, 46*(2), 277–287.

Taylor, I., & Taylor, M. (2014). *Writing and literacy in Chinese, Korean and Japanese: Revised Edition*. Amsterdam: John Benjamins.

Twinn, S. (1997). An exploratory study examining the influence of translation on the validity and reliability of qualitative data in nursing research. *Journal of Advanced Nursing, 26*(2), 418–423.

Tolston, M., Riley, M., Mancuso, V., Finomore, V., & Funke, G. (2018). Beyond frequency counts: Novel conceptual recurrence analysis metrics to index semantic coordination in team communications *Behaviour Research Methods* 1–19.

Watson, B., Angus, D., Gore, L., & Farmer, J. (2015). Communication in open disclosure conversations about adverse events in hospitals. *Language and Communication, 41*, 57–70.

Weigand, E. (Ed.). (2017). *The Routledge handbook of language and dialogue*. New York: Routledge.

Wong, A., Juang, J., & Chen, H.-C. (2012). Phonological units in spoken word production: insights from Cantonese. *PLOSone, 7*(11), e48776.

Yip, V., & Matthews, S. (2017). *Intermediate Cantonese: a grammar and workbook* (2nd ed.). Routledge.

Epilogue

Mapping the Challenges and Opportunities of Translational Health Communication Science and Practice in Asia

The chapters included in this volume have been selected as they each contribute to an expanding of scholarly understanding of how culture informs the processes and context in which health communication is practiced in various locations in Asia. What makes these chapters so compelling as a collective is the various elements of culture that are emphasized throughout. Each chapter makes a unique contribution in a given area, but like stars in a constellation, a new picture emerges when viewed as a whole. Some of the chapters focus on the culture of medicine, specifically how communication practices emerging from biomedical approaches on illness contrast with communication practices grounded in more holistic perspectives on well-being. Other chapters focus on how regional, national, and ethnic cultures shape our interpersonal communication practices and the consequences of those practices for individual physical and mental health in healthcare contexts. A third dimension is the culture of research. The research presented grapples with issues such as applying Western metrics of research rigor to other cultural contexts and how data analytic tools can be optimized to capture the beauty and complexity of various types of languages. In short, the picture that emerges from this volume shows the complexity of creating new knowledge at the intersection of health, culture, and place but also the beauty that is found in exploring uncharted territory.

In addition to exploring issues of health and culture in Asia, this book seeks to enhance the focus in the discipline on knowledge translation. Indeed, special issues of the *Journal of Applied Communication Research* and the *Journal of Language and Social Psychology* have previously focused on the importance of identifying pathways for translational health communication scholarship to change how the art and science of medicine is practiced. In the biomedical sciences, there is a push to

© Springer Nature Singapore Pte Ltd. 2020
B. Watson and J. Krieger (eds.), *Expanding Horizons in Health Communication*,
The Humanities in Asia 6, https://doi.org/10.1007/978-981-15-4389-0

shorten the timeline between medical discovery and clinical implementation. In health communication, we know too little about the translational pathways and timelines for implementing and sustaining evidence-based approaches in various contexts. There are examples of efforts to move in this direction, such as the National Cancer Institute's Research Tested Intervention Programs website. Still, there are far too many important findings that have yet to change practice in a systematic way.

This volume also adds a new and important component to the growing work on knowledge translation. And that is how knowledge translation is influenced by the translation of languages. Recognizing English as the lingua franca of our disciplines presents a persistent problem in terms of diversity and inclusion of scholars from non-English-speaking regions and cultures. As an interdisciplinary group of academics, we need to consider more openly how to translate research from English into other languages as well as how to translate the work being done in other languages into English without losing the socio-cultural nuances and subtleties that shape language itself. Our knowledge base is limited to the extent to which we can globalize efforts for making research accessible to diverse audiences. Next, we will highlight a few of the chapters that demonstrate this important link between knowledge translation and language.

Implications of Language for Knowledge Translation

The research presented in this volume highlights how language influences knowledge translation. For example, how can health communication research be translated in a cultural context in which there is no translation for the English illness or condition? These are some of the issues that Raisa, Bylund, Islam, and Krieger's chapter (this volume) highlight. While many of the chapters in this volume address health communication in Chinese contexts, this chapter reviews health communication interventions in Bangladesh. One of the challenges this chapter highlights is that medical terminology created in English cannot always be clearly or directly translated into other languages. For example, there is no word for "breast cancer" in Bangla, the native language of Bangladesh. This can create challenges when words or phrases are created to approximate the English term. Again, for example, the term for cervical cancer is often translated in Bangla to words meaning an "ulcer in the neck of the womb." This process of language translation may not give women an accurate understanding of their health and limits opportunities for knowledge translation.

Similarly, Ang and Della's chapter (this volume) demonstrates how the convergence of languages and cultures in cosmopolitan areas such as Singapore can pose significant challenges to clear communication in care settings during key processes such as nursing handovers. They describe how nurses in the same unit often speak different languages and rely on the use of slang terms in the process of nursing handovers. As they describe, the process of translating important knowledge for the new nurse about a patient's care and well-being during a handover can be impeded by the process of language translation.

Finally, the work of Yau and colleagues (this volume) draws attention to the issues associated with using software to analyze transcripts of logographic (non-alphabetic) languages. In their chapter, the authors focus on Cantonese which is written in traditional Chinese (logographic) characters. Although current software programs may be theoretically able to analyze non-alphabetic data, there is limited research using untranslated Cantonese data. Given that culture and language are inextricably linked, it is essential that tools be developed or improved so that more work can be done on the analysis of first and native languages. This novel work moves research forward in broadening software development to include Cantonese.

Implications of Knowledge Translation for Language

The close tie between knowledge translation and language can also be reversed, with different implications. In some cases, what constitutes scientific knowledge is simply an understanding of how particular linguistic features are constructed by individuals in a particular cultural context. For example, while active patient participation in consultations is considered ideal in Western medical consultations, Schoeb and Yip (this volume) demonstrate how Chinese patients in Hong Kong are less willing to ask questions of their physiotherapists. Conversely, health communication patterns of Chinese physiotherapists may not be considered patient centered by Western standards. However, when they integrated the use of verbal and non-verbal resources, patients' active participation during exercise therapy was facilitated. This suggests that understanding what type of communication constitutes patient centeredness needs to be contextualized to a particular culture. More broadly, it indicates challenges and opportunities in the realm of knowledge translation for understanding how mechanisms and processes can be transferred (or not) across cultural boundaries.

Another variant on this idea is considering treatment decision-making. Shared decision-making between a patient and practitioner is often considered the gold standard in Western health systems Perhaps one of the greatest areas of need in the health communication arena is understanding communication functions and processes in contexts characterized by non-biomedical approaches to health and well-being. Three of the chapters in this volume describe an important initial step in the decision-making process in terms of understanding which treatment philosophy health service users wish to pursue. To this end, this volume has three chapters devoted to describing the role of communication in Traditional Chinese Medicine (TCM). For example, the chapter by Wong, Loong, and Lee (this volume) describes how the focus of Western medicine on a specific disease site (e.g., colorectal cancer) can be at odds with a patient's conceptualization of illness as being an imbalance within the system. Ying Jin (this volume) found that the individual focus of TCM treatments combined with longer appointment times is attractive to patients in contexts where both TCM and Western approaches are available in Mainland China. Yip and Zhang (this volume) describe the different approaches to communication offered by practitioners of Western medicine and TCM.

It is vital for this knowledge to be translated and explored in other important cultural contexts. For example, many patients and individuals who do not want to seek medical care in the West seek "home remedies" and complementary and alternative medicine (CAM). Diverse opinions are held across different medical disciplines about the effectiveness of such alternative medicine. Thus, it is possible that other approaches to health and well-being outside of the biomedical sphere face similar issues. Next, we explore the value of knowledge and language translation for health communication science and practice.

Translation Helps Us Understand Our Differences

One value of promoting translation is that it helps the scholarly community identify, understand, and articulate our differences. One of the chapters in this volume that is particularly useful for this purpose is Ladegaard's chapter about the traumas experienced by domestic migrant workers in Hong Kong. Through his writing, we are transported into the lived experiences of domestic migrant works and shown how privileged individuals living in Hong Kong can, in some cases, exert extreme power and abuse on these workers. For those of us living outside of Hong Kong, his careful analysis offers a rare glimpse into communication practices that many of us could never be exposed to in any other way. This example can serve as a guide for other scholars who are considering the role of their privilege in shaping the way communication research is conceptualized and conducted. We must, to the best of our abilities, ensure that communication scholarship reflects the diversity of the populations we serve.

Another example is the chapter by Harrison and Lam. These authors use interview data with both counsellors and students to better understand the perspective of each as they journey through the different stages of counselling. They describe how the pressure imposed on young clients in Asian countries to conform may be greater than in comparable Western contexts, where more individualistic cultures are observed. These cultural differences are important because if young people view counselling as aberrant, then they may be less inclined to participate. The importance of conducting health communication research with individuals from every background and every language enriches our understanding of the needs and opportunities for our field.

Translation Helps Us Celebrate Our Similarities

Other chapters help us understand the similarities among people across the globe. For example, although Harrison and Lam identified some cultural differences that were important to young people, they also suggest that the three main themes shared by counsellors and clients in school-based counselling in Hong Kong are universal and central to young peoples' experiences of counselling globally. On that same note, Tay, Huang, and Zeng (this volume) posit that when clients are given a concept on which to focus, it results in more linguistic expression which has implications on how counsellors can use this knowledge to assist clients to learn from and move forward from the issues they are trying to address. Again, this technique is likely to have utility across cultures.

The chapter by Chan focuses on communication in nursing which is generally viewed as a high-pressure occupation. We see patients' perspectives in recorded interview videos and audiotaped nurse responses in nurse–patient communication. Chan's findings suggest that even though nurses work in intense and stressful environments, they are still able to respond appropriately to the emotional needs of their patients.

This idea of measure generalizability extends to methods. Della and colleagues validated a measure for international contexts. Their validation of the 42-item Nursing Home Survey on Patient Safety Culture (NHSPSC) tool for use in Singapore is a significant contribution to recognizing the challenges in patient care when different cultures communicate together but need to achieve a safe patient culture. This work will help researchers conduct important, cross-national comparative studies in the future. Cross-national research is valuable because it can highlight best practices as well as our common failures. Cummings (this volume) describes both the similarities and differences in public health communication in the United Kingdom (UK) and Hong Kong.

A Vision for the Future

The research presented in this volume inspired us to think broadly about the future of field. We have identified two areas which could amplify the influence of health communication scholarship. We hope readers will be encouraged to consider how increasing research accessibility and collaboration can be reflected in their own research program.

Accessibility. In order to advance scholarship in the area of health communication, we need to think about is who is and who is not participating in the dialogue and why. Often, our academic dialogues occur through English-language publications or conferences. It can be difficult to cultivate diverse perspectives on culture and health within these parameters. The most basic level of research accessibility is disseminating research results in various languages. Although there are significant financial barriers to multi-language publication, many journals are beginning to publish abstracts in multiple languages. This is an important intermediary step that can help scholars identify work that may be relevant to their own area of inquiry. To this end, we have made translations of chapters abstracts available on the IRCAHC website with a link to STCC: https:www.ircahc.org.

Collaboration. Increasing accessibility of work will facilitate the ability of scholars to identify others with similar interests. However, we cannot assume that shared research interests with academics in other regions are sufficient to foster collaboration. Indeed, there are many logistical, cultural, and organizational barriers to scholars working jointly to address problems.

Academic centers can have an important role in creating vital bonds and fostering collaborations. Like many others, we are enthusiastic about engaging in international work as an early career scholar. However, the logistical barriers and time constraints made this difficult. However, our passion for connecting with others around health communication research remains. Thus, another goal of this volume was to forge a connection between IRCAHC at The Hong Kong Polytechnic University and STCC at the University of Florida. We want to create a structure that will connect researchers across sites in work that engages clinicians and then translates findings to the public in clear language free from jargon. We hope that many other academic units will create similar partnerships to support scholars in their international endeavors.

We hope that this book, and the collaboration that it represents, will contribute in some small way to the grand goal of making health communication research more accessible and collaborative. In so doing, we will be more prepared to address the big questions that health communication scholars are uniquely trained to answer. Some of those questions that the field is poised to address include:

- How do we communicate about illness in communities where there are no words in the native language? It is important for scholars with a deep understanding of language to be involved in these advancements.
- How do linguistic and visual strategies aid community-based participatory research?
- What is the interplay of culture and our ethical (bioethical) principles?
- The world is more accessible through technology but how do we effectively leverage the use of these tools in healthcare research and practice?

These pressing questions provide opportunities for the next generation of scholars to develop new approaches to understand the deep connection between place, language, culture, and well-being. Our hope is that this book will begin a dialogue about the nature of health communication from Eastern cultural, linguistic, and social perspectives and encourage future work to be more inclusive. We look toward a future where health communication scholars and clinicians across the globe work together to create a healthier world.

CPSIA information can be obtained
at www.ICGtesting.com
Printed in the USA
LVHW011243070621
689564LV00001B/49